OCCUPATIONAL THERAPY LEADERSHIP

Your Pro............. ,
and Your Organization

Grace Emanuel Gilkeson, EdD, OTR, FAOTA
Dean and Professor Emerita
Texas Woman's University
Denton, Texas

 F. A. DAVIS COMPANY • Philadelphia

F. A. Davis Company
1915 Arch Street
Philadelphia, PA 19103

Printed in the United States of America

Last digit indicates print number: 10 9 8 7 6 5 4 3 2

Publisher: Jean-François Vilain
Senior Acquisitions Editor: Lynn Borders Caldwell
Developmental Editor: Marianne Fithian
Production Editor: Stephen D. Johnson
Cover Designer: Louis J. Forgione

As new scientific information becomes available through basic and clinical research, recommended treatments and drug therapies undergo changes. The author and publisher have done everything possible to make this book accurate, up to date, and in accord with accepted standards at the time of publication. The author, editors, and publisher are not responsible for errors or omissions or for consequences from application of the book, and make no warranty, expressed or implied, in regard to the contents of the book. Any practice described in this book should be applied by the reader in accordance with professional standards of care used in regard to the unique circumstances that may apply in each situation. The reader is advised always to check product information (package inserts) for changes and new information regarding dose and contraindications before administering any drug. Caution is especially urged when using new or infrequently ordered drugs.

Library of Congress Cataloging-in-Publication Data

Gilkeson, Grace Emanuel, 1926–
    Occupational therapy leadership : marketing yourself,
  your profession, and your organization / Grace Emanuel Gilkeson.
        p.   cm.
    Includes bibliographical references and index.
    ISBN 0-8036-0253-7 (pbk.)
    1. Occupational therapy.   I. Title.
  RM735.G55   1997
  615.8'515—dc21   96-53182
                                                           CIP

To my family, without whose support
this book would never have eventuated:
my aunt, Emma M. Emanuel, who had the foresight
to direct me into occupational therapy;
my husband, who has endured 45 years of my
absences on behalf of occupational therapy;
and my children, whose understanding and valuing
of service to others made it all possible.

Foreword

As a member of the occupational therapy profession for more than 40 years, I have viewed change from a number of perspectives. There have been changes in the conditions for which occupational therapists provide care for their clients, changes in the venues in which care is provided, and a shift from the primary orientation of occupational therapists as those who engage clients individually in therapy to remote intervention and primary evaluation and assessment.

When one has seen the scenarios projected almost 20 years ago[1] as possible alternatives for future healthcare delivery systems come to fruition, and has observed the ways in which the profession of occupational therapy has met and continues to meet the challenges of the new models, it is heartening to read *Occupational Therapy Leadership: Marketing Yourself, Your Profession, and Your Organization.* This book provides the substance, blueprint, and guide needed for planning and negotiating the known present and the unknown future. It futurizes the profession of occupational therapy.

Dr. Gilkeson proposes that occupational therapy educational programs need to provide learning for students and therapists that will make them competent to plan and implement programs in the managed care environment. She reiterates that more than personal rapport and the desire to work with patients are demanded, stating that "increasingly more complex reimbursement guidelines [must] be learned, data collected, numbers crunched, and cost reductions made without sacrificing quality care." In order to practice with competence, the occupational therapy student today must have knowledge and skills that include "critical thinking, divergent and innovative problem solving, systems management processes, budgeting, securing reimbursement from third-party payers, managed care, Medicare and agency contracts, outcomes documentation, personnel management, productivity management, marketing, networking, and ethical decision making." In a survey of newly graduated occupational therapists, Dr. Gilkeson found five recurring themes in the resulting data. These therapists reported that "change is inevitable, active participation in professional organizations is everyone's responsibility, appreciating the marketing process is essential, understanding cultural differences is critical, and comprehending and negotiating politics are necessary."

This book describes in detail, with wit and humor, the knowledge and skills needed for leadership, marketing, and management. The historical perspective on the changes that have occurred in the practice of occupational therapy over the years gives the reader the opportunity to view the viability of the profession and the many ways in which its practitioners met the challenges presented by change. Dr. Gilkeson's work greatly expands and provides the operational guidelines for models of care described previously in our literature.

Models of care that include action systems of the dyad consisting of the client and therapist as well as the extended group (which may include the family, peers, or client) with the therapist are commonly used when the goal is to assist the individual client in a one-to-one relationship or with a peer group or family group. Direct intervention is the hallmark of this model.[1]

A second model, the auxiliary system, involves the occupational therapist interacting with key persons in the client's life. These may be children, siblings, parents, teachers, counselors, community workers, employers, religious leaders, or caregivers. This model places the therapist in a somewhat removed position and permits direct service to be provided by another person at the direction of the occupational therapist. A third model, which has been called the system for program, structure, and policy alteration, is also somewhat removed from individual "hands-on" therapy but has the potential to reach many potential clients.[1]

To reconceptualize the therapeutic and rehabilitation services provided by therapists, Baum[2] identified proposed programs as products and described the commodity as an occupational therapy product line. Such programs as adapted sports and recreation programs, caregiver training programs, community education programs, exercise and fitness programs for elderly persons, independent living skills centers, programs for injury prevention in the workplace, school and vocational readiness, computer access center programs, driving programs to assess capacity, return-to-work programs, and wheelchair and mobility programs were included. These services just begin to make the transition from the present to the future.

Specific models, guides, frames of reference, and theories are useful in the conceptualization of the profession, but strategies, methods, and procedures are necessary to focus the performance of occupational therapists in the care of their clients. The student and practitioner will find the way paved for them by this book, so that they will be able to challenge the future with confidence and genuine success. Occupational therapy uses an open systems frame of reference that permits practitioners to use existing knowledge and skills and integrate them with new knowledge and skills for problem solving and decision making. The practitioner will employ environmental scanning and incorporate the knowledge and observation gained in that process to create environmental and care management adaptations for desired outcomes. These adaptations then become a part of the new knowledge and skills that permit practitioners to meet the future and fulfill its demands. This represents a continuous cycle, which is embodied in the narrative that makes up this book. It projects a rich, challenging, positive outlook for the future of occupational therapy practice.

Lela A. Llorens, PhD, OTR, FAOTA
Professor Emerita, Occupational Therapy
Former Associate Academic Vice President, Faculty Affairs
San Jose State University
San Jose, California

REFERENCES

1. Llorens, L: Health care systems models and occupational therapy. Occupational Therapy in Health Care 5(4):25–37, 1989.
2. Baum, C: Identification and use of environmental resources. In Christiansen, C, and Baum, C: Occupational Therapy: Overcoming Human Performance Deficits. Slack, Thorofare, NJ, 1991, pp 788–802.

Foreword

The Wheelwright's Shop by George Sturt, first printed in 1923, is a wonderful story of the life and times of three generations of wagon makers in Surrey, England. The book describes the process of wagon making, from felling the tree for lumber to delivering the finished wagon.

In the foreword, Mr. E. P. Thompson speaks about the wagon-making process:

"It is the formation of knowledge, not from theory, but from practical transmission, from the ground up. The skilled craftsman is taught by his materials. Their resources and qualities enter through his hand and hence to his mind. The artifact takes its form from the function it must perform, the shape of the wheel from the motion of the horses, the ruts in the road, and the weight of an average load. These are not finely calculated on paper, they are learned through practice."

So it is with *Occupational Therapy Leadership: Marketing Yourself, Your Profession, and Your Organization,* handcrafted by Grace E. Gilkeson. The book takes its form from the function that it is intended to accomplish. Dr. Gilkeson came by her word-smithing skills through practical application.

Dr. Gilkeson graduated from the occupational therapy program at Virginia Commonwealth University in Richmond. She has started occupational therapy clinics in several states and watched them grow. One began in an abandoned drive-in restaurant in Lorain, Ohio and today is the Lorain Rehabilitation Center. Another program, which she originated in a Quonset hut in a parking lot in Easton, Pennsylvania, is today's Occupational Therapy Department of Easton Hospital.

She became an instructor of occupational therapists at Texas Woman's University (TWU), Houston Center and eventually was selected to be Dean of the TWU School of Occupational Therapy based in Denton. Before retiring, she established the first degree program for the PhD in Occupational Therapy in a public institution.

Dr. Gilkeson developed the popular, innovative postprofessional master's degree program that allows occupational therapists to "fly in" for a weekend of classes once a month and thus earn their master's degrees without leaving homes and jobs. She invited me to be a guest lecturer when the class studied marketing and entrepreneurship. Each year the students seem more ready to accept new roles and more willing to challenge the status quo.

Dr. Gilkeson and I often talked about the need for a book on marketing, but we never followed through. Finally, she decided to do it herself. It is fitting that the wheelwright (master clinician) should be the author of this book.

I predict that this book will make profound changes in the occupational therapy profession. Therapists will learn leadership skills, updated management techniques, and marketing expertise that have been missing from their approaches and attitudes. The writing style elicits action rather than just conveying information. The logical structure of each clearly written, fast-paced section makes the book easy to use. Recent advances in academic preparation of therapists around the world should make this book a global best-seller. Other professions, such as physical therapy, will also find it helpful to extrapolate the information and create their own illustrations.

The book reflects the status of the profession at the end of this century and builds on the past of a profession that is nearing its own century mark. I am honored to play a part in it.

Fred Sammons, OTR, PhD, FAOTA
Sammons Preston

Preface

"The best way to predict the future is to create it."[1]

This is neither a management book nor a scholarly work. It is intended for use by new occupational therapy practitioners as a bridge that demonstrates the feasibility of applying theory and concept to everyday practice. It is designed particularly for faculty members teaching in occupational therapy educational programs and for new occupational therapy practitioners who are venturing forth into a complex and changing healthcare system.

Occupational therapy practitioners are creative; however, this does not mean that they will automatically succeed in their chosen field. It is wise to pause and think about some sage comments made by folks who had already earned reputations for having succeeded. Thomas Edison is credited with saying that "genius is 1 percent inspiration and 99 percent perspiration," and Henry Ward Beecher wrote that "if a man can have only one kind of sense, let him have common sense. If he has that and uncommon sense, too, he is not far from genius."

This book uses common sense, based on concept and theory, to introduce the entry-level occupational therapy practitioner to the world of current practice, where preparation and intelligence will not make it happen without that "99 percent perspiration." Theoretical and conceptual references are followed by examples taken from current business and healthcare news sources. The book culminates in a graphic summary that illustrates the convergence and parallels among the processes of occupational therapy, marketing, management, and leadership. Each of these processes is essential to the future of occupational therapy. Each requires analytic thought, constant planning, feedback, and use of that feedback to make revisions in planning.

Listening is basic to successful occupational therapy as well as to marketing, management, and leadership. Covey[1] emphasized that one needs to seek first to understand, then to be understood. One should listen with the intent to empathize, not with the intent to reply. Schön[2] stressed that the practitioner of the future needs to be reflective, to conduct reflective conversation with the client, and thus to be directly accountable to the client. A marketing attitude, made up of active listening while encouraging expression of another's thoughts and preferences, can be developed by systematically and empathetically investigating the needs of all with whom daily transactions are conducted. Responding to those individuals' expressed needs will, in turn, enhance most personal interactions and mutual satisfaction regardless of job specialty.

The aim of this book is to recognize and describe concepts, processes, and skills that can amplify the capabilities of occupational therapists as leaders in today's healthcare delivery system. It is a blend of concepts and practical guidance, a collection of historical observations, practical reality, and strategies that guide new therapists toward professionalism and leadership.

The idea for this book originated while I was observing how some occupational therapy practitioners were approaching clients today. Like most healthcare providers, many occupational therapists in recent years too often deliver services that they themselves deem necessary as professionals. This could be interpreted as a nonmarketing approach, exactly opposite to a true marketing approach. Both marketing and nonmarketing approaches are based on meeting needs, but each has a different definition and method of measuring needs. In this book, the differences between marketing and nonmarketing attitudes are clarified, and readers gain an understanding of how marketing principles and techniques can guide today's occupational therapists on their way to becoming leaders. Bennis[3] observed that many successful people never said they wanted to be leaders or aspire to a certain kind of success. Instead, they found needs to fulfill and were exceptionally proactive in looking for opportunities.

Current issues have been addressed constructively and objectively. Furthermore, the intent of this book is not to repeat what has been already perceived and recounted about the straying of occupational therapy from its founding beliefs.[4] Rather, its purpose is to recognize some of today's healthcare delivery problems and to suggest a way of approaching and resolving them.

Occupational therapy students completing the didactic phase of education deserve adequate preparation for fieldwork education and for entry into practice in today's real world. The functions of this book are to supply a missing link between academe and practice and, at the same time, to suggest a means of developing leadership within the profession. The beginning of the book provides a background and foundation in leadership, marketing, relevant aspects of management, and collaboration, as well as an appraisal of the occupational therapy profession today. Transformations in the world of work, as well as the nature of change itself, are described. A discussion of interdisciplinarity, globalization, and futurism follows, and the book concludes with examples of occupational therapy leadership and a comparative analysis of processes.

This book is presented in nine parts, each containing two to four chapters. Leadership, the primary focus, is discussed in Part One. Its theoretical foundation is highlighted, and strong occupational therapy leaders past and present are recognized. However, by definition and example, leadership is exemplified throughout this book as being found throughout the profession and at all levels of practice, whether local, state, national, or international.

In Part Two, marketing is introduced only as a social process. Readers are referred to multiple publications written by individuals who are professionals in the field of business marketing. It must be clearly understood at the outset that this book purports only to introduce a marketing perception and not to presume expertise in the field. Marketing professionals, who are educated and experienced in finance, business and organizational theory, and statistics, should be called on for expert consultation. Therefore, the concept and role of marketing in this book are presented from Bing's[5] view that the more we learn from others, the less time we waste in the present in proving what already has been proved.

Part Three discusses the collaborative process. It reviews aspects of the individual's collaboration as a therapist and as a healthcare team member. Part Four demonstrates that parallels exist conceptually among the processes of occupational therapy, marketing, management, and leadership, and Part Five introduces the idea of change—its nature, the forms that resistance to change can take and how they can be addressed, and how occupational therapists can and do cope with change.

Part Six looks at the changing world of organization and management and explains how occupational therapists can join in the transition by understanding the transformations taking place. Entrepreneurship, managed care, and the role of information technology are among the topics addressed. Strategic planning, or anticipating the changes and emerging as leaders, constitutes Part Seven. Occupational therapists are admonished to become familiar with systematic risk taking, strategic decision making, and the futurity of decision making.

Worldwide healthcare service delivery trends and issues are shown as relevant to broadening the scope and locations of occupational therapy practice everywhere as Part Eight addresses futurism and work in today's world. Part Nine concludes with a comparative analysis of the processes described in the book and with examples of occupational therapy practitioners who became leaders by using a marketing approach to achieve success.

This book integrates the conceptual and the practical because the well-prepared, thoughtful, proactive occupational therapy practitioner requires this kind of introduction to effective occupational therapy practice. The uniqueness and strength of occupational therapy can then be found in their rightful place—as the star in the crown of healthcare services—because occupational therapy practitioners approach it that way. This is a time of challenge and opportunity in the world of healthcare delivery, and occupational therapists must enter that world with an attitude similar to the one expressed in the quotation that opened this preface: "The best way to predict the future is to create it."[1] It is up to you.

REFERENCES

1. Covey, SR: The Seven Habits of Highly Successful People. Simon & Schuster, New York, 1989.
2. Schön, DA: The Reflective Practitioner: How Professionals Think in Action. Basic, New York, 1983.
3. Bennis, W: Why Leaders Can't Lead. Josey-Bass, San Francisco, 1989.
4. Shannon, P: The derailment of occupational therapy. Am J Occup Ther 31(4):229, Apr, 1977.
5. Bing, R: Occupational therapy revisited: A paraphrastic journey. Am J Occup Ther 35(8):499, 1981.

Acknowledgments

The author is indebted to all those who had a hand in the development of this book: my aunt, Miss Emma M. Emanuel, who shared her years as an English teacher to offer grammatical advice; my daughter Susan, who skillfully prepared all tables and figures; F. A. Davis Editor Lynn Borders Caldwell, who never thought it would happen, then did everything possible to bring it about; and my occupational therapy colleagues, who gave invaluable observations and suggestions. Gratitude is expressed to those who reviewed the original proposal and manuscript for this book and furnished suggestions for its improvement:

Carol Leonardelli Haertlein, PhD, OTR, FAOTA
Associate Professor
Occupational Therapy Program
University of Wisconsin-Milwaukee
Milwaukee, Wisconsin

Liane Hewitt, MPH, OTR
Assistant Professor and Program Director
Occupational Therapy Assistant Program
Loma Linda University
Loma Linda, California

Lela A. Llorens, PhD, OTR, FAOTA
Professor Emerita, Occupational Therapy
Former Associate Academic Vice President, Faculty Affairs
San Jose State University
San Jose, California

Helen Nodzak, MOT, OTR
Program Director, Occupational Therapy Assistant Program
Southwestern Community College
Sylva, North Carolina

Sharan L. Schwartzberg, EdD, OTR, FAOTA
Professor and Chair
Boston School of Occupational Therapy
Tufts University
Medford, Massachusetts

Kristin Seidner, MSW, OTR
Associate Professor and Program Director
Occupational Therapy Department
Louisiana State University
Shreveport, Louisiana

Contents

xviii

PART ONE

LEADERSHIP

When the best leader's work is done, the
people say, "We did it ourselves."
Lao-Tzu, 604–531 BC, *Tao Te Ching*

CHAPTER 1

Leadership Explored

CHAPTER OBJECTIVES

- To define and explain leadership.
- To compare manager and leader roles.
- To recognize the forms that power can take.
- To trace the evolution of leadership theory.
- To identify traits, skills, and behaviors for tomorrow's leaders.

Regardless of where an occupational therapist is employed, the potential to become an effective leader is always present. In the last analysis the single factor that actually and universally defines a leader is the acceptance of leadership by followers. The participative style of leadership is more likely to be acceptable to the majority of today's workers than autocratic behavior; however, no single pattern of leadership behavior is appropriate to all situations at all times. If your employees are mostly professionals, you may use mostly the participative style, but there still may be times when the situation calls for an autocratic approach, that is, making a decision, issuing an order, and expecting results. Also, there may be times when bureaucratic behavior is needed, when strict interpretation and application of rules are required.

Each successful leader is unique, yet all possess traits in common: values, vision, communication skills, persistence, self-confidence, optimism, empathy, and observation. You can improve your own skills in each of these areas, for leadership can be learned. As a manager, do not doubt or underestimate the fact that history and common sense tell us that people in any organization respond to the atmosphere created by the person at the top.

Leadership expert Warren Bennis[1] found that many of the successful people he interviewed never said they wanted to be leaders; rather, they found needs that required fulfillment and were very proactive in their search for opportunities. During periods of challenge and assessment in an organization, the nonleader is likely to expend too much energy trying to restore the organization to its previous way of operating. A true leader recognizes the same situation as an opportunity for organizational innovation. Positive energy plus the ability to recognize the relevance of seemingly unrelated facts signify a leader.

▨ The Manager vs. the Leader

Braque, the great French painter, is credited with having said that the only thing that really matters about painting cannot be explained. Bennis had a similar thought about leadership, that books by and about leaders are more interesting than books about leadership. He found the difference between managers and leaders to be fundamental, supporting this assertion by noting that:

The manager administers.	The leader innovates.
The manager maintains.	The leader develops.
The manager relies on systems.	The leader relies on people.
The manager counts on control.	The leader counts on trust.
The manager does things right.	The leader does the right thing.

Bennis also said that leadership involved questioning the routine. In unsettled times, managers have to be leaders and integrators besides managing their organizations for performance. Managers spend their time coping with change; leaders cause change and make their competition cope with it.

The views of Boyett and Conn[2] agree with those of Bennis. They asserted that the focus of a leader's attention and interest differs from that of a manager in still other ways. Although managers are mainly focused internally, leaders are politically adept, building consensus on a vision of the future and the steps needed to achieve that vision. At the same time these leaders are taking care of their internal management responsibilities. Managers think and act from a short-term view, while leaders operate for the long term. Managers have employees, but leaders have followers. Managers control and command as leaders inspire and empower. Leaders do not try to avoid or minimize change, as most managers do, but encourage and take advantage of it. Managers recognize and solve problems for their employees; leaders operationalize a vision and direction and empower and clear the way for their followers to make decisions and solve the problems.

From these perspectives you can readily see how management and leadership differ. You can also see why some individuals are considered to be *both* managers and leaders, while others succeed in doing solely the job of management, albeit very well. Managers' reliance on business as usual has led in many cases to their failure to meet, match, and beat competition because they possessed no gifts for changing, much less responding and improving. Without vision, the ability to build a network of people, and the resources to implement a strategy, a manager will not emerge as a leader. It is more difficult to develop leaders than to develop managers, and hardest of all is developing managers who can lead.

In his *Why Leaders Can't Lead,* Bennis[3] wrote that at least part of the reason why American business did not fare well in the 1980s was its "elevation of obedience over imagination. . . . The very businesses that have suffered the most, such as the auto industry, were founded by people who were far more imaginative than they were obedient. . . . America itself emerged out of simultaneous disobedience and vision. But in the current climate, vision is a fragile thing and needs to be nourished and developed in executives as well as employees and co-workers."

Bennis[3] took to task not only those in the major businesses of America but also each of us as individuals, declaring that few of us use even 50 percent of our potential. His further contention was that the best qualities found in all Americans (which most do not choose to use) are also the basic ingredients of leadership: *integrity* (standards of moral and intellectual honesty on which conduct is based), *dedication* (a passionate belief in something), *magnanimity* (noble of mind and heart; generous in forgiving; above revenge or resentment), *humility* (self-possessed, gracious winners and losers, who take more pride in what they do than in who they are), *openness* (willingness to hear and try new ideas, tolerance for ambiguity and change, rejection of prejudices, biases, and stereotypes), and *creativity* (thinking for yourself, truly seeing, hearing, understanding, connecting, and comprehending).

TWO MANAGERS WHO ARE ALSO LEADERS

One example of a manager who is also a leader is Herb Kelleher, chief executive officer of Southwest Airlines, noted for his vision, his unorthodox ways of achieving goals, his interest and concern for employees, his ability to identify what customers want and to then provide it, his skill in locating resources, and his endless enthusiasm and energy. Another recognized leader and doer, coincidentally also in the airline industry, is Jan Carlzon, who turned around two airline subsidiaries and then Scandinavian Airlines System itself by finding out what customers wanted and giving it to them. At age 32 he became president of an SAS subsidiary that offered tours, moved on at age 36 to be president of the SAS domestic airline, and in 1981 at the age of 38 took over SAS itself.

Like Kelleher and all leaders, Carlzon first of all *listened.* Also as leaders do, he took risks based on sound information coming out of that listening. In that way he turned SAS around in 1 year. Instead of relying on surveys, he put his marketing people behind ticket counters, face-to-face with buyers. New SAS planes were designed to suit passengers rather than simply using the latest technology. Wrong decisions did not cost employees their jobs, but right decisions did win praise and rewards. A typical response to an employee who made a costly mistake might be "No, why should I fire you? We have already invested $100,000 in you, and you have now learned a valuable lesson that will enable you to make better decisions in the future." Failure itself helps to mold leaders, and excellence comes from making more knowledgeable choices.

OCCUPATIONAL THERAPISTS AS MANAGERS WHO ARE LEADERS

Occupational therapists can be managers, leaders, or managers who are also leaders. Occupational therapists who are both managers and leaders are those who remain alert and aware of multiple trends and who subsequently attune themselves and adapt to changing circumstances. One example of adaptation to a trend is recognition of the differences between American workers in their 20s and those in their 30s and 40s, dubbed the generation Xers and the baby boomers. The former have been stereotyped in too many cases as cynical underachievers with dilatory work habits and ambitions. This is, of course, a generalization, and the manager-leader of today must recognize that generation Xers are individualistic and that they come with computer literacy, an understanding of diversity, a more global mindset, and constructive rebellion. Rather than perceive only adverse characteristics the leader-manager sees potential and develops it. Giving small teams of overachievers the freedom to break traditional management rules by providing them with moral support can stimulate creativity. Still another approach might be to realize that there is a difference between tolerating slackers by being "nice" and demanding achievement, which is truly being charitable.

▨ Power

Two important considerations are inextricably bound with the notion of leadership: power and acceptance by followers. A leader's ability to influence, persuade, and motivate followers is based largely on the *perceived* power of the leader. The forms of power a leader may possess are as follows:

> *coercive*—power based upon fear. A follower perceives that failing to comply with the request initiated by a leader could result in some form of punishment: a reprimand or social ostracism from a group.
>
> *reward*—power based upon the expectation of receiving praise, recognition, or income for compliance with a leader's request.
>
> *legitimate*—power derived from an individual's position in the group or organizational hierarchy. In a formal organization, the first-line supervisor is perceived to have more power than operating employees. In the informal group, the leader is recognized by the members as having legitimate power.
>
> *expert*—power based upon a special skill, expertise, or knowledge. The fol-

lowers perceive the person as having relevant expertise and believe that it exceeds their own.

    referent—power based on attractiveness and appeal. A leader who is admired because of certain traits possesses referent power. This form of power is popularly referred to as charisma. The person is said to have charisma to inspire and attract followers.[4]

This explanation of power can be applied specifically to an understanding of *leadership*, defined here as "interpersonal influence directed through communication toward the attainment of some goal or goals." With this definition in mind and because leadership involves use of influence, all interpersonal relationships—whether a football team or a committee—can involve leadership. The clarity and accuracy of what you communicate to potential followers can affect their behavior and performance. A leader may have to deal with individual, group, and organizational goals. Effectiveness is usually considered in terms of how effectively one or more of these goals are accomplished.[5]

In a far earlier place and time, Sophocles said in *Antigone,* "It is hard to learn the mind of any mortal, or the heart, till he be tried in chief authority. Power shows the man." An aspiring potential leader will do well to heed this thought.

Leadership Theories

THE GREAT MAN THEORY

Years ago it was believed that a person was "a born leader," inheriting the genes necessary to be a leader. The word *leader* first appeared in the English language in the year 1300; the word *leadership* itself did not appear until about 1800. In his *Handbook of Leadership* Stogdill[6] produced an organized inventory of all the research findings published about leadership up to 1974. For those readers wishing to study in depth the evolution of the subject, Stogdill offered an excellent compilation and summary of definitions based on 3000 studies conducted since 1902.

TRAIT THEORIES

Early theoretical studies of leadership focused on attempting to identify the traits effective leaders had in common. Most of the research was designed to identify intellectual, emotional, physical, and other personal characteristics of successful leaders. Stogdill found a general trend for leaders to be more intelligent than followers; however, extreme intelligence differences between leaders and followers may be dysfunctional.[6] Extensive research suggested that personality traits such as alertness, originality, personal integrity, individuality, and self-confidence were associated with effective leadership. Above-average height and weight were not disadvantages but at the same time were not necessary.

PERSONAL-BEHAVIORAL THEORIES

Several style or personal-behavioral leadership approaches hypothesized that a particular style of leadership brought about end results such as high production and satisfaction. They are represented by research done at Ohio State University and the University of Michigan, the Blake and Mouton managerial grid, and the four-factor methodology of Bowers and Seashore.

Many of the University of Michigan studies used effectiveness criteria including person-hour productivity, job satisfaction of organization members, costs, turnover, absenteeism, grievance rates, and employee and managerial motivation. Results of this research identified two distinct styles of leadership, known as *job-centered* and *employee-centered.* Job-centered leaders practice close supervision to ensure that subordinates perform their jobs according to strict procedures; they rely on coercion, reward, and legitimate power to influence the behavior of their followers. Employee-centered leaders, by contrast, delegate decision making and aid followers by creating a supportive work environment. These leaders are concerned with the personal advancement, growth, and achievement of their followers. Overall results of this body of research suggested that employee-centered leader behaviors are more effective.[7]

From the Ohio State studies emerged the *two-factor theory of leadership.* One independent leadership factor is *initiating structure,* which means that the leader organizes and defines the relationships in the group, establishes well-defined patterns and channels of communication, and specifies how the job is to be done. The other factor is *consideration behavior,* which indicates friendship, mutual trust, respect, warmth, and rapport between leader and followers. Early results implied that leaders above average in both consideration and initiating structure were more effective; however, researchers then began to find increasingly more complex interpretations, such as instances in which those supervisors who scored higher on structure had high ratings from superiors for productivity but more employee grievances and absenteeism. At the same time, higher consideration scores were related to lower productivity and less absenteeism. Final results indicated that leadership behavior has different effects on employee satisfaction depending on differing organizational climates.[6]

Although it lacked empirical support, the Blake and Mouton managerial grid was popular because it enabled leaders to identify their own leadership styles. The authors assumed that people and production concerns are complementary rather than mutually exclusive and therefore believed that leaders must integrate these concerns for effective performance results.[8]

Bowers and Seashore,[9] from the University of Michigan, saw four behavioral factors that define leadership behavior:

1. *Support:* behavior that builds followers' self-esteem and personal worth

2. *Interaction facilitation:* behavior that encourages close, mutually satisfying relationships in the group.

3. *Goal emphasis:* behavior that motivates enthusiasm for achieving high performance levels

4. *Work facilitation:* behavior that works toward goal achievement through scheduling, coordinating, planning, and providing resources

CONTINGENCY AND PATH-GOAL APPROACHES

Contingency theories suggest that leadership effectiveness depends on how personality, task, power, attitudes, and perceptions fit together in given situations, groups, and kinds of leaders. The three main leadership approaches that represent this school of thought are the life-cycle theory, the contingency model, and the path-goal theory.

Hersey and Blanchard's[10] *life-cycle approach* is based on the assumption that as the followers' level of maturity increases, appropriate leader behavior requires less structure (task) and less socioemotional support (relationships). Therefore, if a leader's followers are below average in maturity (i.e., achievement motivation, willingness or ability to take responsibility, education, and experience), the best style of leadership provides the most structure and the most interpersonal relationship. As followers reach the highest level of maturity, the least amounts of direction and relationship are required.

The conclusions of Hersey and Blanchard were that the maturity level of a group, or the stage of group development, is an important consideration in deciding how to lead. They suggest that leader behavior, to be effective, must change as followers mature. The occupational therapist can learn an important lesson here by keeping in mind that many more employees today are educated, motivated, and technically competent, so these employees potentially have more self-direction and self-control. Consequently, the most effective style of leadership, after initial orientation to the new job or task, usually has minimal structure or direction and relationships. The occupational therapist has the responsibility to evaluate the situation and make an appropriate choice of leadership style.

Fiedler[11] developed the *contingency model* of leadership effectiveness, which theorizes that group performance depends on the interaction of leadership style and favorableness of the situation. Fiedler stated that three situational factors influence a leader's effectiveness: leader-member relations, task structure, and position power.

Interpersonal *relationships* between leader and followers are likely to be the most important variable that determines power and influence, as they reflect the degree of confidence, trust, and respect followers have in the leader—their acceptance of the leader. The dimension of *task structure* includes goal clarity (how clearly stated and known the tasks and duties of the job are to those performing the job), goal-path multiplicity (the variety of procedures available to the worker to solve a problem), decision verifiability (how hard it is to get feedback that a solution or decision made by the worker is "correct"), and decision specificity (the degree to which there is more than one correct solution to a problem). *Position power* refers to the amount of power inherent in the leadership position: whether the leader can recommend rewards and punishments, independently punish and reward, or recommend promotion or demotion of subordinates.

The leader's power and influence seem most dependent on whether leader-member relations are good or poor, whether the task is relatively structured or unstructured, and whether the leader's position power is relatively strong or weak. It is easier to be a leader in a group in which you are liked, have a structured task, and hold position power.

Data accumulated from contingency model research indicated that a first step is to determine whether leaders are task- or relationship-oriented. Leadership style is then matched to the job and the environment and situation modified, if possible and if necessary.

The *path-goal theory* hypothesizes that leaders are effective because of their positive impact on followers' motivation, ability to perform, and satisfaction.[12] It is called *path-goal* because it centers on how a leader influences the followers' perceptions of work goals, self-development goals, and paths to goal attainment. Underlying this supposition is the expectancy motivation theory, which states that an individual's attitudes, job satisfaction, behavior, and effort on the job can be predicted from the degree to which each person feels that his or her behavior or performance will lead to various outcomes (expectancies) and how much the person values the outcomes. In other words, followers are motivated by leader style or behavior to the extent that it influences expectancies (goal paths) and valences (goal attractiveness). An important part of a leader's job is to clarify for followers the kinds of behaviors that are most likely to help them reach their goals.

This early path-goal work led to a more complex theory that involved four specific kinds of leader behavior: directive, supportive, participative, and achievement. A *directive* leader lets subordinates know what is expected of them, whereas the *supportive* leader treats subordinates as equals. *Participative* leaders consult with subordinates and use their suggestions and ideas in reaching decisions. An *achievement-oriented* leader proposes challenging goals, expects a high level of performance from subordinates, and continually looks for improvement in performance. House and Mitchell suggested flexibility in their conclusion that these four styles can be practiced by the same leader in various situations, in contrast to Fiedler, who thought that altering a leader's style is difficult.

Such research is valuable to today's practitioner, as are the concepts of stage of group development and the leader role. The leader role in the formation stage of a group is critical in this time of rapid turnover and change in the healthcare environment, a good illustration of contemporary group leadership in action.

AN INTEGRATED LEADERSHIP MODEL

Tannenbaum and Schmidt's[13] research model showed a continuum of leadership styles, each style related to the amount of authority used by the superior and to the degree of subordinate involvement in actually making decisions. The model supported the idea that no one style of leadership is better than another. The chosen type of leadership depended on each situation, keeping in mind the leader's own personality, the individual characteristics, needs, and behavioral patterns of the subordinates, the type of organization, the development and effectiveness of the group itself, the type of task being presented, and the pressure of time. Finally, external forces—the environment surrounding the situation—were taken into account.

Because in practice leaders are usually not totally participative, considerate, or directive, and because many situational, personal, and group variables influence leadership effectiveness, there is no "one best" style or theory of leadership. Aspiring occupational therapy leaders should diagnose their individual job situations in light of group characteristics, situational variables (related to the group), group behavior, their own characteristics, leader-related situational variables, their own behavior, and group effectiveness.

With this introduction to leadership research as a foundation, the occupational therapist who aspires to leadership should make a habit of reading current business-related literature. For example, words and phrases currently in popular use, such as *stretch goals* and *benchmark organizations,* are more readily understood and put into context with knowledge of the theoretical underpinnings from which they have evolved. Then the challenges of today's ever-changing healthcare delivery scene become more understandable and surmountable.

▓ Styles or Types of Leadership

There are multiple ways to categorize styles of leadership, each one depending on the words used by a particular writer; however, in the last analysis the only differences are semantic. Liebler, Levine, and Rothman[14] categorized styles of leadership as *autocratic, bureaucratic, participative, laissez-faire,* and *paternalistic.* Autocratic leadership is also considered authoritarian, boss-centered, or dictatorial and is characterized by close supervision. Employees are given direct, clear, and precise directions telling them what is to be done and how and leaving no room for employee initiative. Autocratic leaders use their authority as their principal, or only, method of getting work done.

Like the autocratic leader, the bureaucratic individual tells employees what to do and how to do it, with the institution's rules and regulations as the basis. He or she strictly enforces rules, allows employees little or no freedom, and rarely takes chances.

Participative leadership emphasizes the contribution of the group to the organizational effort. Employees are involved in the decision-making process and in the maintenance of cohesive group interaction. The leader acting as facilitator makes full use of the talents and abilities of the group members. A leader's formal authority is not weakened because the leader retains the right to make the final decision.

Laissez-faire or "free rein" leadership is based on the assumption that employees are self-motivated and so receive little or no supervision. As individuals or as a group, they identify their own goals and make their own decisions. Acting primarily as a consultant, the leader allows the employees to lead themselves.

Paternalistic leaders treat employees as children in the belief that employees do not really know what is good for them or how to make decisions. The "benign dictator" watches over the employees and encourages them to become dependent on their paternalistic boss.

▨ Leadership Traits, Skills, and Behavior

Leadership theory can be useful in situations that are encountered upon entry to practice. Leadership is both a function of personality structure and situational interaction, not a position inherited "by divine right" of birth or personality. True, common sense dictates that certain traits such as intelligence, risk taking, flexibility, and verbal facility may prove valuable in identifying some individuals capable of developing leadership potential, but leadership itself is too complex to be limited by one list of universal criteria.

Boyett and Conn,[2] in analyzing the revolution reshaping American business, gave their prophecy of what will be needed by leaders going into the next century. These authors added their own particular version of personal attributes for leaders to those previously cited: positive regard for self as well as others, optimism, lifelong learning enjoyment, an orientation to action and change, empathy, a clearly defined set of values, and a need to achieve.

Besides attributes, some of which are genetic (e.g., intelligence) and most of which are learned (personal and interpersonal), Boyett and Conn believed that with heuristic encouragement most people can learn the skills of leadership. Among the skills they considered necessary were:

- Communication skills—the ability to read rapidly with high comprehension, to write clearly, to speak persuasively, and to listen effectively.
- Political skills—negotiation, conflict resolution, and consensus building.
- Motivation skills—use of cognitive and behavioral approaches to change people's behavior.
- Trust-building skills—expression of commitment, demonstrating self-confidence, sharing values, and sensitivity.

- Empowerment skills—delegation, exacting responsibility and account-ability, building teams, facilitating problem solving.
- Skills to evaluate current trends and foresee long-term significant de-velopments that could affect the organization. Of particular importance is a global awareness of economics, science and technology, and cul-tures other than one's own.

Intellectual or cognitive skills needed by a leader might be the ability to fig-ure out a problem, to handle abstract ideas and see a broad perspective, to make a plan and follow through, and to project into the future and see the con-sequences of decisions. The personal skills of leaders enable them to judge ap-propriateness of decisions, directions, or suggestions, cope with unpleasant-ness, absorb interpersonal stress, and tolerate ambiguity, delay, and frustration. Interpersonal or group behaviors for a leader include listening to and recogniz-ing the abilities of others, interacting easily with others and inspiring confi-dence, perceiving and handling unstated feelings, following well, supporting group members, accepting responsibility, determining appropriate courses of action, organizing others, directing activities, delegating responsibility, and es-tablishing the mood of the group.

Tomorrow's Leaders

Leadership in the changing healthcare organizations of today does not differ from that of other business corporations. It is influencing human behavior in an environment of ongoing uncertainty. Major corporations today have acknowl-edged that the "hard and soft" sides of management must be melded as young leaders are developed. They must be helped to grow, listen, and become more intuitive. Leader-managers of these organizational environments focus on re-moving barriers in the way of creative, constructive persons and minimizing constraints that inhibit their productivity. The idea of "management by walking around," an expression credited to Sam Walton of Wal-Mart, could be taken one step further and labeled "management by getting out of the way," for today's leader is apt to be not defensive or egotistical but rather open-minded, focused, and committed to nurturing the potential in employees.

Ongoing examples of research about leadership characteristics can be read in current business publications. These offer illustrations of leadership research concepts at work. For example, the Campbell Soup Company, formerly a strong and steady success over the years, at the close of the 1980s was beset by falling earnings, weak marketing, and internal feuding.[15] New CEO David Johnson brought the company back by 1995 to rival benchmark companies by exempli-fying the aforementioned leadership characteristics in clearly identifiable ways. Emotional and quantifiable factors were the answer, as Johnson used rational thinking, charisma, and a clear, tough analysis of the financial aspects of the com-pany. Experts asserted that many CEOs fail at two crucial tasks: communication strategy and aligning their followers behind a vision. Johnson, in his own estimation, succeeded fully in achieving both of these tasks by thinking like a small company, diminishing bureaucracy and the power games, rewarding successful risk taking, and empowering and building confidence among employees.[15]

Leadership can also be regarded as character that requires growth and personal change. The variety of leadership found among those who "bloom where they are planted" is as essential to the growth of the profession as that of the "Alexander the Great" type, and occupational therapy literature is replete with examples of both.

▓ Summary

This chapter has introduced the concept of leadership and emphasized its importance and relevance for occupational therapists. The history and evolution of theories of leadership were described to provide a foundation for understanding this complex and timely subject. Several recognized authorities' observations on the subject of leadership were shared and their value for occupational therapists explained. The varied kinds of power were explained, as was the importance of perceptions of power in the dynamics of leadership. With this discussion as a basis, Chapter 2 more directly relates the leadership concept to occupational therapy practice.

REFERENCES

1. Bennis, W: Leadership from inside out. Fortune, Jan 18, 1988, p 173.
2. Boyett, JH, and Conn, HP: Workplace 2000. Dutton, New York, 1991.
3. Bennis, W: Why Leaders Can't Lead. Jossey-Bass, San Francisco, 1989, pp 109–110, 117–120.
4. French, JRP, and Raven, B: The bases of social power. In Cartwright, D, and Zander, AF (eds): Group Dynamics, ed 2. Row, Peterson, Evanston, Ill, 1960, p 607.
5. Fleischman, EA: Twenty years of consideration and structure. In Fleischman, EA, and Hunt, JG (eds): Current Developments in the Study of Leadership. Southern Illinois Univ. Pr., Carbondale, 1973, p 3.
6. Stogdill, RM: Handbook of Leadership. Free Press, New York, 1974.
7. Likert, R: New Patterns of Management. McGraw-Hill, New York, 1967.
8. Blake, RR, and Mouton, JS: The Managerial Grid. Gulf Pub., Houston, 1964.
9. Bowers, DG, and Seashore, SE: Predicting organizational effectiveness with a four-factor theory of leadership. Administrative Science Quarterly, Sept, 1966, p 238.
10. Hersey, P, and Blanchard, KH: Management of Organization Behavior. Prentice-Hall, Englewood Cliffs, NJ, 1972.
11. Fiedler, FE: A Theory of Leadership Effectiveness. McGraw-Hill, New York, 1967.
12. House, RJ, and Mitchell, TR: Path-goal theory of leadership. Journal of Contemporary Business, Autumn 1974.
13. Tannenbaum, R, and Schmidt, WH: How to choose a leadership pattern. Harvard Business Review, May–June, 1973.
14. Leibler, JG, Levine, RE, and Rothman, J: Management Principles for Health Professionals, ed 2. Aspen, Gaithersburg, Md, 1992.
15. Grant, L: Stirring it up at Campbell. Fortune 133(9):56, May 13, 1996.

CHAPTER 2

Occupational Therapy Leaders: From the Student Perspective

CHAPTER OBJECTIVES

- To recognize a continuing need for leadership in occupational therapy.
- To know what occupational therapy leadership means.
- To identify an effectively led organization.
- To value the power of charisma in leadership.
- To consider new career roles for occupational therapy leaders.
- To offer perspectives and advice for beginning occupational therapists.

For every occupational therapist who feels that he or she is not a leader, be reminded that Abraham Maslow said, "Each time one takes responsibility, this is an actualizing of the self." With that in mind, *any* responsibility you assume is also the first step toward taking charge, and that is becoming a leader! What responsibilities have you assumed lately? In the past year? Are you further along the path to being a leader than you realized? In only 10 two-letter words, *leadership* can be defined: If it is to be, it is up to me.[1]

Through explanation and example, this chapter guides the reader toward a leadership role. It defines sometimes misunderstood terms to assist you in developing a growing awareness of personal potential.

▨ Leadership Begins with the Past

Beginning occupational therapists are blessed with a rich heritage of leaders who have laid the foundation and set the standards through their effective work to establish this profession. It is always dangerous to begin naming names, for the list of valued leaders is long, illustrious, and still growing; however, students need to familiarize themselves with the extraordinary accomplishments of those who have preceded them.

Students, if you have not yet done so, read as much as possible of the history of occupational therapy, as one leader after another proactively laid the groundwork of this field. Begin with the earliest pioneers—Adolf Meyer, Susan Tracy, Herbert Hall, Eleanor Clarke Slagle, William Rush Dunton, George Edward Barton, and Susan C. Johnson—and then follow the continuing achievements of outstanding leaders such as Clare S. Spackman and her evaluation and treatment of patients with physical disabilities, Gail S. Fidler and the psychodynamic approach to occupational therapy, A. Jean Ayres with a neurobehavioral orientation, Wilma West and her proposal for prevention and movement of practice into the community, Anne Cronin Mosey with frames of reference for psychiatric occupational therapy, and Mary Reilly with an occupational behavior orientation. Leadership and progress are rooted in history, so today's beginning occupational therapy practitioner is urged to develop a strong sense of continuity, gain a broad perspective of the present environment, and maintain that special attribute of creativity.

A LEADER FOLLOWS TO LEAD

Effective leaders take more risks, encourage others to be creative, are respected by their peers, and are sought by others for their ideas. A good leader is, at the same time, a good follower. An effective leader leads a group in setting and achieving goals but additionally listens to and values the opinions of each individual and arrives at mutually satisfactory decisions with the group. As noted in Chapter 1, much helpful research has been conducted to determine how a person becomes a leader; however, leadership experts all agree that you can reinforce your inherent leadership abilities by recognizing what they are and how you can use them. Growth begins when individuals objectively understand their own strengths and weaknesses and take responsibility for their own development.

Climate of an Effectively Led Organization

As managers, occupational therapy practitioners should assume responsibility for effective organizational leadership. When envisioning an organization with effective leadership, such as that described by Bennis in *Why Leaders Can't Lead,*[2] one pictures a satisfying environment. Leadership of this kind can be felt throughout the organization. Work is given pace and energy through an empowered work force. Bennis contends that "empowerment is the collective effect of leadership" and that in organizations with effective leaders four themes are present:

1. People feel significant, that what they do has meaning and makes a difference.
2. Learning and competence matter, and there is no failure, just mistakes that provide feedback to be used in future performance.
3. People are part of a community with a close-knit feeling.
4. Work is exciting, challenging, fascinating, and fun with a style of influence that attracts and energizes people.

Bennis observed that the basic ingredients of leadership are integrity, dedication, magnanimity, humility, openness, and creativity and that few of us use even 50 percent of our full potential. Imagining the result if occupational therapists fully applied these ingredients of leadership is a heartening prospect indeed.

Current management literature extols the value of the manager who is able to lead with empathy and perception. It is time that occupational therapists, already endowed with these characteristics and more, cease being reticent and instead emphasize using their special attributes of empathy, nurturance, creativity, and perception of human needs. Charisma is discussed next because understanding its role in leadership provides added strength to potential occupational therapy leaders.

Leadership and the Power of Charisma

Rose's[3] opinion was that charisma is the most powerful form of leadership, the kind that inspires and involves people in a dream or vision. The word *charisma* comes from the Greek, is translated as "gift of divine grace," and continues to be rather esoteric, admired, and difficult to understand. Rose envisioned charisma as an individual quality that enables persons to empower themselves and others. She further thought that the title of her book, *Charisma: Power, Passion and Purpose,* describes what is actually meant by the word. An explanation of *power,* as interpreted by French and Raven, was presented in Chapter 1. Rose thought that a leader also imparts power through the ability to put things in order or to make sense of a chaotic world. By *passion* she meant a deep belief presented by the leader, a belief so intense and truly felt that it seems somehow obtainable; *purpose* is a clear and definite future vision.

Of most potential help to new practitioners is Rose's contention that *everyone* has some power to attract, motivate, and inspire others. As a result, she developed a five-rung charismatic ladder with which individuals can assess their current status and plan for future charismatic growth. The five-rung continuum begins with the individual who has potential but is not acting on it, moving on to the next level to one who has charm or glamour. (Rose's personal experience has been that physical appearance actually has very little to do with charisma.) At the third step, individuals have well-developed self-esteem, and they project confidence. Charisma that is perceived as a result of achievement is fourth, with these persons having gone beyond competence and self-confidence to really making a dent in their own cultures. At the highest level, rarely reached, individuals through their mere presence exude power, passion, and purpose.

Students should strive to add order to their lives, find a worthy role model to emulate, improve their vocabularies, begin to work toward accomplishments and achievements, and develop problem-solving skills. The process can begin today.

▓ Occupational Therapists in New Roles

In 1967 one of occupational therapy's outstanding leaders, Wilma West, foresaw four emerging roles for occupational therapists as evaluators, consultants, supervisors, and researchers. The 1990s find occupational therapists indeed in those roles and more as they have moved forward in the community and in academe.

The premiere issue of *OT Practice* in 1995 illustrated the amazing diversity of choices in occupational therapy practice today. To demonstrate the potential for leadership in infinite forms within occupational therapy today, a few examples of current achievements are cited here.

Mary Sadler, COTA, has established a medical records business in New Mexico that specializes in serving only therapists and whose mission is to provide therapists with high-quality documentation of services to improve the reimbursement process. Following 10 months of community research to determine what services were needed, Susan Swindeman, OTR, BCP, SII, SIPT, opened Wee Care Therapy, Inc., in Indiana, to offer occupational therapy, physical therapy, and speech-language pathology with emphasis on the family's and the child's goals. She uses much cotreatment, close communication, and high-quality care that is child-directed but therapist-guided.[4]

Partners in Play was founded in Florida by Catherine Theiss Feyerabend, OTR. This is a new, developmentally based program for parents and their children that, because of Feyerabend's occupational therapy background, offers more than the traditional developmental play program. In Maine the Arthritis Foundation sponsored Diane Robarge, OTR, to lead a special exercise class for persons with arthritis at a local hospital: People with Arthritis Can Exercise (PACE).[4]

In Pennsylvania, Joseph Padova, OTR, established the Monitor Neuro Fitness Program for patients whose treatment for stroke was ended for varying reasons. Rather than sending them home with a customary exercise regimen, Padova devised a program that focuses on the stroke patients' upper extremities and follows through on what the patients were doing in their original therapy programs.[4]

Ann Burkhardt, MA, OTR, president of the New York State Occupational Therapy Association, uses alternative therapies routinely in her private practice. She notes that "at one time what the Bobaths were talking about was considered pretty radical. Today it's second nature."[4] A few major medical centers are now trying non-Western healing methods. A renowned cardiothoracic surgeon uses alternative therapies in some cases because conventional medicine is not sufficient to relieve the depression and stress experienced by cardiac patients.[5]

Florence Gold, MA, OTR, a home health occupational therapist in California, is part of a team that provides antepartum home care to women experiencing a multitude of complications during pregnancy. The high-risk antepartum home-care program filled a need for service for women with high-risk pregnancies who were discharged home and ordered to wait out their preconfinement in bed. Any woman confined to bed rest for more than 4 weeks receives occupational therapy.[6]

In 1984 Engel wrote of the horse as a modality for occupational therapy.[7] Since that article appeared, a growing body of literature has reinforced the contention that hippotherapy is an appropriate area for occupational therapy practice. One example is the Therapeutic and Recreational Riding Center Inc. (TRRC) in Glenwood, Maryland, a 55-acre complex that, when complete, will offer occupational therapy, physical therapy, speech and language pathology, aquatic therapy, hippotherapy, and riding lessons. The unique facility was founded by Helen Tuel, EdD, in response to people with special needs who could be helped with therapeutic riding. In addition to children, patients of all ages with cancer, head injuries, cerebral palsy, amputations, heart conditions, strokes, autism, mental retardation, and emotional trauma are among those benefiting from Tuel's initial response to a recognized need.[8]

Steve LaBossiere of Peterborough, New Hampshire, was diagnosed with multiple sclerosis in 1990. He lost his communications job. Recognizing the need for people with disabilities to network with peers, doctors, and allied health professionals to learn more about their disabilities, he founded Disabilities Connection, an online bulletin board that enables people with disabilities to communicate. LaBossiere's wife, Carolyn, an occupational therapist, and Virginia Younie, another occupational therapist from Keene, New Hampshire, serve as moderators for this 24-hour service. They offer a wide range of topics, from diagnostic categories to leisure activities and beneficial information about the healthcare professions. LaBossiere focuses on his goal to make the network informative and entertaining while he and his staff offer individual guidance to participants new to the system.[9]

Among the current and potential roles in mental health occupational therapy practice, Jane Lipscomb, OTR, suggests that occupational therapists make ideal leaders in improving psychiatric outcomes through directive group treatment. Because occupational therapists have backgrounds in both physical disabilities and psychosocial skills, she thinks that they can achieve most effectively the objectives of such groups.[10]

Peggy Swarbrick and Diana Hunt, in New Jersey, have developed a health promotion model to extend the role of occupational therapists into community health care while introducing the perspective of wellness and health promotion. Realizing that this perspective is an integral part of occupational therapy, the two secured a grant from the Council of State Association Presidents (CSAP) and evolved their idea.[11]

▓ Organizations Widen Their Boundaries

Many organizations continuously adapt and widen their boundaries. At the Texas Institute for Research and Rehabilitation (TIRR) in Houston, all occupational therapy treatment program planning begins with the questions "What can't you do?" and "What do you want most to do?" This is as it has always been. Widening boundaries has been the goal since William Spencer, MD, established TIRR, an independent center.

Today the finding and filling of needs goes on as Barbara Nelson, OTR, coordinates the Challenge Program, an outpatient community reintegration program for clients who have suffered traumatic brain injuries, brain tumors, anoxia, and other conditions and for clients with severe spinal cord injuries. For many years TIRR has been noted and respected for its successful treatment of spinal cord–injured clients. The Challenge Program was developed when leaders realized that clients leaving the intense rehabilitation program at TIRR found barriers to transferring their learned skills to community and home settings. As a result, work continues with clients in the home and at work, including travel on city buses.

Across the country this form of successful adaptation takes place as creative occupational therapists expand their boundaries of thinking and practice. Shoshana Shamberg, OTR, and Aaron Shamberg, MLA, teamed up in Baltimore with their business, Abilities Occupational Inc., a consulting firm specializing in independent living services. Clients such as those who have had brain injuries can maximize their independence at home with environmental modifications, adaptive equipment, and caregiver training.[12]

Jill Spokojny, OTR, owner of VOCA Rehabilitation in the Detroit area, specializes in home accessibility, works with the building industry, and recognizes a huge potential market for occupational therapy practitioners who will work with seniors who wish to "age in place." She asserts that frequently the environment prevents people from staying in their homes. Jacqueline Dobson, COTA/L, an access design and resource consultant who founded Solutions for Accessibility in Framingham, Massachusetts, concurs. She adds that, for example, occupational therapy practitioners can bring a knowledge of disability and product resources and can predict what a client's function will be in 5 years. Both agree that occupational therapy practitioners must learn the language of the construction industry as a start toward successful teamwork with the builder. The occupational therapy practitioner often knows what result is needed, but it is the contractor or architect who know how to get there. Spokojny notes that occupational therapy practitioners in home accessibility cannot be passive and wait for people to come to them. They need to get out into the community and explain what they do, so the community begins to realize that they are not limited to medical rehabilitation.[13]

Adams described the work of burn team members (nurses, physical therapists, and occupational therapists) at Saint Barnabas Medical Center in Livingston, New Jersey. They recognized the need to produce home healthcare professionals who are better educated in the treatment of survivors of severe burns in their home settings. Team members share their experience with their peers through their course, "Home Care for Burns."[14]

Hospice care is still another opportunity to which occupational therapists have responded. Nancy Griffin, EdD, OTR, of Denton, Texas, is an example of an occupational therapist who responded in the early 1980s by joining with several professionals and clients to form a local hospice. Griffin continues to serve as a board member of this highly successful organization, Ann's Haven Hospice of Denton.

■ Beginning a New Career

Entry-level occupational therapy practitioners are particularly fortunate in that they have already been taught in their educational programs those core values and skills that are the essence of the "soft" side of leadership and management. Courses that include information about leading groups, the psychology of working with clients, and clinical reasoning help occupational therapists relate to and motivate individuals. Those in business are the first to recognize that human interactions are harder for most leaders to manage than the business "hard stuff." At the same time, the student must realize that tough standards of accountability, an understanding of profit and loss, and the hard realities of business are essential for success today. With that realization firmly in place and while working toward its achievement, occupational therapists can rejoice in the fact that they already understand the other essential part of leadership, the "soft side," for which many others must work to add and integrate.

When embarking on a career today, any individual should expect to be employed and valued for her or his contribution to the organization, not for a particular level in the hierarchy. Many of today's organizational charts consist of often-shifting project groups that are led by the group members possessing the professional background and competencies needed to address the problem assigned to those groups. Growth in your chosen profession will be a goal as your career evolves.

With leadership goals in mind, employees should not always rely on convention but rather question it constructively. Become aware of globalization and its consequences and opportunities. Never stop trying to grow; lifelong learning is becoming increasingly essential for success. Benchmark your skills regularly by checking the want ads to see what employers seek and what you may need to learn to enhance your personal and therapeutic abilities and thus your future potential. Be constantly aware of what you are contributing in your current position and of your marketable skills.

▓ Summary

This chapter has shown how an entry-level occupational therapist can begin to develop the skills and attitudes of a leader. Recognizing opportunities and welcoming the accompanying responsibilities should become part of a developing leader's personality. Organizations that have climates of effective leadership were described. Examples of occupational therapists who have successfully moved into leadership positions in new roles across the country are meant to be representative of the hundreds who are today's creative role models. Chapter 3 introduces the possibilities that are awaiting the potential occupational therapy professional leaders of tomorrow.

REFERENCES

1. Simon, M: Unpublished material, 1995.
2. Bennis, W: Why Leaders Can't Lead. Jossey-Bass, San Francisco, 1989.
3. Rose, LH: Charisma: Power, Passion and Purpose. Bearly Limited Press, Buffalo, 1991.
4. Stancliff, BL: Innovative occupational therapy practitioners. OT Practice, Premiere Issue, Nov 1995, p 11.
5. Stahl, C: Dealing with doctors. Advance for Occupational Therapists 11(45):12, Nov 13, 1995.
6. Marmer, L: Antepartum home care saves lives and money. Advance for Occupational Therapists 11(23):13, June 12, 1995.
7. Engel, BT: The horse as a modality for occupational therapy. Occupational Therapy in Health Care 1(1):41, 1984.
8. Adams, R: Therapy center offers diverse treatment options and much more. Advance for Occupational Therapists 11(41):10, Oct 16, 1995.
9. Kerr, T: Getting the right connection. Advance for Occupational Therapists 11(41):22, Oct 16, 1995.
10. Lipscomb, JM: Improving psychiatric outcomes. OT Week 9(44):14, Nov 2, 1995.
11. Kerr, T: Opening the door to prevention. Advance for Occupational Therapists, May 8, 1995, p 20.
12. Shamberg, S, and Shamberg A: Reentry begins at home. Rehab Management 8(5):124, 1995.
13. Hettinger, J: Beyond building codes. OT Week 10(27):12, July 4, 1996.
14. Adams, RC: Treating patients with burns at home. Advance for Occupational Therapists, May 22, 1995, p 10.

CHAPTER 3

Potential Occupational Therapy Leadership: An Entry-Level View

CHAPTER OBJECTIVES

- To understand the balance between opportunity and responsibility.
- To value the options for leadership open to occupational therapists today.
- To offer admonitions for wise progression through the levels of leadership.
- To recognize the potential options in career development.
- To perceive the power and potential within occupational therapists.

Adaptable, flexible, innovative occupational therapists are responding enthusiastically to today's many challenges and new possibilities. When an occupational therapy student recently asked, "What is the future of occupational therapy?" the immediate response was "That is up to you." An old Army Air Corps acronym says it even better: CAVU, or ceiling and visibility unlimited. Opportunity abounds in education, research, practice, public service, industry, and new niches still undiscovered. Students are encouraged to become aware of the multiple avenues for leadership awaiting them within occupational therapy.

This chapter introduces the student to a wide variety of choices for practice. It includes admonitions for avoiding certain areas of practice that require advanced expertise.

▨ Beginning on the Road Toward Leadership in Practice

Students may still feel perplexed at this point about the available avenues for leadership. One systematic way to begin deciding on a direction is to consider the potential roles of occupational therapists as listed by the AOTA Occupational Therapy Roles Task Force, approved in 1993 by the AOTA Representative Assembly. The suggested roles are OTR practitioner, COTA practitioner, educator (consumer, peer), fieldwork educator (practice setting), supervisor, administrator, consultant, fieldwork coordinator (academic setting), faculty, program director (academic), researcher, and entrepreneur. While gaining practical on-the-job experience during fieldwork education, the student can observe occupational therapists who are employed in each of these categories.

Graduating students should carefully choose fieldwork placements and first jobs, preferably in structured, supervised situations—or at the very least with an experienced mentor or role model—in order to gain experience and self-assurance before venturing into positions requiring more independent performance. The time invested in such positions will be rewarding in the long run because improved self-confidence will then enable therapists to feel more comfortable in new and innovative roles and progress into leadership situations. In addition, each therapist is representing occupational therapy and should be demonstrating the high quality of service that professionals can provide and that clients expect. Each person is therefore responsible for being sufficiently prepared. Following are several examples of areas of practice that graduates may choose. The demands and complexities of each are often not apparent to the neophyte, and unfortunately common sense often is the most needed but least available commodity among the inexperienced.

PRIVATE PRACTICE

Occupational therapists began to venture into private practice roles in the 1970s. *Private practice* is defined here as a sole proprietorship in which independent contracting therapists provide direct services in a private practice office. Shriver[1] described an added dimension for this role as that of the private practice occupational therapist in evaluation, treatment, consultation, and testimony for workers' compensation or personal injury cases. Extensive experience in management and in treatment are among the skills needed for assuming control of any private practice enterprise.

WORK HARDENING

There appears to be a continuing demand for work hardening. Before venturing into this specialty with leadership as a goal, occupational therapists need more business and in-depth marketing skills. *Work Hardening: State of the Art* by Ogden-Niemeyer and Jacobs[2] and numerous publications written more recently describe this potential specialty area of practice and its opportunities for leadership.

SCHOOL SYSTEMS

Employment in school systems is a steadily maturing area of practice for occupational therapists. There are leaders in classrooms, state education agencies, transition program planning in the public education system, and in many other roles depending on local, state, and federal regulations. The value and potential of occupational therapy to enhance service provision for children within age-appropriate natural life environments and to advocate for a comprehensive integration of adaptive skills with the child's and family's specific environmental needs become steadily more evident. This occupational therapy leadership role can be conducted as a therapist in direct treatment, as part of an educational team, in a group format, or as a consultant.

CONSULTANCY

Occupational therapy consultants are found in many areas of leadership in education and practice today. Consultation is a complex process that includes elements of helping, interaction, problem solving, resource identification, and systems analysis. Occupational therapists employ varying degrees of each of these skills, depending on the level of consultation in which they are involved. Levels of involvement range from case-centered consultation to educational consultation to program or administration consultation. There are models of occupational therapy consultation practice in school settings, long-term care, developmental centers, acute care, geriatric psychiatry, hospitals, community facilities, adult day care, business and industry, academe, and in many other types of facilities.

Consultation is obviously an intricate process into which a new therapist without extensive personal experience should never consider entering. *Occupational Therapy Consultation* by Jaffe and Epstein[3] makes clear the theory, principles, and components that must be studied and understood well before venturing into this challenging, demanding role.

▓ Academic Leadership

Lecturers, instructors, fieldwork educators, professors, program directors, department chairs, deans, and vice presidents are leaders, and occupational therapists can be found across America and internationally holding these positions in occupational therapy education. Not only are these leaders important in the institutions employing them but also their contributions are critical to the survival and future of the profession. They are expected to transfer the profession's core knowledge to students and at the same time remain updated on all trends and changes in practice, then integrate this information into the coursework, for graduating students should be prepared to enter today's world of work.

Faculty members who have been rewarded by their educational institutions for their outstanding teaching are often found in occupational therapy programs. Educational program directors are additional evidence of the leadership within the profession, as nearly 100 new OTR programs have been developed and successfully accredited since 1944, and from the first three COTA educational programs begun in 1960 there are today more than 140.

Leadership is evident among the newest and in the more seasoned occupational therapy educators such as Gail Fidler, a prominent name and guiding force in occupational therapy for more than 50 years. Known for her vision and innovation, she embodies the spirit of leadership. The list of educator-leaders is too long and illustrious to detail here. The rewards to be found in an academic career may differ from those of other areas of practice, but nevertheless the dividends are many. Therapists are encouraged to watch for continuing education offerings from AOTA in *OT Week*. Presentations at state and national conferences also offer guidance in how to make transitions from clinical practice to academe.

▦ Leadership in Management

Whatever the location of employment, occupational therapists daily show leadership in management. To do this effectively, though, requires thorough familiarity with managerial functions and an awareness of key business trends. These are among the skills of manager-leaders who are proactive in their adaptation to changes.

With the introduction of managed care and product-line management have come project teams and often-daily committee meetings, as task groups seek to resolve assigned problems. A competency needed by both new and experienced managers is skill in conducting productive committee meetings. Chairing meetings affords opportunities for anyone to experience and demonstrate leadership acuity.

Occupational therapists who already have experience in management can never stop learning, either. In this they are not alone. Admission to executive master's in business administration (EMBA) programs, such as those offered at the Wharton School of the University of Pennsylvania, University of Chicago, Purdue University, or Columbia University, requires that students be already-experienced managers and in midcareer. The guiding premise is that management development must be regarded as a continuum that begins with a person's first job and continues to career end.[4]

Research Leadership

Validation of occupational therapy is one of the most essential challenges and needs within the profession today. It is therefore the responsibility and privilege of therapists to contribute to the body of knowledge, whether they are employed in the academic community or in another area of practice. The quality and quantity of occupational therapy research grows daily, thanks to the hard work and interest of many professionals. Role models among occupational therapists in research leadership are those who have been elected to be members of the prestigious Academy of Research and the leaders honored by being selected to present the Slagle Lectures. The profession is proud of the accomplishments of each of these outstanding professionals and appreciates the validating knowledge they have contributed.

Contributions to research are not limited to those individuals, however. Growing numbers of grants and contracts are awarded after rigorous competitions to occupational therapists who conduct valuable studies in support of occupational therapy. Researchers use both quantitative and qualitative methodologies for theory development, outcomes studies, or work on the efficacy of specific treatment modalities. Quantitative methods of measuring results are essential and widely used. At the same time, qualitative methods can lead to equally effective and useful clinical practice. There is an exciting breadth in the possibilities open to those occupational therapists whose primary interests and talents lie in research careers.

Students must learn research skills and thus be better able to engage in studies of the effectiveness of the treatments they are providing. Such research is essential not only to the future of occupational therapy but also to gain remuneration for services in a cost-conscious healthcare environment. The processes and tools of research provide practitioners with a valuable means through which they can represent occupational therapy in collaboration with their professional colleagues. Research results effectively demonstrate the efficacy and productivity of occupational therapy and ultimately improve the quality of care itself.

Leadership in Wellness and Health Promotion

Educated and attuned to the integral power of activity, occupational therapists are prepared to move naturally into health promotion and disease prevention. Articles in popular and scientific publications attest to the growing recognition of health promotion attitudes and activities as wise and logical approaches to health care. The profession for years has had visionaries, two of whom are Wilma West and Jerry Johnson, who have urged colleagues to move into health promotion roles. Here, then, is still another option to be considered by the beginning therapist; however, a receptivity to wellness and to health promotion should be integrated into an occupational therapist's attitude regardless of specialty choice.

Ethical and Moral Leadership

Even a mention of this aspect of occupational therapy would seem unnecessary, yet it is critical to remind new occupational therapists to be fully conscious of how to integrate ethical and moral conduct into every day. All occupational therapists have encountered ethical and moral dilemmas on more than one occasion. The inevitable future complexities and pressures of healthcare service delivery will not lessen this challenge. It is therefore the responsibility of all occupational therapists to keep themselves apprised of how to make ethical and moral decisions in education or in community practice.

An illustration of the importance of ethics to everyone is the presence on the AOTA staff of an ethics program manager, Penny Kyler-Hutchison. Her frequent articles, sharing new information and citing experiences as examples, can be found in *OT Week*. Members are encouraged to contact the ethics program manager with their questions. Another valuable resource is the book *Ethical and Legal Dilemmas in Occupational Therapy* by Bailey and Schwartzberg.[5] The authors used a format developed by Hutchison and Hansen to analyze and resolve questions of ethical behavior typically faced by occupational therapists, whether students, clinicians, or managers.

Assuming leadership in ethical and moral behavior is within the power of every occupational therapist. It is not easy, and some dilemmas are infinitely harder to resolve than others. At the same time, all therapists are called on to make value-laden judgments in their professional lives, and there is no true leader who does not act with the highest of ethics and morals.

Leadership in Professional Association Service

Commencing as students in occupational therapy programs, here is an area in which everyone can and should participate and assume leadership. National, state, district, and school occupational therapy associations offer opportunities to serve and lead. The profession values and supports student leaders, for they are tomorrow's association leaders and are the future of occupational therapy. The rewards of serving one's professional association are many, for this is a readily available training ground for progression to higher levels of leadership. The efforts expended directly benefit everyone, most of all the participant.

Leadership in Client-Centered Treatment

Peloquin[6] brought to our attention the importance of reaffirming commitment to the *art* of occupational therapy, to the central caring element of treatment. One method she suggested was to read fiction "to provide occupational therapists with sustaining images: images of relationships, images of qualities that make relationships meaningful, and images of the meaning of occupation in a life." She decried the tendency to reduce occupational therapy "to a sterile science of occupation" and away from the caring elements in collaborative treatment planning and relationships. This assertion is reminiscent of Spencer's[7] observation that "the dark area" of practice is the *art* of practice in contrast to its *science*.

Since its inception, occupational therapy has enfolded the notion of collaborative treatment. The word *client* throughout this book denotes this collaboration of therapist with the person for whom the treatment plan is created. The objective of the remainder of this book is to provide multiple perspectives through which leadership in client-centered, collaborative performance can be viewed and achieved.

▓ The Potential Within Every Occupational Therapy Practitioner

To the student who does not feel that an opportunity for leadership has yet been made available, begin with these questions: Have you led a class group project? Assumed leadership of a student committee? Spoken up at a class meeting? Volunteered to be a student representative to a professional or university organization? The entry-level therapist could be asked: Did you present and defend your treatment plan in a staffing? Chair the last total quality management (TQM) meeting? Express your opinion in a letter to the editor? Of such first steps is professional leadership born.

Once on the way, progression toward higher levels of leadership is a developmental process that requires the acquisition of skills and attitudes through experience, continuing education, reading a broad range of literature, and advanced study related to specific goals. In addition, access to a mentor and use of professional networks, directly and through computerized opportunities such as listservs and bulletin boards, help the new therapist develop.

▓ Summary

Occupational therapists continue to achieve new heights in leadership. Examples of the ever-growing number of options for leadership have been introduced in this chapter, from careers in traditional treatment and in education to creative new niches. These are only representative of what is out there, which includes working with children with visual deficits, mental retardation, cerebral palsy, or conduct disorders; adolescents with depression, chemical dependency, or burns; young adults with spinal cord injuries, schizophrenia, AIDS, or rheumatoid arthritis; older adults with multiple sclerosis, muscular dystrophy, or strokes; or the elderly with Parkinson's disease, Alzheimer's disease, hip arthroplasties, or hearing and visual impairments. Perhaps your choice will be to engage in health promotion or research or policy formation. Occupational therapists should simultaneously become leaders in local, state, and national professional associations to thus ensure the future of their chosen profession.

Regardless of the career choices made, occupational therapists entering practice are urged to think carefully about these options and suggestions. The wisdom and experience of occupational therapy leaders who have preceded them will go far in preparing them to adapt, to understand both continuity and innovation, and to assume positions of leadership in this profession.

REFERENCES

1. Shriver, DJ: A new arena for private practice in OT: Workers' compensation and personal injury. OT in Health Care 2(2):25, 1985.
2. Ogden-Niemeyer, L, and Jacobs, K: Work Hardening: State of the Art. Slack, Thorofare, NJ, 1989.
3. Jaffe, EG, and Epstein, CF: Occupational Therapy Consultation. Mosby–Year Book, St. Louis, 1992.
4. Hoffman, E: E.M.B.A.s. USAir Magazine 2(10):63, Oct, 1995.
5. Bailey, DM, and Schwartzberg, SL: Ethical and Legal Dilemmas in Occupational Therapy. FA Davis, Philadelphia, 1995.
6. Peloquin, SM: Occupational therapy as art and science: Should the older definition be reclaimed? American Journal of Occupational Therapy 48(11):225, 1994.
7. Spencer, JC: The usefulness of qualitative methods in rehabilitation: Issues of meaning, of context, and of change. Presented at John Stanley Coulter Lecture, American Congress of Rehabilitation Medicine, San Francisco, Nov 15, 1992.

PART TWO

BASIC CONCEPTS IN MARKETING

*Marketing encompasses exchange
activities conducted by individuals and
organizations for the purpose of satisfying
human wants.*

Enis

CHAPTER 4

The Marketing Process

CHAPTER OBJECTIVES

- To differentiate between marketing as logic and marketing as a profession.
- To demonstrate the association between leadership and marketing.
- To learn how a social perspective of marketing evolved.
- To recognize the presence of marketing in good management.
- To realize that marketing makes selling superfluous.
- To explain the marketing process.
- To compare managerial and social perspectives of marketing.
- To recognize exchange relationships as the basis of marketing.
- To identify the role of constituencies or publics.
- To see the importance of environmental factors.
- To understand how a market analysis or audit is conducted.
- To categorize constituencies and plan individual strategies.
- To recognize the components of a marketing strategy.

The link between leadership and marketing, according to Bennis, is that "the leader knows what we want and what we need before we do and expresses these unspoken dreams for us in everything he or she says and does."[1] Because marketing is based on the mutually satisfying results of transactions between parties, the leader as described by Bennis can be said to have engaged in the process of marketing as well as in the process of leadership. The leader has obviously assessed the needs and wants of the followers and integrated them with universal goals. The marketer employs the same methodology.

Part Two acquaints the reader with marketing as a social process that holds great promise for occupational therapists. Chapter 4 begins with an explanation of the concept and its direct link with leadership, followed by an explanation of the components of the process itself. Chapter 5 shows how the process can be broken down into tools and techniques that are used to implement the marketing plan. Chapter 6 selects one marketing tool, selling, as an example of what the occupational therapist can use to achieve certain goals.

Applied Logic vs. Professional Marketing

To the occupational therapist who reads this book and as a result develops a marketing attitude, the distinction between marketing as logic and marketing as a competence cannot be stressed too often. Anyone can benefit from applying marketing logic to a problem; however, he or she is not a professional marketer. A professional marketer works regularly with specific marketing problems and has specialized knowledge in marketing. A person can master the logic of marketing, but to master a particular market requires additional education and experience.

This book presents marketing from the perspective that marketing *logic* is a highly effective tool available to the occupational therapist for effective daily conduct of all job-related responsibilities. The professional marketer is to be consulted in matters requiring *specialized knowledge*. This distinction may be viewed in much the same way as the occupational therapist who, in spite of having mastered anatomy, physiology, orthopedics, and kinesiology, understands and appreciates that the orthopedist must be consulted as the ultimate expert and professional specialist in orthopedically related cases.

A Social Process

Marketing as a social process is the heart and soul of artfully delivered occupational therapy, the maxim of the respected administrator, and the foundation of entrepreneurial success. Once understood, the very richness of the concept of marketing is at once apparent, and its inherent excitement and opportunity are energizing. The possibilities are legion. A new attitude emerges as the occupational therapist realizes the full potential of an altered perspective, regardless of practice interest or place of employment. At that point another enthusiast for the marketing approach has emerged.

The idea of marketing may at first seem totally alien and negative to an occupational therapist. Nonprofit organizations believe that what they are offering is inherently good and simply needs to be made available to a grateful public. Images of deceptive advertising may leap into the imagination when the word *marketing* is heard. The word *hucksterism* may come to mind. Actually, marketing is simply a system of planning that was previously used primarily in business. In response to the simple question, "Why market?" Kotler and Andreasen's[2] opinion was that all healthcare organizations will be required to do so to survive in an increasingly competitive environment. Their definition of *marketing* should give occupational therapists an initial understanding: "Marketing in the true sense means being sensitive to and responding to the needs of the people as they perceive them."

▓ The Beginnings and Evolution of a Concept

Nickels[3] noted that until 1960 marketing was generally considered a business activity. Marketing was originally founded as the branch of applied economics dealing with distribution. During the 1960s the emphasis was on managing the marketing of goods and services from producer to consumer. Later it became a management discipline devoted to bringing about sales increases.

Among the first to suggest broadening the concept of marketing were Kotler and Levy.[4] Their inventive proposition was that "marketing is a pervasive societal activity that goes considerably beyond the selling of toothpaste, soap, and steel." They interpreted the meaning of marketing for nonbusiness organizations and the nature of marketing functions such as product improvement, pricing, distribution, and communication in such organizations. They questioned whether traditional marketing principles could be transferred to the marketing of organizations, persons, and ideas and advocated that the marketing discipline become eclectic and widen to include social science. This suggestion did indeed evolve as marketing took on the character of an applied behavioral science concerned with understanding the buyer and seller systems in the marketing of goods and services.

In the 1970s, marketing expanded to include activities of nonprofit organizations, and traditional definitions changed as well. Marcus et al.[5] construed marketing to be "those activities performed by individuals or organizations, either profit or nonprofit, that enable, facilitate, and encourage exchange to the satisfaction of both parties." In 1975 Kotler[6,7] called it "the effective management by an organization of its exchange relations with its various markets and publics" and in 1976 "human activity directed at satisfying wants and needs through the exchange process." Enis[8] envisioned marketing to be "exchange activities conducted by individuals and organizations for the purpose of satisfying human wants"; MacStravic[9] said it was "simply a conscious, systematic approach to the planning, implementation, and evaluation of the exchange relationships of an organization" and "the management of exchanges."

In 1972 Sweeney's[10] opinion was that marketing faced an identity crisis. He examined the implications of conflicting views on marketing education, research, and the crucial issue of the social responsibility of marketing. Of particular interest and value to occupational therapy today was his question, "Is marketing fundamentally a collective social process inherent in the smooth and effective functioning of a society?" After contrasting divergent viewpoints, his conclusion was that marketing as a social process provides a broader, more comprehensive, and more robust concept of the nature of marketing without denying or omitting the valuable insights and technological advances generated at the organizational level.

▨ Perception and Reality: Process and Technology

Sweeney[10] observed that the focus of marketing, from the social system perspective, is on the transaction or the exchange, whereas from the organizational system point of view transactions are accomplished through application of marketing technologies. In other words, the exchange exists independently of the technology that may be employed to execute the exchange: "The process of exchange occurring in a society *is* the marketing process. Marketing is seen not merely as something that is *done*—a management technology—but as something that *is*—a social process."

Sweeney made the point that government, education, and marketing are not merely organizational technologies but also inherently social processes. None of these entities is done *to* individuals but are processes in which members of society *participate* collectively. From the social system perspective, the study of marketing is not limited to only the technologies employed by marketing organizations. "It also includes the study of the relationships among these organizations, the relationships between the marketing process and other social processes, and consequently the roles played by the marketing process and marketing institutions as integral parts of the general social system."[10]

When they became aware that the concept of marketing could indeed be a valuable aid to nonprofit organizations, several writers produced evolutionary —and revolutionary—books and articles on the subject. Notable among them were Philip Kotler and Scott MacStravic.

Kotler advocated a generic concept of marketing. He suggested that his original proposal should be broadened still further to include the transactions between an organization and all of its publics. He saw marketing as a disciplined task that created and offered values to others for the purpose of acquiring desired responses. He urged others to see marketing fundamentally as a collective social process inherent in the smooth and effective functioning of society.[7]

▧ The Concept in Action

There is a tendency to think initially of marketing only in terms of salesmanship. In truth, selling becomes unnecessary if marketing is understood and conducted correctly. The difference between marketing and selling is more than just the words; selling focuses on the needs of the seller, whereas marketing centers on the needs of the buyer. For example, a merchant purchased a large number of sink faucets to take advantage of a special bulk-rate price. His need and his goal were to "move"—to sell—many sink faucets as soon as possible in order to retrieve his investment plus a profit. By contrast, a group planning to build a retirement center surveyed potential clients and their families as to what amenities and options are most meaningful and important to them. Following construction of the facility, which was built to include those features whose importance had been noted, minimal effort was required to attract residents because their needs have already been anticipated and provided. The product, whether a thing or a service, becomes the *consequence* of the marketing effort, not the starting point of the process.

People are seeking solutions to problems and not just making choices among products and services. By being aware of problems and needs, the marketing imagination makes an inspired leap from the obvious to the meaningful, and a solution is born. In this way an organization is prepared to supply the needed solution whenever the public becomes aware of needing it. By making available to the residents the solutions to their problems, the retirement center builders had already developed a successful marketing plan, and selling was unnecessary.

Many healthcare managers profess to know what is meant by a marketing plan, yet actually their marketing strategies are usually sales approaches. They are product oriented rather than market or needs oriented. They seek to *create* demand for unused services, even though these services often do not address even latent market demand. Selling of this sort is highly unlikely to result in successful marketing in the true sense. Awareness and listening are requisite if an organization is to continuously respond to its changing environment, for markets and the competition are constantly in transition.

As for marketing and leadership, what they share in common is that at the completion of these processes the constituencies and followers feel that they accomplished the feats themselves. In both cases empowerment has been skillfully implanted during the transactions and left the participants mutually satisfied.

There is a logical, systematic way to proceed to develop a marketing attitude. First, there is understanding of the concept, as mentioned previously. The next step is becoming familiar with the components of the marketing process itself so as to be able to apply it to a wide variety of situations. The following information explains in more detail how to proceed.

Planned Procedures in the Marketing Process

The marketing process comprises carefully planned procedures that may be given different names by different authors but are similar in purpose. One author, MacStravic,[11] offering primarily a social process perspective of marketing, guided the reader through steps leading to implementation of a marketing plan:

- Identification of constituencies
- Assessment of the marketing environment and its problems
- Selection and evaluation of marketing objectives
- Design of a marketing strategy
- Planning, implementation, control, and evaluation of marketing efforts

Kotler,[12] one of the world's leading authorities on marketing, was an early proponent of broadening the concept of marketing as originally taught in schools of business. His book *Marketing for Nonprofit Organizations* shows parallels with MacStravic's explanations of marketing; however, Kotler used a managerial approach involving analysis, planning, implementation, and control. His purpose was to provide more relevance for managers and administrators.

Occupational therapists will find these two "classics" and the subsequent marketing publications by both authors, one a professional in business and marketing and one with a background in healthcare planning and administration, to be helpful as well as easy to read and understand. They can provide more detailed information about the marketing concepts introduced in this book.

Marketing is simply a set of planning concepts previously used mostly in business. Before occupational therapists can apply marketing principles to their practice, they must understand the concept. In the true sense, marketing is being sensitive to and responding to the needs of people as they perceive those needs. Meeting the needs and wants of markets by using facilities and programs as tools to do this is what marketing is all about. It is part of the social responsibility of healthcare professionals to perceive and respond to their consumers' needs.

Exchange Relationships

Marketing is a framework in which exchange relationships may be examined, predicted, and managed; that is, people think that what they get is at least equal to what they relinquish. Exchanges are planned and managed to gain objectives.

Marketing as an exchange relationship requires two ingredients:

1. A constituency—some person, group, or organization with whom an exchange is to be accomplished
2. A value—that which is exchanged, by an organization or person and by the constituency

Kotler and Clarke[13] offered a succinct explanation of this important concept of transactions or exchanges between two constituencies. Four conditions must be present for an exchange to take place:

1. *There are at least two parties.* In the simplest exchange situation, there are two parties. In health care, because of third party reimbursement, there are often three or more. The marketer is the party more actively seeking an exchange; the marketer is someone seeking a resource from someone else and willing to offer something of value in exchange.

2. *Each can offer something the other perceives to be of value.* If one of the parties has nothing that is valued by the other party, exchange will not take place. In general, three categories of things tend to have value. The first is physical goods—any tangible object that is capable of satisfying a human want. The second is services—any act another person might perform that is capable of satisfying a human want. Services are usually characterized by the expenditure of time, energy and/or skill. The third category is money, a generalized store of value that can be used to obtain goods or services. In the health care field, a fourth category, the utilization of services, has value for provider organizations because of regulatory and political pressures for efficiency.

See Figure 4–1 as an illustration of the exchange of two categories of value: services offered in exchange for money.

3. *Each is capable of communication and delivery.* For exchange to take place, two parties must be capable of communicating with each other. They must be able to describe what is being offered, and when, where, and how it will be exchanged. Each party must state or imply certain warranties about the expected performance of the exchanged objects or services. In addition to communicating, each party must be capable of finding means to deliver the things of value.

4. *Each is free to accept or reject the offer.* Exchange assumes that both parties are engaging in voluntary behavior, there is no coercion. Some exchanges in health care appear not to be voluntary, such as the involuntary commitment of a patient to a psychiatric hospital. However, the decision-maker (a psychiatrist or family member, for example), acting for the patient, engages in the transaction freely, so it is a voluntary exchange.

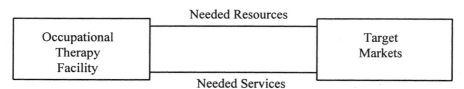

FIGURE 4–1. Organization survival through exchange. (Adapted from Kotler and Clarke,[13] p 46.)

The exchange concept can be further visualized in Figure 4–2. It is helpful to imagine that when two social units are engaged in an exchange transaction the element of mutual needs satisfaction is always present.

The first exchange, example *A*, describes a classic commercial transaction. Money is exchanged for goods or services. The exchange in *B* is a transaction between employer and employee. A civic transaction is illustrated in example *C*, an interaction between citizens and the police department. The interchange between the citizens and a health promotion agency is presented in example *D* to indicate a social marketing transaction, and the exchange between a donor and a charity is shown as an example of a charity transaction.

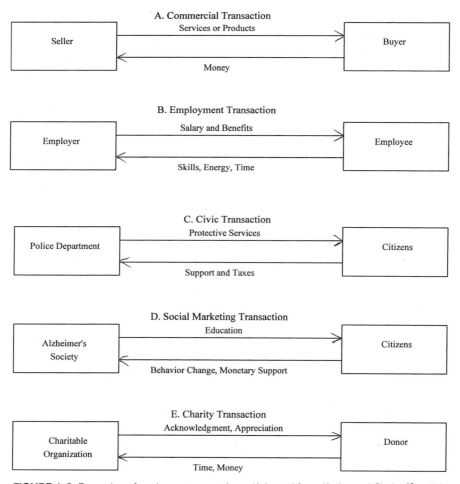

FIGURE 4–2. Examples of exchange transactions. (Adapted from Kotler and Clarke,[13] p 48.)

HEALTHCARE TRANSACTIONS

Many healthcare organizations are involved in more complex exchange transactions, such as that in Figure 4–3.

CONSTITUENCIES OR PUBLICS

The logical starting point for an occupational therapist's marketing approach is to identify each set of people or organizations that can be separately analyzed and considered to be constituencies or publics. A *constituent* in this sense is any supporter, customer, professional colleague, employer, employee, or other indi-

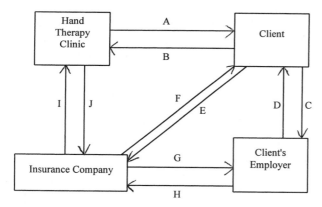

A. The hand clinic provides hand therapy services to the client.
B. The client provides direct payment or guarantee of payment from a third party.
C. The client, as an employee, provides productive work services to the employer.
D. The employer provides wages as payment for work services and also partial coverage of the employee's health benefits.
E. The client makes monthly payments for health benefits coverage, beyond that paid by the employer, to the insurance company.
F. The insurance company provides a guarantee of partial coverage for the client's therapy expenses.
G. The insurance company provides a means through which the employer can guarantee health coverage to the employees.
H. The employer makes monthly payments to the insurance company.
I. The insurance company pays for services rendered to the hand therapy clinic.
J. The hand therapy clinic guarantees that therapy services will be delivered in a cost-efficient manner so that the insurance company will not have to pay out more in reimbursements than it has attracted in payments.

FIGURE 4–3. One patient's transactions with a hospital. (Adapted from Kotler and Clark,[13] p 49.)

vidual with a real or potential impact on an organization. Without constituencies and effective exchange relationships an organization—and a therapist—cannot exist. Kotler and Clarke's[13] synonym for *constituency* is *public*.

MacStravic[11] noted that most health organizations can identify four categories of constituencies: (1) external, those who support, regulate, or impact from outside; (2) internal, those who work in the organization and enable it to operate; (3) client, those who use or benefit from services provided to them by the organization; and (4) colleague constituencies, those who provide similar or relevant services and represent possible competition or collaboration.

Examples of external constituencies are lawmakers, funding agencies, and vendors. Policy-making or advisory boards and committees are internal constituencies, as are employees, team professionals, and referring physicians. Examples of client constituencies are patients, clients, and persons such as the parents of children who are patients who do not directly receive service but do directly benefit from your services. Colleague constituencies are people or organizations that provide similar or related services; they may be competitors or

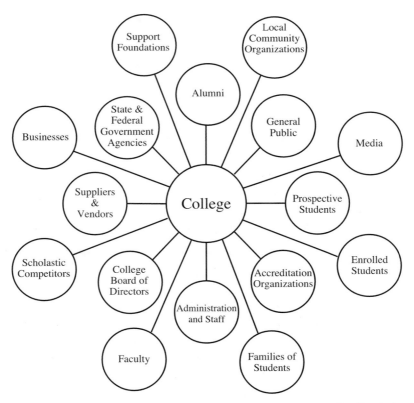

FIGURE 4–4. The college and its publics. (Adapted from Kotler and Fox,[14] p 25.)

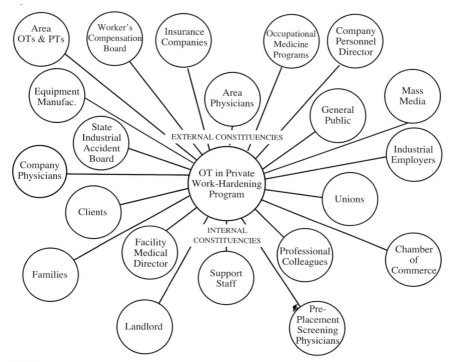

FIGURE 4–5. The publics/constituencies of an occupational therapist in a private work-hardening program.

collaborators, sometimes simultaneously, depending upon circumstances at any given time. For example, the owner of a competitive hand therapy practice may collaborate in joint negotiations with the local union representative. Therefore, constant attention must be paid to each constituent or public, and adjustments or substitutions made when any exchange becomes ineffective or inefficient. Furthermore, *any* constituent or public may occupy a role in one or more of these categories at any given time or may move among them.

Kotler and Fox[14] offered an example of how this visualization of exchanges can be applied in educational institutions. Figure 4–4 shows the publics surrounding a college and its operation. The potential constituencies or publics of an occupational therapist who is planning a work-hardening program could be pictured similarly (Fig. 4–5).

■ Environment

The context or environment within which an organization exists is a vital element of marketing success. Continual awareness and assessment of all internal and external environmental factors are essential. Adjustments in relationships with identified constituents or publics should be ongoing to ensure the position and status of one's organization. Internally there must be awareness of client satisfaction, public acceptance, and constituent support. Outwardly the needs and attitudes of colleagues, clients, and external constituencies must be analyzed and managed so as to achieve organizational objectives.[11]

External environmental factors that affect your organization include:

- Population size and demography
- Local, state, and national economies
- Local, state, and national political, governmental, and legal decisions
- Cultural and behavioral factors
- Technology

These circumstances may affect each one of your categories of constituents in endless ways. To illustrate this statement, following is a description of the multiple potential effects that cultural and behavioral factors alone might have on just a few of your own potential constituencies.

First, external constituencies are affected. Cultural attitudes (as well as governmental income tax changes) regarding charitable donations and obligations have important implications for the nature and extent of healthcare delivery. People's willingness and ability to donate to healthcare organizations and to research are of critical concern to the futures of these entities.

One internal constituency, healthcare employees, particularly women and minorities, has been directly influenced by cultural and behavioral changes. The "glass ceiling" experience has created consternation and dissatisfaction among women as they have tried to climb the administrative career ladder in healthcare institutions. Rising tuition costs coupled with increased admissions competition have brought changes in values and priorities among some students and entry-level healthcare professionals, as more primary importance has been given to higher beginning salaries and employability assurance. Scarcity of certain types of qualified personnel has altered salary demands and expectations among these health services professionals, in many cases straining institutional budgets as a result of the supply and demand factor. Nurses' increased interest in becoming nurse practitioners or others' interest in becoming physicians' assistants have affected and in many cases transformed—subtly and often overtly—the appearance of the culture historically found in medical facilities. Those individuals responsible for initial examinations and treatment are not always physicians, for example.

Client constituencies have been affected by general changes in attitudes toward authority and by increased pressures for consumer input into healthcare decisions. Litigious attitudes have affected behavior of both clients and healthcare providers. Because of the closing of many small hospitals, the lack of healthcare insurance among growing numbers of citizens, and the urgent need of many for any source of health care at all, overuse of emergency rooms at larger hospitals rose dramatically.

Colleague constituencies share these pressures, which may result in stronger competition on all fronts. Expanded advertising and promotional campaigns have resulted. With the scarcity of occupational and physical therapists, among others, behaviors and strategies for attracting healthcare employees have become more evident. Pressures to increase pro bono work directly affect income while creating personal ethical decisions.

From these examples it is apparent that occupational therapists must maintain daily awareness of both the internal dynamics of their organizations and the world around them. They must know what is happening in the economy, what laws are being passed, what cultural shifts are in motion, and what new technologies are being introduced. They must then develop the habit of constantly integrating these facts into their daily thinking to try to foresee the direct effect the happenings will have on their lives and livelihood. Every event affects some constituency, existing or potential exchanges, and the organization. Therefore, to avert crises and recognize opportunities, this personal survey of daily circumstances is critical. In this way, both the therapist and the organization will become responsive, adaptive, and entrepreneurial in attitude and approach to change.

▓ The Market Analysis or Audit

Beginning in 1973 Drucker[15] observed that, for a strategic plan, you should begin with an evaluation of the current position of your organization, estimate what that status *will* be if activities continue unchanged, and finally decide where you *want* your organization to be. With that in mind, a marketing approach becomes obviously logical. A careful, objective analysis of the current constituencies, environment, and objectives of your organization marks the start of an individualized marketing plan. MacStravic[11] suggested beginning with two basic measures: (1) the status of the current market situation of each of your constituencies and (2) a general idea of what that status should be if you are to meet your objectives. Another term for this self-audit is SWOT (strengths, weaknesses, opportunities, and threats) analysis.

OPTIONAL MARKET RESEARCH TOOLS

Necessary information for a market audit or analysis can be gathered by a variety of methods. Decisions about the relative merits of using mail, telephone, or interviews can be made easier through use of a comparison such as that suggested by Hillestad and Berkowitz[16] (Table 4–1).

TABLE 4–1

A Comparison of Market Research Methods

Criterion	Personal Interview	Telephone Survey	Mail Survey	Focus Groups
Cost	Most expensive.	Relatively expensive; experienced interviewers needed.	Potentially lowest costs (if response rate is sufficient).	Relatively expensive.
Interviewer reliability	High likelihood of bias. Appearance a factor.	Less bias. No face-to-face contact. Phone call suspicion to be overcome.	Interviewer bias eliminated. Anonymity provided.	Need trained moderator.
Adaptability	Most flexible method. Responses can be probed. Assistance can be provided in completing forms. Observations can be made.	Cannot make observations. Some probing possible.	Least flexible method.	Very flexible.
Sampling limits	Most complete sample possible.	Limited to people with telephone. No answers.	Mailing list problem. Nonresponse a major problem.	Need careful selection process.

Adapted from Hillestad and Berkowitz,[16] p 166.

BEGINNING THE MARKETING PLAN

To assist in determining where to focus your energies, MacStravic[11] proposed that each of an organization's current constituencies be placed into one of eight categories:

- negative—potential constituents deliberately avoiding exchange
- inert—constituents acting indifferently to desired exchanges
- engaged—constituents engaging in exchanges with other organizations
- unrealized—those wishing to make an exchange which is currently unavailable
- declining—exchange quantity falling from former level and likely to keep falling
- undesired—either quality (who) or quantity (number) of exchanges is different from desired level (e.g., overuse of emergency room)

- fluctuating—quality and quantity of exhanges acceptable but timing is bad
- perfect—that rare occasion when exchange transactions with a constituency are a good balance[11, p 65]

MacStravic followed this categorization with some specific examples of alternative strategies to take with a constituent in one of these classifications.

- negative—ignore potential constituents or overcome their antipathy toward the organization and available exchanges
- inert—get around inactive constituents or stimulate them to make desired exhanges
- engaged—attract all or a share of exhanges from the numbers of constituents desired
- unrealized—make the exchange available, but be prepared to treat as negative, inert, or engaged if it turns out that way
- declining—discover reason for decline; make up with other transactions or reclaim departing constituents
- undesired—either alter the organization to cope with what are now undesired qualities or excesses of exchanges, or change the exchanges themselves
- fluctuating—either alter the capacity of the organization to be closer to the existing rhythm of exchanges or attempt to smooth our variations
- perfect—enjoy it while you can; try to discover how it got to be that way for future reference, and prepare to react as it changes into one of the other situations[11, p 67]

The Plan of Action

Now that the status of actual and potential markets has been identified, marketing objectives can be selected and a marketing plan developed. With constituencies identified, the market is *segmented* or divided into homogeneous, distinctive groups in order to develop separate approaches to each group. The composition of these segmented groups varies according to an organization's specific objectives. For example, the objectives of a hand therapy clinic are probably different than those of a work-hardening program, and the actual and potential customers of each lead to different kinds of groupings within their segmented markets. Segments are determined according to criteria such as location of clients, demographic characteristics, type of injury, behavioral attributes, and age (Fig. 4–5).

SELECTION OF STRATEGY

Each segment is analyzed to determine what type and amount of opportunity it represents. MacStravic[11] advocated approaching these market objectives with a priority strategy (pursuing the best opportunity first), a general strategy (all constituents approached at once with no distinction made in priority among segments), or a mixed strategy (all segments addressed but with exchanges tailored for each one). The selection of which strategies to pursue and to what extent must be carefully considered as you keep in mind the changing internal and external environments, the facts about each constituent, and the goals and objectives of your organization.

FROM AWARENESS TO ACTION

Historically, many healthcare professionals have depended solely on professional judgment and expertise to make strategic decisions on behalf of patients. Some may therefore initially have difficulty in instead first seeking out the needs, wants, and feelings of potential clients, colleagues, and supporters; however, this process is the basis of marketing. Once healthcare professionals have identified these needs and wants, potential constituents must be moved through a series of stages toward successful exchanges. These stages have been described as progressing from a state of being unaware of the existence of a potential service or exchange, to being aware, to being interested, then to the decision to make the exchange, next to actually doing it, and finally to being a satisfied, regular user and to being an agent (one who recommends to friends that they make similar exchanges).[11]

Other authors have advocated a similar process. One source used different terminology and guided the consumer from awareness through interest to a stage of desire and finally action.[17] Another followed successful business sales through the steps of awareness, comprehension, conviction, and ordering.[18] Their common direction and purpose are evident, regardless of individual expertise, terminology, or focus.

IF THERE IS COMPETITION

It is prudent to recognize that a strong competitor may be vying for the attention of your potential constituent. In that case, three alternatives are available: (1) give up if competition appears too strong, (2) compete to secure the desired share of the market, or (3) cooperate with the competitor to accept a reduced share.

■ Components of a Marketing Strategy

Let us suppose at this point that the occupational therapist has now identified the constituents or publics, the potential users of the product or services

(Fig. 4–5). The current interests and needs of each constituent have been determined. Objectives have been set, and awareness of the internal and external environment is ongoing. The occupational therapist looks next at the four components of the marketing strategy, originally classified by McCarthy[19] in 1978 as the four Ps: product, price, place, and promotion.

In a healthcare delivery perspective, the *product* may be a service provided or a tangible product produced. The *price* is, of course, the value of that product, whether in money, time, or satisfaction to the consumer. Variations of *place* center on how you organize and deliver your services, including timing, location, and the amount of space required. Finally, *promotion* takes into consideration all those tools you might need to communicate what you are offering: advertising, publicity, promotions, personal contact, selling. You may not need to use any of these techniques; however, it is well to understand what each entails. Kotler and Clarke[13] referred to the particular blend of these techniques you choose as the *marketing mix*. The objectives and market position you have chosen for your services or product determine which elements of the marketing mix to feature.

PRODUCT

A product in marketing may be a person, place, idea, physical good, service, social cause, or any combination of these. It is not necessarily something that you can see or feel, yet it is something that another person perceives to be of sufficient value to be interested in making an exchange for it.

Following the environmental survey of internal and external target markets and a determination of the needs and wants represented, the occupational therapist takes a hard, objective look at the product or service offered to potential consumers. If it is a service, what is the client to receive in the proposed exchange? In the case of a hand clinic, of what is the initial evaluation comprised? If the transaction is with the local school district, what comprises the 8 hours of occupational therapy service? What is the specific role of the occupational therapist in relation to that of the classroom teacher? If a tangible product is offered, such elements as quality, packaging, and special features must be taken into consideration. How closely do these characteristics meet the needs and wants of the consumer?

For both services and tangible products, the success of the exchange depends on the value the consumer places on the product. Monetary value alone often does not fully account for satisfaction in a successful transaction. For example, rather than just buying 15 minutes of purposeful activity in the form of activities of daily living (ADL) instruction from the occupational therapist, the patient is purchasing a means to become independent and to gain an increased sense of self-worth through becoming able to prepare breakfast. That increased feeling of self-worth is usually not a publicized feature of your service.

High quality in a product is essential if the exchange is to be successful and the demand repeated. When services are performed, the amiability and concern of the occupational therapists who treat the clients may make the critical difference between using your facility or another that purports to offer identical services. Word of mouth continues to be one of the most important means by which the image and reputation of an organization are spread. Negative feelings and comments have been found to circulate exponentially faster and further than those that are positive.

Other aspects of your product or service that require attention include effectiveness, safety, and convenience, each variable given attention as it applies to your particular service or product. At all times you need to remain aware of any need to discontinue, revise, amplify, or add to your service in response to an ongoing survey of internal and external relationships and environments. Also to be kept in mind is the effect of any such change on the size and scope of your services. Do you have limits to either in mind? Is the time right for the changes you are contemplating?

PRICE

The topic of price in providing or purchasing healthcare services is not simple today. Methods of payment are complex, and analysis of costs and benefits associated with delivery of services is equally intricate and perplexing. As can be noted in Figure 4–3, recognition of the exchanges present in healthcare service provision and reimbursement is basic to successful marketing. Direct, out-of-pocket, fee-for-service compensation in health care is becoming unusual, rather than the common method of payment in the United States today.

In addition to the monetary value associated with healthcare delivery are other related costs. For example, there is an expenditure of the patient in terms of time to travel to the site of treatment, transportation problems, psychological toll, and possible sitter dilemmas. The direct provider of services has an outlay for overhead expenses (e.g., space, location, equipment, office staff wages, formal and continuing education), promotional expenses both fiscal and in community service, and all other costs to be acknowledged and included in the "picture." Once again, it is important that the patient or client be accorded friendly, personal care, especially in light of growing competition among providers and of consumer vigilance and demand.

One way of approaching final decisions in pricing is to base fees for service on cost, competitive factors, geographic area, and what the consumer is willing to pay. Major methods usually selected for arriving at fee decisions are unit value system, cost-plus, local survey, and state code.

For guidance in determining the final price for your services, consult a marketing text such as Chapter 13, "Price Decisions," in Kotler and Clarke's *Marketing for Health Care Organizations*,[13] which proposes four steps: First, a statement of pricing objectives must be determined, and then a selection of strategy, whether cost-based, demand-based, or competition-based. Next should be recognition of situations such as self-pay or reimbursement markets, and finally an admonition to be fully informed at all times so as to anticipate changes in future reimbursement procedures and prepared to respond to them.

PLACE

Three things are said to be necessary for a successful restaurant: location, location, and location. A decision about the location of an occupational therapy service is, of course, not approached with exactly the same criteria in mind, but a therapist planning a marketing strategy does have to keep in mind just how much importance must be given to this variable. All details are to be thoughtfully addressed, including the amount of space needed now and in the future. Again, changes in the scope or the type of services offered may affect, and be affected by, the location.

Almost daily the aspect of place (or *distribution*, the term used traditionally by professional marketers) changes in occupational therapy. The location and manner in which occupational therapy services are delivered are altered continually by those external and internal factors noted previously. Because the area in which most occupational therapists are engaged is distribution of services, discussion here will center on physical access, time access, and promotion of services.

If the product to be distributed is a tangible object, the problems are those of physical distribution: warehousing, inventory, flow of goods, retailing, and wholesaling. Consult current business marketing texts for the most reliable and technologically up-to-date information on this topic, as that is not the primary purview of this book.

PHYSICAL ACCESS

Physical access means the channels used for delivery of services, location, and facilities. Traditionally, occupational therapy services were most commonly found in hospital and rehabilitation center departments. Over the years therapists have extended practice into public school systems, home health care, industry, and an infinite number of other actual and potential arenas. As free enterprise has become more and more prominent on the healthcare scene, it has expanded the challenges and opportunities for delivering occupational therapy services. It has simultaneously opened up unlimited career advancement possibilities for occupational therapists to move into greater leadership positions.

For those occupational therapists contemplating new businesses and facilities, first determine the objectives of services, identify and segment the potential consumers, and assess and analyze the needs of each constituent. Analyze your competitors to reveal the strengths and weaknesses of each so that you can determine your own differential advantage. With these facts as a foundation, you can decide on the channels for delivery of services as well as the lo-

cation, size, and type of facility. In view of costs to the prospective patient, locate services to be most convenient for transportation (access). The steady
growth in home healthcare delivery bears witness to still other problems related
to distribution, from both the access and the cost-benefit perspectives.

The third physical access question is facility design. A home health agency
has problems that are obviously different from a facility at a fixed location
whose outside surroundings and building create important first impressions of
aesthetics and safety. Entry ramps provide a realistic accessibility aid as well as
the necessary response to legal requirements. Both the inside and outside surroundings need to communicate to the client general feelings of safety, comfort, and well-being if they are to want to return; you never get a second chance
to make a first impression.

Inside the facility, careful planning for the flow of activities provides the
highest level of efficiency as you go about the operation of your business. Consumers, you, and your employees all benefit.

TIME ACCESS

Time access means not only the stated hours during which your facility is open
but also the time that a consumer must wait for an appointment and, after arrival, in your waiting room. Regardless of the type of organization, the convenience of the consumer must be carefully balanced against the realities of service delivery.

PROMOTION

Promotion refers to decisions associated with how to bring together the provider
and the consumer. For example, in a hospital setting the primary source of referral to occupational therapy services is the physician, although such a referral
may be prompted by the suggestion of a nurse or other professional colleague
with whom the occupational therapist has established a positive relationship.
Hospital discharge planners are liaisons with post–acute care facilities and services in the community. Because a growing number of occupational therapists
find themselves in this community aftercare market, the person (constituent) in
the discharge planning role is very important. Potential constituencies to approach could be the chief occupational therapist at the hospital, the nurse, the
social worker, or whoever holds the responsibility for discharge planning. Chapter 5 outlines specific promotional tools or techniques to consider.

▓ Summary

This chapter described differences between marketing as a management technology and marketing as a social process. How the concept of marketing was

broadened in the 1970s was explained by tracing its evolution through literature. The difference between marketing as a logical concept that may be used by occupational therapists and marketing as a specialized field of knowledge was explained. The notion of an interrelationship between leadership and marketing was introduced. The components of the marketing process were described, as well as the feasibility of occupational therapists' applications of this methodology. It was made clear that the steps in the marketing process must be learned and understood before they can be applied in individualized occupational therapy situations. Chapter 5 explains the tools and techniques available to occupational therapists as they develop plans for using marketing to achieve leadership.

REFERENCES

1. Bennis, W: Why Leaders Can't Lead. Jossey-Bass, San Francisco, 1989, p 159.
2. Kotler, P, and Andreasen, A: Strategic Marketing for Nonprofit Organizations. Prentice-Hall, Englewood Cliffs, NJ, 1987, p 7.
3. Nickels, WG: Marketing Principles. Prentice-Hall, Englewood Cliffs, NJ, 1978.
4. Kotler, P, and Levy, SJ: Broadening the concept of marketing. Journal of Marketing 33:10, Jan, 1969.
5. Marcus, B, et al: Modern Marketing. Random House, New York, 1975, p 4.
6. Kotler, P: Marketing for Nonprofit Organizations. Prentice-Hall, Englewood Cliffs, NJ, 1975, p x.
7. Kotler, P: Marketing Management, ed 3. Prentice-Hall, Englewood Cliffs, NJ, 1976, p 5.
8. Enis, BM: Marketing Principles: The Management Process, ed 2. Goodyear Publishing, Santa Monica, Calif, 1977, p 17.
9. MacStravic, RE: Marketing Health Care. Aspen Systems, Germantown, Md, 1977, p 19.
10. Sweeney, DJ: Marketing: Management technology or social process? Journal of Marketing 36(3):7, Oct, 1972.
11. MacStravic, RE: Marketing Health Care. Aspen Systems, Germantown, Md, 1977, pp 65–67.
12. Kotler, P: Marketing for Nonprofit Organizations. Prentice-Hall, Englewood Cliffs, NJ, 1975.
13. Kotler, P, and Clarke, RN: Marketing for Health Care Organizations. Prentice-Hall Englewood Cliffs, NJ, 1987, p 46.
14. Kotler, P, and Fox, KFA: Strategic Marketing for Educational Institutions. Prentice-Hall, Englewood Cliffs, NJ, 1985.
15. Drucker, PF: An Introductory View of Management. Harper & Row, New York, 1977.
16. Hillestad, SG, and Berkowitz, EN: Health Care Marketing Plans: From Strategy to Action. Dow Jones–Irwin, Homewood, Ill, 1984.
17. Schewe, CD, and Smith, RM: Marketing Concepts and Applications. McGraw-Hill, New York, 1980.
18. Peter, JP, and Donnelly, JH Jr: Marketing Management. Irwin, Homewood, Ill, 1992.
19. McCarthy, EJ: Basic Marketing: A Managerial Approach, ed 6. Irwin, Homewood, Ill, 1978.

CHAPTER 5

The Promotion Mix: Advertising, Publicity, Personal Selling

CHAPTER OBJECTIVES

- To compare the components of a promotion mix.
- To see the differences between marketing and public relations.
- To develop comfort with publicity and public speaking.
- To understand the role research plays in promotion.
- To appreciate the nature of effective personal selling.

Armed with an introduction to the concept of marketing, a growing understanding of marketing terms, and a marketing plan, the occupational therapist is ready to make decisions about the promotional aspects of the plan. For promoting a tangible product, later chapters of this book furnish general assistance in the form of examples and cases. References such as *Marketing Management* by Peter and Donnelly[1] furnish the business principles and specific procedures for movement of goods to guide your efforts.

Advertising

Because of its visibility, advertising is probably the best-known method of promotion. More often than not, a person asked for a definition of *marketing* erroneously responds that it is either selling or advertising. The forms that publicity and advertising may take are many and depend on the requirements of the occupational therapist to satisfy the needs of the constituent (public) and the environment.

Advertising is an impersonal kind of promotion for which a sponsor pays. It is communicated through mass media (e.g., newspapers, magazines, television, radio, direct mail, billboards, and new avenues such as the Internet). Peter and Donnelly defined *advertising* as "any paid form of nonpersonal presentation of ideas, goods, or services by an identified sponsor."[1] Because it is impersonal, there is no attempt made to match the message to the individual needs, wants, or interests of the receivers of the message. Few attempts have been made to survey the consumers of the advertising, nor has market segmentation focused on homogeneous characteristics of those seeing or hearing the information. Because it is difficult at best to accurately determine the effectiveness of advertising, it is usually one of the most expensive methods of communicating services. Advertising may reach a large audience; however, compared with personal selling, it provides no opportunity for the immediate reactions and adaptive responses of a face-to-face situation.

Public Relations

Public relations as a management and staff function has grown rapidly over the past five decades. It is a promotional activity devoted to communicating a favorable image of an organization. Mature public relations practice involves empathic listening, counseling management, imaginative planning, and persuasive communication. No two programs have the same objectives or tasks. To be effective, a public relations program must be tailored to the institution it serves. Public relations goes beyond the basic needs of marketing; however, a favorable image certainly helps occupational therapists fulfill needs and provide satisfaction to target markets. Because of overlap of responsibilities and objectives, public relations and marketing departments are sometimes related and often mistaken for each other in institutions. The task of earning and getting public good will is constant, but, for the purposes of this book, public relations is considered to be an entity separate from marketing.

One helpful explanation of the relationship between marketing and public relations is that public relations is "primarily a communications tool, whereas marketing also includes needs assessment, product development, pricing, and distribution."[2] The primary purpose of public relations is to influence attitudes; marketing aims at eliciting specific behaviors. Furthermore, public relations is a support function, whereas marketing sets the goals and is involved in defining the organization's mission, customers, and services to be offered.[2]

Publicity

Compared with advertising, personal selling, and sales promotions, one has little control over publicity. Nonetheless it is a vital part of marketing efforts. Publicity is information about an organization that is disseminated through the mass media but for which the organization does not pay money. Publicity is information communicated through newspapers, magazines, radio, television, or public speaking engagements. Negative as well as positive facts and stories may be made public, and it is obviously in the best interests of an organization to have positive news circulated.

CREATING POSITIVE PUBLICITY

Occupational therapists should be constantly aware of opportunities for favorable publicity about their organization and profession. Informing the general public about the value and benefits of occupational therapy is a professional responsibility and adds to the visibility and credibility of you, your organization, and your profession.

There are many possibilities for positive publicity. Inviting the local newspaper editor to send a photographer and reporter to cover an event at your facility spreads the word about occupational therapy and your efforts. Inviting a reporter from *OT Week* to attend the 50th anniversary of your program shares that celebration with professional colleagues. Items written about interesting activities or accomplishments within your organization or on a helpful topic within your area of expertise may be sent to appropriate newspapers, newsletters, magazines, or journals. You yourself may take pictures of important happenings and include them with your article writeup. At best, the publication will welcome the news, share it with an interested public, and give you appreciated exposure and visibility. At the very worst, you may have to try again. More probably, other reporters or editors will notice your pieces and may contact you for further articles or for quotations to be included in articles they are writing.

Unless you make an effort, the public—specifically, potential clients and professional colleagues or sponsors—may never be made aware of your valuable services and successes. There is no reason that good, high-quality performance should not be appreciated by the public. Begin by contacting the health editor of the newspaper or magazine with a suggestion for a story, or send a query letter, a short letter describing the subject of your article, the angle you will take, and some information about yourself.

When you receive a positive response and an invitation to submit a press release, be sure to include the following items:

- The name of the person to contact for more information
- Release date (usually immediate)
- Headline (short descriptive summary of what is in the release, 4 to 12 words)
- Body of the item: who, what, where, why, and when, given in the first paragraph

The press release should be double-spaced, one to two pages at most. Be prepared for an interview.

OCCUPATIONAL THERAPISTS AND PUBLICITY

There are countless examples of occupational therapy colleagues who serve as representatives in ways that bring pride and recognition to their profession. *OT Week* and *Advance* are good sources for up-to-date news of those who are providing positive publicity for occupational therapy. For example, watch the regularly featured column "OT Practitioners in the News" in *OT Week*. The July 6, 1995, issue told of three occupational therapists who appeared on major television networks: Eve Taylor, PhD, OTR/L, on ABC's *20/20;* Jacque Burgum, OTR, on NBC's *Today Show;* and Joyce Yeary, OTR/L, CHT, on CBS's *Rescue 911.* Each one of these occupational therapists provided fine examples of professionalism in practice by being willing and able to share experiences with the public. Others have brought attention to the value of occupational therapy by being mentioned in biographies of famous people or through personal interviews on radio shows. The possibilities are infinite and require only willingness, an open mind, recognition of opportunities, and creativity.

Public Speaking

Public speaking is an excellent means to spread the word about occupational therapy and your organization. Anyone can master the art of speaking in public. The first time is the most difficult, but it becomes easier with practice. The first rule is to prepare your speech well in advance; never go unprepared to "wing it." That may be not only a disastrous experience for you but also not the positive impression you had intended.

The ability to speak well in public is the most important skill any political or business leader can have. In making a first impression, your appearance can raise expectations, but what you say and how you say it determine how people evaluate you. Good speaking is also a key to leadership, for your degree of speaking skill determines to a great extent how seriously people take your ideas and whether they will follow your lead.

WHERE TO LOOK

Social, civic, and professional associations regularly seek speakers for their meetings who can bring interesting information and fresh insights to their members. In addition, these service organizations look for worthwhile projects to which they can lend their support and endorsement. To begin, request the name of the program chairperson and indicate your willingness and your area of expertise. A letter to the person with a list of potential topics, their potential benefits and interest to the group, and highlights of your background introduce you. Follow up your letter in a few weeks with a phone call.

Before making your presentation, find out from the program chairperson some background information about your audience in order to focus on a topic of interest to them. Consider the listeners' age, sex, educational level, and occupations, and then use examples in your speech that relate to their background and experience. Prepare your speech carefully with a strong beginning and ending, and emphasize personal benefits to the members of the audience. It is wise to rehearse the speech and to use minimal notes. Slides work well, as you can use them as your prompts.

PREPARING THE SPEECH

Begin by drafting an outline consisting of five parts: topic, objective, opening, body, and closing. The objective of your presentation should be what you want to happen as a result of your speech—what the audience can gain from listening to you. Ask yourself what you hope to gain through speaking to them, as well. For example, two key objectives of your talk might be that the members of the audience will learn a new approach to pain control, and at the same time you want those same attendees to tell their physicians to refer patients to your services.

Your opening statement should get their attention; it should usually be written last. In the body of your speech, don't try to say too much. Your audience can absorb only so much information before their attention begins to wander. Concentrate on making two or three main points. In closing, restate the main points, make a statement related to the opening, make your conclusions and recommendations, and call for action.

Add variety by using visual aids to emphasize key points. Carefully check your equipment before your speech to make sure it is in working order. Handouts can also add interest. Distribute them at the end of your presentation so that listeners are not distracted from your talk by reading them. Notes should be kept to a minimum. The worst thing a speaker can do is try to read a speech. To use cue cards as an assist, write clearly and limit each card to one thought, so that a quick glance triggers your thoughts.

Allow time at the end for any questions from the audience, followed by time to answer personal questions afterward. A helpful suggestion for those who wish to develop their speaking skills is to locate the local chapter of Toastmasters. In an informal, yet structured, approach and in a social setting, either over lunch or dinner, the group guides members through a series of speechmaking skills that ease fears and build speaking expertise. For concern about stage fright, John Wolfe, author of *Miracle Platform Power,* advised that with practice the butterflies may not be removed entirely, but they may be made to fly in formation.

Research has shown that the usual characteristics of occupational therapists preclude a natural interest in activities such as making speeches. However, therapists who think of gaining positive and well-deserved publicity that furthers their profession and organization will profit from the effort.

▦ Research and Publishing

Another professional responsibility that offers a valuable additional source of publicity is conducting research and publishing results. After reading your articles, peers will be aware of the effective service you and your organization give to the profession. As a student or entry-level therapist, it is your professional responsibility to develop a research attitude. Begin by becoming part of studies designed to validate occupational therapy efficacy. The results will surprise and encourage you.

▦ Personal Selling

According to Drucker,[3] selling is not necessary if the process of marketing has been conducted successfully. However, there may be instances when knowing how to go about promotional activities, including personal selling, may be valuable.

Personal selling may be defined as direct, face-to-face relationships between the seller and the customer. An occupational therapist can also think of this as personal influence used to promote services. Using creativity in personal selling is as important as having mastered the sequence of stages or steps to be followed to increase the likelihood of making the intended sale.

FEATURES VS. BENEFITS

Probably the most basic rule of selling is that what is being sold is benefits; it is also often the most overlooked as the salesperson tries to overwhelm the buyer with features. A *benefit* is what the customer gets or gains from buying from salespeople or from following their recommendations. A *feature* is a characteristic of the product that produces the benefit. To be effective at selling benefits, a salesperson must have a thorough knowledge and understanding of the product and its applications; at the same time, there must be a complete understanding of the customer and of the customer's needs and wants.

An example is the farmer who is trying to sell a cow by extolling the virtues of the cow's placid nature, the strong contours of the animal, and the strength of her teeth. The prospective buyer, however, cares little for any of these features, preferring to learn whether the cow gives milk and how much, the benefit that satisfies a buyer's need and want. For a retailer seeking to sell a new splinting material to a prospective acute-care occupational therapist, emphasizing the features of finish and color instead of the light weight, strength, coolness, and rapid setting capabilities for use at bedside is another example.

When planning a presentation, begin with benefits (e.g., by using occupational therapy less nursing care is needed because patients are more functionally independent). Make a list of the four or five benefits that best meet the customer's needs. Opposite each, list the product features that produce that benefit. Add ideas and exhibits that prove or dramatize them. Photos of customers enjoying the product, testimonial letters, fact sheets, statistical summaries, demonstrations, and samples are a few ways to illustrate the benefits that you offer. Sell customers what they want and show them how they can be sure you can really satisfy the wants they have—that's selling benefits.

LISTENING

Perhaps the most surprising fact to learn about being an effective salesperson is that today's sales training teaches would-be salespeople to be:

- Good listeners and questioners who are sensitive to the needs of others
- Knowledgeable about what they are selling
- More of an adviser than a seller

As a matter of fact, some experts have gone so far as to declare that there is no greater asset in selling than the ability to listen. Would-be salespeople who buy a pocket dictating machine and record themselves on a sales call get to hear what their customers hear.

Listening is a skill that can be improved. In addition to instruction already received in school, the student may wish to add to this skill by reviewing some suggestions:

1. Attitude profoundly influences the success or failure of your listening. In all cases the listener should assume an attitude that he or she is about to learn something original rather than feel already fully knowledgeable and informed and not likely to add anything new.

2. Do not assume that you already know what a person means or where the words are headed; do not jump to conclusions or complete a statement. Make no judgment until you are certain that you fully understand the communication.

3. Particularly in communications with persons whose primary language is not English, be careful that there is a mutual understanding of the meaning of the words being used. Even among those who share English as a primary language, there is much room for misunderstanding, as the same word can have quite a different meaning to different people.

4. Ask questions, if necessary, to be certain that you fully understand what a person means by a word or statement.

5. Do not intimidate by assuming or inferring a superior-inferior position; instead, listen solely for ideas or information.

6. In tandem with this thought, do not form a preconceived opinion or judgment of the person that can affect your reception of the information about to be received.

For detailed information on the psychological aspects of selling as well as suggestions on how to view the actual process of selling, see Chapter 6.

Comparative Effectiveness of Promotional Efforts

Schewe and Smith[4] offered a comparison of the effectiveness of promotional activities. They saw advertising as highly effective in creating awareness, but it had less impact on the subsequent stages of interest, desire, and action. Personal selling, by contrast, was of less help in creating awareness but was valuable in creating desire and action. Publicity and public relations assisted in fostering general awareness.

Closing the Perceptual Separation

McInnes,[5] a recognized authority in marketing, suggested another way to understand the marketing approach. He declared the existence of a "perceptual separation" between producers and consumers as compared with geographic, spatial, or time separations. He asserted it is due partially to a lack of knowledge and partly to a lack of interest, thus requiring that steps be taken to ameliorate the situation. *Perceptual separation* seems to be a particularly apt way to describe some of the occupational therapy service delivery problems. To close this separation, the therapist can consider bringing information to the attention of potential consumers through such tools as brochures, presentations, or whatever other promotional or public relations tools are deemed best. Different objectives and content must be developed to accomplish different purposes after first carefully identifying the status of each target consumer. For example, the target markets or constituencies or publics could be those who need but lack knowledge of occupational therapy or those who currently have no interest in knowing. In that case the promotional materials begin with the assumption that the constituencies have no knowledge of occupational therapy.

Another differentiation made by McInnes that is helpful to occupational therapists is that of *value separation*. He defined this term as the value placed on a product and noted that this value varies among individuals. Until the producer and the consumer find the cost and product (occupational therapy services) of a value that is mutually satisfactory, no exchanges are made. Unless the occupational therapy practitioner satisfactorily fulfills the client's need for unique, individual attention and for the benefits of the therapist's skills and techniques, a value separation exists, for it is unlikely that therapists in turn will receive the respect and remuneration they need and deserve.

Effect of Gender on Communication

Finally, the occupational therapist should be aware of the potential role that gender plays in daily communication. Knowing in what ways there may be miscommunication between men and women, in what should be simple conversations, may help. Both men and women can learn why they failed to meet someone's expectations and what might in the future be improved. Research has shown that men and women have different goals in communication that, if understood, can greatly improve relationships with colleagues and clients.

Linguist Deborah Tannen, in her book *You Just Don't Understand*,[6] addressed these differences. What sets both sexes immediately on edge derives from the facts that women find security in closeness and connection while men find their security in maintaining their status among others. Conversations reflect this difference. Within small groups, women consider all members equally important; men tend to compare themselves with others with the goal of receiving respect. To women, agreement is essential to self-esteem, and men find independence or even disagreement more important. Overall, women feel more obligated to listen, giving audience rather than advice or comment, whereas men tend to lecture or to give the information. Women lean more toward valuing relationships, not achievement, as their main focus, but men proclaim their accomplishments and themselves. Basically, male body language communicates power and high status; women typically imply affiliation and connectiveness.[6]

Understandably, these are generalizations; however, simply being aware of gender-driven responses can be of value in managing mutually satisfactory exchanges. One's own gender tendencies can be adjusted to fit different situations in which certain kinds of communication seem most effective. Whether you are part of a committee, an interdisciplinary team, or in any aspect of management, knowing what to anticipate in exchange transactions from a gender perspective is invaluable.

Perhaps most important is being accepting of each other and of differences, knowing that difference is not a deficiency, making allowances for those differences, and maintaining a good sense of humor to lighten any situation. If you are a female manager working with a male subordinate, be direct, concise, and to the point in a conversation, remembering that men often will not say they need help or that they do not understand. Also keep in mind that men may not particularly care for working with a female manager, and do not take that personally unless a man's attitude interferes with performance. If you are a male manager working with a female subordinate, be sure that she is given the same opportunities—interesting projects or difficult tasks—as the men with whom you work. Realize that you do not need to be excessively polite, but you do need to be aware of and perhaps avoid language or jokes you might customarily use in male company. Keep in mind that your first reaction to a female colleague's concern should be to listen and to ask rather than to immediately dispense advice unless it is requested. Men and women both need and appreciate positive comments, but stay with genuine compliments about performance rather than appearance.

▓ The Marketing Plan

Regardless of specific environment, objectives, and promotional mix, a marketing plan is usually developed in a similar fashion. Elements common to most marketing plans include:

1. An executive summary
2. Situation analysis (i.e., background, forecast, opportunities and threats, strengths and weaknesses)
3. Objectives and goals
4. Marketing strategy
5. Programs to put the strategy into action
6. Budget
7. Methods of control

Every organization's marketing plan will be different. For example, the marketing communications part in the marketing plan of a community hospital might well include development of a corporate logo, public information control and image enhancement, advertising in selected media, direct-mail marketing, promotional incentives, and publications. All of these components of the marketing communications program are planned to assist in achieving previously developed strategic marketing objectives.

Internally the hospital develops specific services in the same manner. For example, the needs of women are met through offering a group of services that include general surgery, mammography, cosmetic surgery, cardiology, cancer care, gynecologic surgery, orthopedics, arthritis care, parenting workshops, obstetrics, stress management, diabetes treatment, fitness lessons, mental health consultation, osteoporosis care, and physical checkups. The market needs of older adults are met by providing services such as health information, mental health consultations, home health care, geriatric assessment, retirement services, nutrition counseling, arthritis and osteoporosis care, podiatry, respite help, urology, cancer care, hospice care, a pharmacy, skilled nursing, fitness training, and diabetes treatment.

EXAMPLE OF AN OCCUPATIONAL THERAPY MARKETING PLAN

Figure 4–5 depicted the potential constituencies of a work-hardening program being developed by an occupational therapist. Using that situation as an example, the occupational therapist might develop a marketing plan along the following lines:

- Internal business environment

  Strengths: Adequate space and equipment

                  Well-developed teamwork among staff

  Weaknesses: Continuing education needed for some employees

                  Assistance needed to reach referring physicians
- External business environment

  Opportunities: Area businesses need and want this service

                  Local occupational and physical therapists see the need

                  Local hospital and HMO are interested

                  Several insurance companies have expressed interest

  Threats: Unions at local businesses are not convinced

                  Work-hardening program already in beginning stages 50 miles away

                  Two managed-care corporations do not perceive need
- Three major goals for the first year:
  1. Reach break-even point within 1 year
  2. Increase client referrals rapidly
  3. Raise visibility among general public as well as among professionals
- Two marketing objectives to meet these goals:
  1. Expand information about all aspects of the potential market
  2. Select promotional tools to increase awareness
- Priority for implementing marketing objectives: Examine status of each identified constituency and bring about changes

- Survey techniques to use to achieve objectives:
  Telephone surveys
  Demographic analysis
  Personal interview
- Determine methods for evaluation and monitoring of plan

This is an elementary and simplistic outline intended to guide an initial attempt to develop a marketing plan. References for this chapter and Chapter 4 provide detailed information.

Summary

This chapter introduced the reader to promotional aspects of the marketing process. Differences among advertising, publicity, public relations, and selling were explained. Specific steps were suggested for creating positive publicity, making effective speeches, becoming an empathic listener, and understanding selling. Examples of how and why promotional tools are assembled to form marketing plans were given. Chapter 6 introduces one approach to functional selling used in training marketers in a major U.S. corporation.

REFERENCES

1. Peter, JP, and Donnelly, JH Jr: Marketing Management: Knowledge and Skills. Irwin, Homewood, Ill, 1992, p 142.
2. Kotler, P, and Clarke, RN: Marketing for Health Care Organizations. Prentice-Hall, Englewood Cliffs, NJ, 1987, p 471.
3. Drucker, PF: Management, Tasks, Responsibilities, Practices. Harper & Row, New York, 1973.
4. Schewe, CD, and Smith, RM: Marketing Concepts and Applications. McGraw-Hill, New York, 1980.
5. McInnes, W: A conceptual approach to marketing. In Cox, Reavis, Alderson, and Shapiro (eds): Theory in Marketing. Irwin, Homewood, Ill, 1964, pp 51–67.
6. Tannen, D: You Just Don't Understand. Ballantine Books, New York, 1991.

CHAPTER 6

Functional Selling

CHAPTER OBJECTIVES

- To interpret one promotional tool, selling, in greater detail
- To explain the functional selling approach
- To recognize categories of behavior in communication
- To discuss interactions and adaptations of achievement and affiliation motivators
- To consider means to change behaviors
- To discern differences among persuasive techniques

A primary purpose of this book is to introduce the marketing process as a logical methodology that occupational therapists can use to develop leadership skills. With that in mind, this chapter is devoted to a discussion of one promotional tool used in marketing, functional selling, a concept used by a major corporation for the purpose of assisting sales employees to become better communicators.[1]

What Is Functional Selling?

Functional selling was defined, by the marketing department representatives of the corporation that originated this term, as a means to mentally categorize both participants in a sales transaction. A salesperson can adjust a sales presentation and make adaptations to accommodate personal differences. If selling is one of the promotional tools selected to implement a marketing plan, familiarity with this methodology may be helpful.

A great number of resources on the topic of selling are available. Many originated earlier than this one, and numerous publications, workshops, and tapes have appeared since. This particular method, functional selling, was selected because it combines a conceptual approach to the selling process with practical application, and it has been used successfully by many salespersons over the years. Furthermore, the functional selling process entails sociological and psychological aspects for which occupational therapists already are educationally prepared. Because this approach is focused on the interpersonal relationships of persons involved in the buying and selling process, it appears to be compatible with an occupational therapy background. Following is a brief introduction to the ideas that comprise functional selling.

Social Motivators in Successful Salesmanship

The functional selling process has the premise that there are three social motivators related to success in sales performance: achievement, affiliation, and power. Of the three, achievement and affiliation are the two of primary concern, with power at an intermediate level in a sales interview environment. To gain maximum value from the following discussion, envision yourself in the position of a salesperson approaching a potential customer. By being familiar with the functional selling perspective, the salesperson is better prepared to make an assessment of the primary motivation of the prospective customer, to adapt the sales presentation, and to expect a successful outcome. Figure 6–1 forms the foundation for discussion of how a salesperson should proceed.

Characteristics of Individuals

To explain the components of Figure 6–1, following are comparative descriptions of behaviors that are characteristic of persons possessing high and low achievement motivation and explanations of what may be expected of individuals with high and low affiliation motivation.

HIGH ACHIEVEMENT

QUADRANT 1
TASK ORIENTED
PROBLEM SOLVING
MUTUAL BENEFITS

QUADRANT 4
SELF-CENTERED
PUSHY/DEMANDING
DOMINEERING

HIGH _____LOW
AFFILIATION   AFFILIATION

QUADRANT 2
FRIENDSHIP SELLS
LIKABLE
AMIABLE/OPTIMISTIC

QUADRANT 3
SUBMISSIVE/PASSIVE
SUSPICIOUS
SECURITY ORIENTED

LOW ACHIEVEMENT

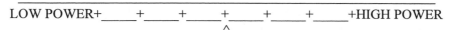

LOW POWER+_____+_____+_____+_____+_____+_____+HIGH POWER

FIGURE 6–1. Two-dimensional social roles model of sales communication. (Courtesy E. I. du Pont de Nemours Inc., Wilmington, Del.)

ACHIEVEMENT MOTIVATION

Individuals demonstrate *high* achievement motivation with the following behaviors:

- Taking personal responsibility
- Engaging in active problem solving
- Seeking recognition
- Taking calculated risks
- Setting and achieving realistic personal goals
- Seeking feedback on performance

These behaviors are reinforced in their everyday lives.
Low achievement motivation is demonstrated by the following behaviors:

- Avoiding any personal responsibility
- Attempts to increase anonymity
- Avoiding problem solving or active decision making
- Small risk taking (or extremely unrealistic risk taking with assured failing results)
- Avoiding feedback on performance

These individuals have a history of failure and frustration in achievement situations. Often they belong to subgroups in which achievement is either not valued or is specifically denied.

AFFILIATION MOTIVATION

Individuals demonstrate *high* affiliation motivation with the following behaviors:

- Concern for the outcomes of others
- Seeking company of others
- Recognition of needs of others
- Helping and aiding behaviors
- Strong group memberships and personal loyalty
- Sharing behaviors

Individuals with high affiliation needs have learned that elements of high affiliation are satisfying to them.

Low affiliation motivation is demonstrated by the following behaviors:

- Hostility in human interaction
- Suspiciousness of needs and outcomes of others
- Self-centered evaluation of environment
- Lone-wolf behavior (everyone for themselves)
- Limited sharing, helping, aiding

Those demonstrating low affiliation motivation perceive the world to be full of hostile "others."

POWER THEME

Although the power role is not considered useful in sales performance, the components of the power theme are included here to make the picture complete. *High* power motivation is evidenced by:

- Seeking positions of leadership and authority
- Directing the activities of others
- Planning and organizing the behavior of others
- Distributing rewards and punishments
- Evaluating the behavior of others
- Deciding and setting group goals

Power is a word that raises negative emotions for many individuals, but in organizations the power functions must be exercised. None of these functions is inherently evil.

Low power motivation is demonstrated by the following behaviors:

- Avoiding all positions of leadership and authority
- Docile acceptance of the direction of others
- Slavish attendance to group or social rules
- Few or no control attempts over environmental stimuli

Power motivation in either its high or low states is considered detrimental to effective sales. It plays little part in the selling-communication situation because few people recognize the legitimate right of a salesperson to exercise authority while trying to close a sale.

Interestingly, the use of power motivation may become necessary if the sales*person* becomes a sale *manager*. In that case, inability to assume the power role can create problems. For example, if the accomplished salesperson fails as a sales manager or a highly competent occupational therapist does not succeed as a manager, an inability to understand and use the power role may well be the reason. Although the power role is not considered useful in sales, it is important for other reasons and is discussed in Chapter 1.

▓ Adaptive Strategies to Be Taken During Sales Transactions

Figure 6–1 depicts four social roles often assumed by both participants during sales presentation situations. These roles are formed by the interaction of affiliation and achievement motivations. Few people fit exactly into a single one of the four quadrants, as each individual has some of the other characteristics as well.

QUADRANT 1: HIGH ACHIEVEMENT–HIGH AFFILIATION STRATEGY

The high-high combination of affiliation and achievement roles has proved to be the most effective sales strategy. The high achievement orientation is tempered by the high affiliation theme. The person with a drive to succeed also recognizes the needs and wants of others. This results in a strategy that seeks to succeed by working with others, bringing them along, and seeking mutual benefits. Although this strategy is not correct for every situation, in the sales situation it is maximally effective (assuming that the buyer has some choice of products, will need continuing service or technical advice, and will be a repeat customer). Most customers fit into the last category.

Behaviors that demonstrate a quadrant 1 (high achievement, high affiliation) role are:

- Mutual goal setting (participation)
- Mutual benefits and outcomes

- Respect for inputs of others (even if in disagreement)
- Strict honesty about differences in goals, inputs, outcomes
- Problem-solving approach (accepts helpful criticism)
- Cooperation and feedback

This can be a difficult social role behavior to identify because needs for both affiliation and achievement are present. Once this behavior has been determined to be present, a quadrant 1 customer can be approached by the salesperson through quadrant 1 behaviors. Such individuals respond to expressions of concerned interest in their goals and needs.

QUADRANT 2: LOW ACHIEVEMENT–HIGH AFFILIATION STRATEGY

The quadrant 2 strategy, although not as effective as quadrant 1, is not totally without merit. Depending upon the situation and the people involved, there are times when a friendly, low profile can be a successful strategy. The success of the quadrant 2 combination of roles usually depends on matching this strategy to the complementary role in the receiver. Behaviors that typify the quadrant 2 (low achievement, high affiliation) role are:

- Has genuine liking for people without regard for benefits, goals, outcomes
- Ignores decision making (it gets in the way of easy companionship)
- Attempts to "belong"
- Feels that "things will work out"
- Avoids task-related communication (talks exclusively about family, vacation, and so on)
- Is somewhat unwilling to face realities of business demands (schedules, quotas, and the like)
- Becomes overinvolved with clients

The quadrant 2 individual responds best to a friendly, low-profile approach. Once the friendship is established, the sales situation should be strengthened by developing a need for achievement in the customer. If this is not done, the customer is vulnerable to the next friendly salesperson who calls.

QUADRANT 3: LOW ACHIEVEMENT–LOW AFFILIATION STRATEGY

The quadrant 3 strategy is the least useful for sales personnel. The quadrant 3 salesperson is only a marginal success in any situation. This role emphasizes security, passiveness, and retreat from the challenges of both tasks and people. This role ensures minimum effectiveness because it limits the individual from actively seeking out task problems or people problems. Behaviors that typify the quadrant 3 (low achievement, low affiliation) role are:

- Security and safety above all else
- General aloofness and isolation
- Suspicion of others' motives
- Fear of incompetence and discovery by others
- Rigid adherence to all rules and regulations
- Never volunteers, never takes a chance

QUADRANT 4: HIGH ACHIEVEMENT–LOW AFFILIATION STRATEGY

Like the quadrant 2 strategy, the quadrant 4 strategy has drawbacks but is not completely without merit. This role emphasizes task problems while ignoring people problems. As in quadrant 2, certain role combinations would make this strategy a viable one. Behaviors that typify the quadrant 4 (high achievement, low affiliation) role are:

- Self-centered goals, benefits, outcomes
- Individualistic and competitive interactions with others
- Win-lose approach (instead of problem-solving approach) to interaction
- Little cooperation, restriction of information
- Suspicion of others' motives and exploitive use of others

Interactions Between Salespersons and Customers/Clients in Different Quadrants

The following discussion should be read in conjunction with the preceding information. It provides descriptions of what can be anticipated during the interactions of persons identified as being in the various quadrants shown in Figure 6–1.

QUADRANT 1 SALESPERSON (HIGH ACHIEVEMENT, HIGH AFFILIATION)

Quadrant 1 client interaction produces the most effective sales communication. Neither task problems nor people problems hinder clear presentation of necessary information. Both parties are goal-oriented and supportive.

Quadrant 2 client interaction also produces the most effective sales communication. Although the client is not goal oriented, the salesperson's task-oriented presentation and obvious affiliation role carry the presentation through. The salesperson has to overcome some impatience with the client's nongoal behavior, but this can easily be accomplished.

Quandrant 3 client interaction is not likely to produce any highly effective communication. The quadrant 3 client is a problem to any salesperson. The quadrant 1 role is likely to meet with at least average success for two reasons:

- The affiliation theme helps reduce suspicion and neutralize isolation and fear
- The achievement theme neutralizes excessive safety and security behaviors

Quadrant 4 client interaction produces higher than average sales communication. The quadrant 1 sales role interacts favorably with the quadrant 4 client. Both individuals express task orientation and, although the salesperson may not like the self-centered tactics of the quadrant 4 client, this does not have to be a barrier to good sales communication. There is little warmth in the relationship, but both sides should benefit.

QUADRANT 2 SALESPERSON (LOW ACHIEVEMENT, HIGH AFFILIATION):

Quadrant 1 client interaction is warm and fairly productive, thanks to the client. The quadrant 2 salesperson is perceived as wasting time, never getting to the meat of the communication. Eventually the client draws out the salesperson, discovers if the salesperson can fill any needs, and *gives* an order. All in all, the sales communication is average, with the client prying out necessary information.

Quadrant 2 client interaction is warm. The interaction at this level is excessively friendly and *does* result in sales (perhaps, if no other influences interfere, high sales) but only by default. When all other things are equal, friendship is a powerful social motivator. The sales communication effectiveness is average.

Quadrant 3 client interaction resembles ships that pass in the night. The quadrant 3 role player often responds with sarcasm and open hostility to the salesperson. The salesperson at least does not threaten the client. This role interaction usually results in lower than average sales communication.

Quadrant 4 customer interaction is a disaster. The client regards the salesperson as a time-wasting babbler. Because the quadrant 4 role has no recognition of people orientation, the two have no common bridge. The salesperson is likely to attempt to avoid this client (and the client is happy to keep it that way). Sales communication effectiveness in this situation is very low.

QUADRANT 3 SALESPERSON (LOW ACHIEVEMENT, LOW AFFILIATION):

Quadrant 1 clients must attempt to dig information out of this salesperson (and without even the help of a common affiliation theme). This process not only wastes time but also can be irritating. Only the client's achievement interest saves communication from being a total loss.

Quadrant 2 clients usually make the quadrant 3 salesperson nervous. Neither is interested in goals and tasks. Again, the only saving grace in this situation is the *client's* interest in the salesperson. Communication effectiveness is well below average.

Quadrant 3 client interaction becomes an apathetic interaction between two people who could care less. The salesperson is an order taker. If there is a specific need at the time, the salesperson can have the order as well as anyone else. Information is not exchanged; no personal relationships are constructed. Sales communication effectiveness is very low.

Quadrant 4 client interaction becomes a most painful experience for the quadrant 3 salesperson. Expecting hostility, the salesperson finds the worst imaginings come true. The customer takes control of communication interaction and attempts to pry information out of the salesperson in as brutal a means as possible. The salesperson often retorts in kind. Sales communication effectiveness is as low as possible.

QUADRANT 4 SALESPERSON (HIGH ACHIEVEMENT, LOW AFFILIATION):

Quadrant 1 client interaction becomes a tug-of-war situation, with the customer asking more than the salesperson wants to give in terms of long-term service, common benefits, and trust. The quadrant 1 client, being a match for the salesperson's task presentation, has the ability to demand these people-oriented benefits. Sales communication is of only average effectiveness.

Quadrant 2 clients often respond very favorably to the high achievement themes presented by the quadrant 4 salesperson. Unfortunately, this client is ripe for exploitation. The quadrant 4 role allows exploitation in order to advance achievement outcomes. If the interaction is a continuing one, sales communication effectiveness can drop from a before-exploitation above-average rating to a post-exploitation below-average rating.

Quadrant 3 client interaction becomes a scene of complete domination by the salesperson and smoldering submission by the client. Unfortunately for the salesperson, if the quadrant 3 client does not *have* to buy the product, there is no sale. In this case the client can always escape. Unlike the salesperson, these clients do not have to subject themselves to discomfort. The sales communication effectiveness is generally quite low.

Quadrant 4 client interaction becomes a wary standoff. Both actors are out for immediate profit, suspicious of each other's motives, and careful not to give away points. Usually both actors enjoy the encounter, but communication suffers so that only average effectiveness results.

▨ Summary of Salesperson and Customer Communication Outcomes

Figure 6–2 is an analysis of the comparative effectiveness of salesperson-client interactions. These designations are presented within the context of the preceding discussion.

Most salespeople have all four quadrant roles at their disposal. Depending on time, place, and customer, any role can be played. Usually, humans have one role that becomes a "preferred" method of interacting with others. Participants should use the role matrix to identify their behaviors and the behaviors of the people with whom they communicate in order to:

		Salesperson			
		Quad 1 High Ach High Aff	Quad 2 Low Ach High Aff	Quad 3 Low Ach Low Aff	Quad 4 High Ach Low Aff
C l i e n t	Quad 1 High Ach High Aff	5	5	2	3
	Quad 2 Low Ach High Aff	5	3	2	4/2
	Quad 3 Low Ach Low Aff	3	2	1	1
	Quad 4 High Ach Low Aff	4	1	1	3

Sales Communication Ratings:

Effective	5
Above Average	4
Average	3
Below Average	2
Ineffective	1

FIGURE 6–2. Summary of salesperson and customer communication outcomes. (Courtesy E. I. du Pont de Nemours Inc., Wilmington, Del.)

- Allow for prediction of outcomes
- Allow for preparation of behavior to counter inappropriate outcomes
- Point out possible changes in sales role behavior for better effect
- Suggest possible cause-and-effect relationships between behaviors and outcomes

Behavior Change

One chapter in a book obviously does not change a person's behavior. Often inappropriate behaviors are well entrenched; many habits are simply not perceived. Several techniques may be helpful to a salesperson: using tape recordings or videotapes to evaluate communication patterns, arranging with a friend to give objective feedback in a communication situation, accepting constructive criticism in a nonemotional, problem-solving manner, and beginning with and building on personal strengths. Occupational therapists may also get feedback from supervisors, peers, and colleagues.

PERSUASIVE TECHNIQUES

1. Increase your credibility as a communicator.
   - □ Demonstrate expertise and proven competence
   - □ Ensure objectivity—the ability to deal with matters factually and not be swayed by subjective involvement
   - □ Develop ability and authority to act
   - □ Be constantly aware that there is similarity between your predictions and outcomes (what you say will happen happens; what you say you will do, you do)
2. Give two-sided rather than one-sided messages. (Giving both sides of a story is a powerfully persuasive tool.)
   - □ Openly compare both positions, not just one side
   - □ Point out "problem areas" with the other position
   - □ Be knowledgeable about the opposing position
   - □ Stabilize your position by being critical first
3. Use methods that demand cooperation and are perceived to be in the individual's best interests rather than forced upon the person.
   - □ Find common ground and common reality
   - □ Demonstrate common goals and outcomes
   - □ Arrange for the individual to "discover" the usefulness of the communication outcome

      □ Make the act of closing the sale an easy behavior to perform, with some immediate reward

4. If the individual's position is far removed from yours, move toward your goal in slow steps over time.

      □ Attempt to move your position only slightly in the desired direction first

      □ Allow time intervals for behavior to become set in the new position

      □ Reward and reinforce the new behavior

■ Functional Selling and the Occupational Therapy Practitioner

Functional selling was described here because of its potential usefulness to occupational therapists who find themselves needing to use selling as one promotional tool for implementation of their marketing plans. This particular approach to selling was selected because its components most closely approximate what an occupational therapist already has learned: the psychological aspects of interpersonal exchanges and transactions. Knowing that you have already mastered and are comfortable with both the feeling and methodology of a sales transaction helps assuage your anxiety about using selling as a marketing tool.

■ Summary

This chapter has described functional selling, an approach suggested as one way to visualize and plan as a salesperson for interactions with prospective clients. A graphic representation of a methodology for analysis of communication patterns helps you plan ahead and ensure successful sales outcomes. Following this analysis of participants in a sales exchange, strategies for achieving the intended goal were furnished, as well as techniques for changing behaviors.

REFERENCE

1. Live Communication, Vol IV, Social Role Theory and Communication. E I du Pont de Nemours Inc, Wilmington, Del, 1974.

PART THREE

COLLABORATIVE
RELATIONSHIPS

Something we were withholding made us
weak until we found out that it was us.
Robert Frost, The Gift Outright, 1942

CHAPTER 7

The Client as Collaborator

CHAPTER OBJECTIVES

- To reemphasize the primary importance of client-centered care.
- To recognize the multiple perspectives of collaborative treatment.
- To realize that effective treatment can result from collaboration.
- To understand the convergence of program management, marketing, and total quality management.
- To recall how occupational therapy literature supports client-centered care.
- To appreciate the value of active listening and empathy.
- To recognize the differences among models of client-centered care.
- To illustrate how standardized tools may be used to set mutual goals.

During opening ceremonies at the 1995 American Occupational Therapy Association (AOTA) annual conference in Denver, Lex Frieden, prominent advocate for the disabled and member of the board of directors of the American Occupational Therapy Foundation, shared a memorable dialogue with AOTA President Mary Evert. Among his observations was an admonition that, to support independent living for the disabled, occupational therapists must become partners with patients, listen to them, and facilitate filling their needs.[1] That the customer has become, almost universally, number one in any service organization—in business in general or in healthcare services delivery in particular—should, by now, be fairly evident.

This chapter discusses client-centered care and why it is timely, essential, and logical for occupational therapists, whether in hospitals, rehabilitation facilities, or the community. The parts played in client-centered care by active listening, empathy, collaboration, and standardized tools are explained.

▓ Customer Perception and Product Marketing

Media promotions on television or in a newspaper have been planned to respond to previously identified wants and needs. The idea is to strike a responsive chord in the observer and thus serve as a reminder that product X is exactly what can satisfy that need or want. Corporations engaged in global marketing have done so successfully by individualizing and tailoring their messages to those customers. Mike Quinlan of McDonald's noted, "If you watch one of our commercials in Argentina and another in England, you'll always see a local touch."[2]

A similar move toward individual need satisfaction can be found in U.S. hospitals today. In this chapter, the word *patient* is intentionally used at the outset and then gradually replaced by the word *client*. The purpose of the difference is to symbolize the changes in attitude of those who receive healthcare services, evolving from passive recipients into active, collaborative participants.

▓ Patient-Centered Care in Hospitals

Patient activism is changing the way hospital care is delivered. In the past, hospital administrators treated physicians as their primary customers because physicians were nearly autonomous in deciding where patients were to be hospitalized. Growing numbers of patients now report that they are actively involved in hospital choice; others first choose a hospital or health plan before choosing a doctor from among those affiliated with a facility or plan. Accordingly, hospital administrators now ask consumers what they want and try to give it to them.

Patient-centered care means more than "being nice" to patients; it means meeting patients' needs as they themselves, not doctors, nurses, or administrators, perceive them. In contrast to the usual patient satisfaction survey, patients are being asked for more concrete details: How long after you asked for pain medication did you get it? Did someone explain why that test was being done? Did they explain how much discomfort you would have during or after the test?

More than just hospital survey data are being gathered, though. Patients judge the quality of care by its impact on their lives. They want to know whether a procedure will restore their ability to see, hear, walk, dress, or feed themselves, for example. Because these outcomes are rarely measured, that is the next step being undertaken by hospitals: using new technology to assess patients' symptoms, functional status, and sense of well-being.

Collaboration of patients with physicians in making decisions about their own care is an ethical imperative because what are called medical judgments are more often actually value judgments. To assist both physician and patient when, for example, a choice must be made between "watchful waiting" or having a prostatectomy, an interactive videodisk dramatizes the fact that there is no right or wrong decision. Based on information input about the patient's age, symptoms, and other illnesses, the computer tailors the probabilities of each outcome to the patient's particular subgroup. Programs are available on treatment options for hypertension, low-back pain, breast cancer, angina, arthritis of the hip and knee, and postmenopausal problems.[3]

THE PATIENT IS NUMBER ONE

In 1988 attention was drawn to the need for prioritizing patient satisfaction with services when Rosenbaum[4] wrote *The Doctor*. One of his assertions was that he wanted his doctors to understand his illness and his feelings and what he needed from his physicians. He knew that they could have done those things, but some of them did not.

Delbanco,[5] a physician in Boston, reported results of a 4-year project to evaluate and improve health services by focusing on the needs and concerns of clients as they themselves define them. Through systematic use of a review of their preferences, values, and needs, he learned that clients do not focus on prettier waiting rooms, better hospital food, or problems with parking. Instead, they want to be able to negotiate the healthcare system, be treated with dignity and respect, understand how their sickness or treatment will affect their lives, learn to care for themselves away from the clinical setting, and often fear that their doctors are not telling them everything they know. Delbanco shared having always known that patients have their differences; however, he thought he could judge what they felt and wanted. During the systematic review, the issues that surfaced surprised and enlightened him. The result was his determination that collecting clients' perceptions and suggestions for change can address clinically significant aspects of their experiences, foster their active involvement in their own care, and help assess and improve the quality of the care delivered.

The founders of the Planetree Model Hospital Project[6] felt that medicine must go beyond crisis care to a shared responsibility for client health. Realizing that many clients perceive doctors and nurses to be uncaring and uninterested and hospitals to be intimidating, impersonal institutions, the founders of Planetree established first a resource center and then a hospital to counteract these client perceptions. The goal was a hospital with staff who would be effective at treating disease and at the same time listen and respond to the needs of healthcare consumers; they would thus supply both the art and science of medicine.

In 1985 Planetree opened a 13-bed medical-surgical unit at Pacific Presbyterian Medical Center in San Francisco, here combining the best of modern technology with the most ancient concepts of nurturing and supportive care. Traditional barriers that separate staff from clients have been removed, with clients becoming active participants in the healthcare team. There is an open chart policy, and clients are encouraged to add comments to the charts themselves. Called *care partners*, family members are encouraged to stay overnight, assist in the physical and emotional care of the clients, and learn how to care for them after discharge.

Many more surveys have been made of the perceptions of those who have used hospital services recently. Because of the results of these studies, hundreds of U.S. hospitals are changing the way they deliver healthcare services to their customers. Common to all of them is renewed focus on the client rather than continued focus on the system.

▨ Raising Client and Staff Satisfaction in Healthcare Organizations

When the Joint Commission on Accreditation of Healthcare Organizations revised its requirements and mandated that all accredited facilities be responsible for devising competency standards for their staffs, this was a new way of doing business. The purpose for introducing this measure was to increase both staff and client satisfaction levels. One facility, Greater Southeast Community Hospital (GSCH) in Washington, D.C., developed such standards in compliance with the order.

Frank E. Gainer, MHS, OTR, director of the GSCH rehabilitation services department, described the initial reaction to the standards that were developed.[7] Clients were asked to rate satisfaction in 11 areas, which included staff courtesy, ease of scheduling appointments, inclusion of family in services provided, and cleanliness and comfort of treatment areas. Staff members were hesitant at first about having clients rate them, but now that the system is in place, client satisfaction has already improved, and staff members are continuing to seek ways to do things better.

Not only did this facility institute the practice of having every client fill out the survey, but also supervisors rate the therapists, discipline-specific peer review is in place, and staff members have the opportunity to evaluate their supervisors annually. Aspects of their jobs on which supervisors are rated include clarity of job descriptions, availability of supervisors, level of supervisor support for professional growth, and the provision of counseling on strengths and weaknesses. The element of responsiveness to consumer needs can be clearly seen in all these transactions, whether client-staff, staff-supervisor, or colleague-colleague in peer review.[7]

The Veterans Health Administration (VHA) medical system has also undergone changes, announcing a new way of thinking about how patient-care services are delivered. A more interdisciplinary, patient-focused VHA with more emphasis on strategic planning and quality improvement had been envisioned. A continuum of care, expanded clinic hours, more points of access, decreased waiting times, and more timely processing of admissions were among the improvements announced. Empowering employees at the local level was another feature, with occupational therapists among those who develop programs around clients' needs.[8]

CONSUMER-CENTERED HOSPITAL-BASED CARE IN THE COMMUNITY

Some examples of hospital-based care in transition are in the area of pediatrics. Karen Fisher, OTR, in Akron, Ohio, has worked in pediatric home health care for the last 3 years under the direction of Saundra Redding, MEd, OTR, manager of occupational therapy at Children's Hospital Medical Center of Akron. Fisher treats medically fragile children not yet strong enough to use outpatient services, such as children with cerebral palsy, cardiac problems, arthrogryposis, bronchopulmonary dysplasia, Prader-Willi syndrome, edema, orthopedic anomalies, and respiratory problems who are dependent on ventilators, tube feeding, and sometimes IVs. Fisher considers early pediatric home health care vital to the children's lives and home environments.

Anita Thrasher, OTR, is one of two hospital occupational therapists employed by Children's Hospital of the Kings Daughters in Norfolk, Virginia, to work with children in their homes. Most of the children she treats have diagnoses of cerebral palsy, spina bifida, or other birth defects. Because many were premature, they are still on respirators, oxygen, and apnea monitors. Thrasher agrees with Fisher that the home is the ideal place to work with infants.[9]

Delivering high-quality rehabilitation services means placing client needs above those of the professionals involved. Kreitner, Hartz, and Pflum[10] shared results of a 1992 experiment at their place of employment, Reading Rehabilitation Hospital, in which a staff member with a simulated medical condition was admitted for a 2-day inpatient trial. Afterwards her comments indicated that as a patient she felt that she had to ask permission to do even the simplest activities—completely unempowered—and that "we just assume we know what is right for patients without even soliciting their opinions."[10]

Kreitner et al. noted the presence of three assumptions on the part of a patient: The patient is the customer; the patient is sole owner of his or her body, mind, and spirit; and services should be delivered with the patient's convenience and desires in mind, not the caregivers'. The authors concluded that client-centered, customer-driven approaches by caregivers emphasized ongoing partnerships with clients that extend beyond their current needs. Well-designed client-centered rehabilitation also encourages families to participate and be empowered.

In light of these and other sources, clearly similarities, parallels, and even a convergence of goals are at work here: program management, marketing, and total quality management (TQM), all based on a client-centered approach. Familiarity with and integration of the techniques of each of these processes promise effectiveness as a result. If occupational therapists are to successfully progress along with other rehabilitation professionals into the next century, services must expand from primarily treatment-centered programs into human-centered programs.

STAYING CURRENT IN REHABILITATION PRIVATE PRACTICE

Physical therapist Bob Doctor[11] described how he developed his 10-office Denver physical therapy practice by noting repeatedly that basic to his success is having listened carefully to what his clients said they wanted. Located in "a wellness atmosphere," his business includes such services as babysitting and reception facilities and has convenient parking and neighborhood locations. Further, he feels that in today's market therapists must be flexible and innovative, stay current, and keep an open mind. Reflecting further on his original premise that customers' wants are primary, Doctor asserted that "listening to patients will affect a practitioner's marketing approach, clinic hours, billing systems, location, parking, and everything that is based on what is best for them. It sounds simple, but if you build around that, it's a real key. It's number one on our mission statement."[11]

▌ Remember Who You Are Treating

Effective occupational therapy relies on a collaboration between therapist and client. This collaboration requires a therapist who listens carefully to what the client relates about personal life tasks and roles. A treatment plan can then be devised with the best potential for a successful conclusion

Many leaders in the profession have cautioned, advised, and admonished about the importance of this aspect of occupational therapy in recent years. Christiansen[12] warned against disregarding patients' life tasks and roles when assessing function, in that decisions related to intervention and program evaluation are only as good as the data upon which they are based. In her discussion of functional assessment, Dunn[13] recommended that an occupational therapist select what is to be evaluated based on the view of the person who would benefit from the services. She further advocated that approaching assessment within a context allows the therapist to identify what the person needs and wants to do. By beginning assessment at this level, Dunn thinks that the therapist can then go on to plan goals for services based on those expressed needs and know what the persons and families being served want to do in their lives.

Peloquin[14] reminded us how essential it is to listen to, and hear, what the client has to say. She used narratives to demonstrate that healthcare professionals often fail to recognize that illness and disability are situations laden with personal meaning. Instead of communicating with their charges, helpers insert a distance that diminishes those they are helping. Information is withheld in a way that eliminates hope. Brusque manners are prevalent, and power is misused. Unnoticed by the professionals, to the client each of these behaviors appears unreasonable, impersonal, and discouraging.

Increasing numbers of occupational therapists practicing in home health have reported successful interventions when treatment is built on client empowerment, what the client most needs and wants, and what is most important to the client. For example, research as well as experience has shown that older persons can most successfully live and recover when they have control over decisions affecting their daily lives. Factors that promote satisfaction among these and other clients are most likely to result in successful occupational therapy outcomes.

Professionals often forget, at least momentarily, that the client is not only the central focus but also the collaborator in the occupational therapy processes. Scenarios such as that reported by Rondalyn Varney Whitney, COTA/L,[15] illustrate the point. Hospitalized for surgery after a fall, Whitney poignantly described her experiences as a client. Following several incidents in which her needs and priorities were ignored, causing her frustration and pain, she was helped by an occupational therapist who worked with her collaboratively. Whitney's concluding remarks encapsulate the meaning here: "The experience has taught me that OT practitioners can overlook symbols and clients' priorities—even shifts in priorities—but we're more effective when we don't. For me, being able to look well was the equivalent of being well. Helen is a British therapist highly specialized in shoulder and hand treatments, but her real gift as an OT practitioner is that she has the ability to look beyond the categories on the evaluation forms and see a person—someone with priorities and preferences and a deep need to regain normalcy. She has helped me become a better COTA."[15] The very title of Whitney's article made the point to be remembered: "Don't Say You Know How I Feel."

OCCUPATIONAL THERAPY AND CAREGIVER COLLABORATION

Klepitsch[16] provided an example of caregiver collaboration in an account of her experience as the mother of a premature baby. She concluded that for effective results the role of an occupational therapist must be collaborative, not only with the premature infant but also with the parents or caregivers. Their unmet expectations for a healthy baby, their feelings of loss of control and helplessness, the tremendous stress, and the overwhelming demands require that the occupational therapist develop a treatment plan to help the entire family. Assisting the parents or caregivers with their needs for time management skills, supplying referrals to respite care and to parent and child play groups, and simply listening to their expression of their needs assure the occupational therapist of better follow-up and compliance by the family whose needs have been heard and met.

The same is true at the opposite end of the age spectrum. Clark, Corcoran, and Gitlin,[17] seeking to learn how occupational therapists develop therapeutic relationships with family caregivers, examined how therapeutic interactions can evoke different caregiver responses and influence collaborative therapeutic relationships. They found four primary types of occupational therapist–caregiver interaction: caring, partnering, informing, and directing.

They also concluded that "therapeutic interaction can enhance client participation in all areas of occupational therapy practice, but in home health care, where environmental influences are more numerous than they are in the controlled hospital setting, the nature of the therapeutic relationship is even more likely to affect treatment outcomes." To build effective partnerships, occupational therapy practitioners working with older clients should implement strategies that involve family members in the therapeutic process, according to study results. Finally, the authors exhorted occupational therapy practitioners to adopt collaborative and empowering treatment techniques. This research is not alone in its recognition of the importance of family caregivers.

RESEARCH IN THERAPEUTIC CAREGIVING

Not only does the literature reveal that family members already do assume primary responsibility for the care of elderly persons[18-20] but also the value and need for healthcare professionals to actively guide and engage family caregivers in treatment of older persons has been documented.[21-28] In two separate studies, Neistadt[29] found that "clients in long-term settings who collaborated on their treatment goals made statistically and clinically significant gains in their abilities to perform or direct self-care and community-living skills. . . . In both of these studies clients had previously reached plateaus in occupational therapy programs where the therapists had unilaterally set treatment goals to improve component skills like perception or fine motor coordination."[29]

Fall 1995 initiatives of the Robert Wood Johnson Foundation (RWJF) encouraged more active consumer participation in health care. RWJF invested $2.2 million in a $4 million demonstration project being conducted by Healthwise, a not-for-profit organization. Rather than following the trend of containing costs by reducing the supply of care and managing what providers can offer patients, RWJF is supporting programs that aim to curb unnecessary use and wasteful practices by coupling community education strategies with self-care tools. The Healthwise Communities Project was judged to be one such initiative, proposing to study how increased consumer involvement in medical decision making affects patient attitudes, satisfaction, and patterns of health services use and costs. According to the director of the project, putting information into the hands of consumers results in the quality of care going up, health costs going down, and satisfaction growing. Through this and other funded projects, RWJF exemplifies growing acknowledgement of the commonsense wisdom of listening and empowerment.[30]

Zejdlik[31] urged professionals to increasingly and actively seek input from consumers by using as an example the movement within rehabilitation research toward participatory action research, which stresses consumer and interdisciplinary participation in research design and formulation of questions. Because the ultimate success or failure of rehabilitation of the spinal cord–injured (SCI) individual is determined by his or her ability to enjoy a productive life, the author suggested that rehabilitation professionals join SCI consumers to together overcome barriers to independence. Such a continuum of teamwork is not only ideal but also possible.

DESIGNING OUTPATIENT PROGRAMS THAT TARGET CONSUMER NEEDS

In the past occupational therapists used the charismatic personality of the program representative to attract referrals to their outpatient services. Once clients were referred, the payer assumed payments for services the medical team deemed necessary. All that has now changed. The needs of the consumer are now central, and the services are developed around the needs of the consumer.

The constituencies and publics of outpatient programs are no longer solely physicians and clients. The circle has widened and now also includes preferred provider organizations, health maintenance organizations, physician-hospital organizations, payers, community employers, business coalitions, and program employees. Alliances with other providers are developed based on geographic accessibility. (Again, review Part Two to renew understanding of the changeability of constituencies into simultaneous or different configurations.) By identifying services that are lacking, new programs may be added to your organization, and thus business will grow.

Customer focus groups can help build business projections and provide input regarding use expectations. Expected outcomes should be identified at the beginning. Once an appropriate new program has been identified, complete your environmental survey, marketing audit, and marketing plan, and choose the marketing mix that best serves your needs.

Collaboration in Action

Among the successful collaborations and mutually satisfying exchanges is Functional Abilities Inc., which has built a progressive network of rehabilitation programs at 12 sites in long-term facilities and outpatient clinics in Florida and employs 100 persons. Credit for this success has been given in great part to founder Vanessa Dazio's responsiveness to the needs of both patients and employees. For example, the Mobility Garden fills the need of low-vision clients to learn to walk safely in a realistic outside environment containing a variety of gravels, grasses, terrain, and surface textures.

Dazio recognized an internal need for more feedback and communication between her staff colleagues and herself. She subsequently revamped the business using TQM principles and developed self-managing teams among the occupational therapists, physical therapists, speech pathologists, and audiologists, rehabilitation aides, and student affiliates.[32]

There are skills and techniques that the occupational therapy practitioner can use to collaborate more effectively with clients and their families, as well as with other healthcare professionals. Active listening and empathy are discussed here as aids toward achievement of that goal.

ACTIVE LISTENING

Advice about the value of listening has been given for many years. Plutarch, for example, admonished people to "know how to listen, and you will profit even from those who talk badly." Too much of people's listening is passive; that is why *active listening* is not an oxymoron. Being an active listener means being alert, paying close attention to the speaker, and thus stimulating him or her. The more closely you listen, the better you can evaluate what was said and act on it. Effective listening requires concentrating, giving full attention to the speaker, and analyzing and assimilating thoughts.

To improve your ability to follow a conversation or idea, first be impartial by not allowing bias, prejudice, or anger to interfere. Concentrate on *what* is being said in place of *who* is saying it. Ask questions for clarification. Paraphrase the central thought as you understand it, either aloud or to yourself. If it is appropriate to the situation and does not interfere, take notes.

Good listening requires work. It is as important as good reading, and both demand complete concentration.

TRUE EMPATHY

Whether the focus of therapeutic attention is a premature infant and her or his family, an elderly client and caregivers, or a developmentally delayed adult, an empathetic approach to individuals requires valuing their personal dignity and entering into their personal worlds. Peloquin reflected this truism when she noted that "when practitioners use skill components to make superficial connections, they substitute social chitchat for empathy."[33]

Students do earnestly wish to learn how to empathize yet often are taught instead only the elements of communication skills and how to play the role of a professional. Katz[34] dubbed healthcare practitioners who underidentify with their clients as "rationalistic empathizers." By this she meant those who say the words and make the gestures of empathic communication, while the personal element of the exchange is missing. Communication skills training holds much value for the learner, but it cannot develop the value called empathy, the exchange between client and therapist that promises mutual satisfaction.

Through thought-provoking examples, Peloquin[33] reminded us of the too-often weak link in the spectrum of care provided by occupational therapists: primary regard for the client as a collaborator in treatment. Her opinion was that three forces negatively affect true caring expression: (1) emphasis on "fixing" problems, (2) overreliance on protocols and methods, and (3) business, efficiency, and profit as the forces driving the healthcare system. Katz said that the preference for fixing causes a helper to neglect feelings and makes it easier to justify being silent, curt, or aloof, resulting in impersonal care.[34] As for overdependence on methods and protocols, Baum reminded occupational therapists that "we are nothing more than a bystander in the life of that individual until a relationship is formed."[35]

Meanwhile, do not be so naive as to fail to acknowledge and deal simultaneously with the practical realities encountered in daily business operations. The pressures and stress caused by urgency of protocols, responsibilities for efficiency, the requirement to make profits, and adaptations required for making necessary transitions into managed care understandably compete with clients' needs for time and compassion. The dilemma is not restricted to occupational therapists; all truly caring professionals share the quandary. Occupational therapists can and must not only adapt to rigorous rules and mandates but also move forward as leaders and show how all parts of successful practice can be effectively handled.

Models of Client-Centered Care: Defining Terms

The preceding discussion has introduced some aspects of today's healthcare delivery as well as indicators of agreement about the values and common sense of client-centered health care. Gage[36] categorized these emerging models of client-centered care into four types: client-centered, patient-focused, case management, and client-driven. *Client-centered care* is a term broadly applied to any model that centers care around what are believed to be the client's needs. It has many different meanings and a different model of care associated with each meaning.

The term *patient-focused* might seem to be just one more form of client-centered care: however, the patient-focused care unit is a unique type of unit that is increasingly found in hospitals. It results in major changes in organizational reporting relationships and staff job functions, documentation procedures, broadened caregiver qualifications, and grouping of like patients on one unit.

The *case management model* emerged in response to the need for a client advocate. There is no one case management model, but the underlying principle in all models is that one primary person interacts with the client. Sometimes the case manager determines the client's needs and finds the required services; in other instances the client plays a more active role in defining his or her needs.

The term *client-driven* first appeared in the literature in 1986. Based on a philosophy of client empowerment, client-driven practice is a relationship between the professional and the client that places decision-making control in the hands of the client. Rather than the professional assessing the client, preparing a treatment plan, and presenting the plan to the client for approval, in a client-driven model the provider spends time with the client determining what the client expects to achieve and eliciting ideas from the client about how to reach this outcome. Table 7–1 outlines the salient features of each model.

▨ The Consumer, Managed Care, and Occupational Therapy

All occupational therapy practitioners can carve out and preserve niches within the managed care model by thinking about who the consumer is, understanding what the consumer wants, and giving it to him or her. The consumer wants high-quality care at a fair and reasonable price. That is what must be given. The next, equally essential step is to prove you are giving it. Ask yourself, "Am I measuring my results? Am I looking at outcomes?" These results, the outcomes of your treatment, can in turn be used to prove that you did, indeed, provide effective treatment and so deserve compensation for your good work.

Prospering in the managed care system begins with *attitude*. Instead of wasting time by reacting indignantly and making excuses, try perceiving the insurance companies and new participants in the healthcare delivery process as consumers or constituencies in the marketing process. Stop and say to yourself, "These people are my constituencies, my publics. How can I improve my relationship with them? How can we become partners?" Your attitude and the way you approach doing business dictate more than anything else whether you prosper in a system in transition.

▨ Using Standardized Tools to Set Mutual Goals

The occupational therapy literature suggests standardized tools for setting treatment goals that are satisfactory to the client. Among them are the Occupational Performance History Interview,[37] Goal Attainment Scaling,[38] and the Canadian Occupational Performance Measure.[39] These and all other standardized measures must be evaluated carefully. Each assessment tool must be looked at in light of its ability to evoke sufficient and accurate information. When using an informal interview to set mutual goals with a client, take care to word questions to elicit responses that depict exactly what the client needs and wants.

TABLE 7–1
Summary of Emerging Models of Care

Item	Client-Centered	Patient-Focused	Case Management	Client-Driven
Perceived need of client	Varies according to the specific use of the term. Could be a perceived need for better hotel services, perceived need to center care around identified needs of client, or perceived need to leave control in the hands of the client.	Belief that the client should come in contact with fewer different employees during the course of the stay.	Belief that the client requires assistance accessing and in some cases identifying the services required.	Belief that leaving decision control in the hands of the client will result in better health outcomes.
Benefits	Varies according to the specific use of the term. If term is used to indicate a need to explore client perception of need, there is more likely to be beneficial outcome.	Client sees fewer new faces and thus, is not as confused about who is who. Multiskilling results in less duplication for the patient. Good client satisfaction, good staff satisfaction.	Client has an advocate who knows his/her particular needs and understands the context of the client's life. If client is encouraged to be active in the assessment and decision-making roles, he or she is more likely to perceive his or her needs are being met.	Client sets and evaluates the outcome of care and thus is more likely to believe he or she has derived the desired benefit from the interaction. Increased control has been found to be related to better health outcomes.
Weaknesses	Depending on application of term, may not meet the healthcare needs of the client any better than the medical model due to the concentration on environmental factors other than health care needs.	It is still possible to work within the medical model in a patient-focused environment. Although there are fewer contacts with different providers, the providers who are in contact with the patient may not interact any differently with the patient than previously.	Some forms of case management are still based on the paternalistic medical model and thus may not change the ability of the system to meet the perceived needs of the client.	Some clients may not be ready or able to be responsible for health decisions.

From Gage,[36] p 203, with permission.

Finally, occupational therapy practitioners must guard against being too quick to explain away perceived failures of their occupational therapy interventions as the fault of their clients. Abberley[40] noted two general kinds of outcomes criteria: client satisfaction and performance. The client satisfaction criterion seems to rely on the client's having "correctly" understood his or her situation, which was part of the occupational therapy practitioner's responsibility to perceptively understand and explain in the education portion of the treatment regimen.

▓ Summary

This chapter centered on the customer as number one, a concept that has permeated the business world, including healthcare services delivery. Confirmation of this transition of focus was illustrated by global product marketing, hospital care delivery, changing professional competency requirements, outpatient care adaptations, and private practice. The rationale and urgency for occupational therapists to practice truly collaborative, client-centered treatment were emphasized with examples of such actions by physicians, by rehabilitation colleagues, and by occupational therapists. The concomitant urgency of business practicalities was recognized. Models of current client-centered care were shared as well as standardized tools available to occupational therapists for setting mutual goals with clients. The value of also providing caregiver support and collaboration was demonstrated. Evidence of increased funding of collaborative therapeutic interaction studies provided added validity. Occupational therapists were admonished to approach practice in the managed care arena with the right attitude, building upon the marketing process and using the client-centered approach already basic in their profession. Part Seven looks at strategic planning as a systematic, visionary synthesis of the tenets preceding it in this book.

REFERENCES

1. Frieden, L: Dialogue with Mary Evert. AOTA Annual Conference, Denver, 1995.
2. Sellers, P: To avoid a trampling, get ahead of the mass. Fortune, May 15, 1995, p 201.
3. Silberman, CE: Providing patient-centered care. Health Management Quarterly 14(4):12, 1992.
4. Rosenbaum, EE: The Doctor. Ballantine Books, New York, 1991.
5. Delbanco, DL: Enriching the Doctor-Patient Relationship by Inviting the Patient's Perspective. Ann Intern Med 116:414, 1992.
6. Orr, R: A new design for modern healthcare: The Planetree project. World Hospitals 23(3 and 4):38, Oct, 1987.
7. Marmer, L: Can you measure the competency of your staff? Advance for Occupational Therapists 12(3):15, Jan 22, 1996.
8. Stahl, C: VHA restructures for consumer-driven care. Advance for Occupational Therapists, May 22, 1995, p 19.
9. Joe, BE: Prepared for anything. OT Week 9(49):12, Dec 7, 1994.

10. Kreitner, C, Hartz, AJ, and Pflum, RD: Patient-centered care. Rehab Management, Apr-May 1994, p 25.
11. Wade, J: The road less traveled. Rehab Management 5(4):113, 1992.
12. Christiansen, C: Continuing challenges of functional assessment in rehabilitation: Recommended changes. Am J Occup Ther 47(3), 1993.
13. Dunn, W: Measurement of function: Actions for the future. Am J Occup Ther 47(4), 1993.
14. Peloquin, S: The patient-therapist relationship: Beliefs that shape care. Am J Occup Ther 47(10), 1993.
15. Whitney, RV: Don't say you know how I feel: A client's perspective. OT Week, July 6, 1995, p 20.
16. Klepitsch, LW: Having a preemie changed my outlook as a therapist. Occupational Therapy Forum 10(13):4, 1995.
17. Clark, CJA, Corcoran, M, and Gitlin, LN: An exploratory study of how occupational therapists develop therapeutic relationships with family caregivers. Am J Occup Ther 49(7), 1995.
18. Anastas, JW, Gibeau, JL, and Larson, PJ: Working families and eldercare: A national perspective in an aging America. Soc Work 35:405, 1990.
19. Biegel, DE, Sales, E, and Schulz, R: Family Caregiving in Chronic Illness. Sage, Newbury Park, Calif, 1991.
20. Cutler, NE: Functional limitations and the need for personal care. In Bonder, BR, and Wagner, MB (eds): Functional Performance in Older Adults. FA Davis, Philadelphia, 1994, p 210.
21. Baum, C: Addressing the needs of the cognitively impaired elderly from a family policy perspective. Am J Occup Ther 45:594, 1991.
22. Bonder, BR: Family systems and Alzheimer's disease: An approach to treatment. Physical and Occupational Therapy in Geriatrics 5(20):13, 1987.
23. Bowers, BJ: Intergenerational caregiving: Adult caregivers and their aging parents. Advanced Nursing Science 9:20, 1987.
24. Chenowith, B, and Spencer, B: Dementia: The experiences of family caregivers. Gerontologist 26:267, 1986.
25. Clark, NM and Rakowski, W: Family caregivers of older adults: Improving helping skills. Gerontologist 23:637, 1983.
26. Corcoran, M: Collaboration: An ethical approach to effective therapeutic relationships. Topics in Geriatric Rehabilitation 9:21, 1993.
27. Hasselkus, BR: Meaning of family caregiving: Perspectives on caregiver/professional relationships. Gerontologist 28:686, 1988.
28. Hasselkus, BR: Working with family caregivers: A therapeutic alliance. In Bonder, BR, and Wagner, MB (eds): Functional Performance in Older Adults. FA Davis, Philadelphia, 1994, p 339.
29. Neistadt, ME: Methods of assessing clients' priorities: A survey of adult physical dysfunction settings. Am J Occup Ther 49:428, 1995.
30. Cantor, C: New RWJF initiatives encourage more active consumer participation in health care. Advances 8(4):2, 1995.
31. Zejdlik, CP: Managing SCI. Rehab Management, Apr/May 1992, p 59.
32. Narod, S: Focus on Function. Rehab Economics 3(4). In Rehab Management 9(4):97, 1995.
33. Peloquin, SM: Fullness of empathy. Am J Occup Ther 49(1):24, 1995.
34. Katz, RL: Empathy: Its Nature and Uses. Free Press of Glencoe, London, 1963.
35. Baum, CM: Eleanor Clarke Slagle Lecture: Occupational therapists put care in the health system. Am J Occup Ther 34:505, 1980.
36. Gage, M: Re-engineering of health care: Opportunity or threat for occupational therapists? Can J Occup Ther 62:197, 1995.
37. Kielhofner, G, and Henry, AD: Development and investigation of the Occupational Performance History Interview. Am J Occup Ther 42:489, 1988.
38. Ottenbacher, KJ and Cusick, A: Goal attainment scaling as a method of clinical service evaluation. Am J Occup Ther 44:519, 1990.
39. Law, M, et al: The Canadian Occupational Performance Measure: An outcome measure for occupational therapy. Can J Occup Ther 57:82, 1990.
40. Abberley, P: Disabling ideology in health and welfare. Disability & Society 10(2):221, 1995.

CHAPTER 8

Occupational Therapists and Teams

CHAPTER OBJECTIVES

- To describe the nature of organizational teams.
- To understand what happens when traditional hospital structures are reorganized.
- To outline different team configurations that include occupational therapists.
- To describe the attributes expected of a team member.
- To see what constitutes the role of team leader.
- To acknowledge the variability among team leaders' roles in decision making.
- To recognize the presence of teamwork among professional associations.
- To suggest ways in which interdisciplinarity can be integrated into health sciences educational programs.

Drucker's[1] viewpoint on the ubiquitous presence of teams is that "we will increasingly see organizations operating like the jazz combo, in which leadership within the team shifts with the specific assignment and is independent of the 'rank' of each member." He further contended that the word *rank* could soon be replaced by *assignment*.[1]

▨ The Team Is In

Major players in the game of healthcare marketing today are team members and leaders. Depending on where the occupational therapist is employed, the structure of the organization, the circumstances of the treatments given, and other variables, "the team" has unique characteristics to which the occupational therapist must adapt if a successful exchange is to take place. However, the very fact that the number of organizations resorting to team delivery of healthcare services is growing exponentially is all the more reason for occupational therapists to enhance and amplify their group interaction skills and their knowledge of teams for effective marketing and leadership. As a foundation, this chapter provides an introduction to the nature of teams and interdisciplinarity, including some specific aids and suggestions for succeeding in this all-important aspect of healthcare delivery today.

TEAMS IN BUSINESS AND SPORTS

Drucker,[1] in describing the difficulties associated with organizational restructuring, observed the presence of three basic kinds of teams: (1) Everyone plays on the team but not *as* a team, with each having a fixed position, similar to a baseball team or a surgical team at work; (2) all members play on the team *and* also are flexible to work *as* a team, exemplified by a soccer team or by the emergency room force; and (3) members have preferred positions, but adjust, adapt, and cover for each other in a manner similar to doubles tennis players, understanding and accommodating for each other's strengths and weaknesses.

Called by many companies the productivity breakthrough of the 1990s or the wave of the future, teams in business are known by many names: self-managed teams, cross-functional teams, high-performance teams, or even superteams. The rule of thumb in these businesses is that the more complex the work, the better suited it is for teams.[2]

▨ Interdisciplinarity

Interdisciplinarity is neither a subject nor a body of content; it is a process for achieving integration that usually begins with a problem, question, topic, or issue. Health professionals must work to overcome problems created by differences in disciplinary language and worldview. There is no specific linear progression, but some general steps can be discerned in the process.[3]

One place to begin is with some rudimentary definitions. *Multidisciplinary* or *pluridisciplinary* signifies a juxtaposition of disciplines; it implies essentially that the relationship is additive and not integrative. Even if they are located in a common environment, educators, researchers, and practitioners continue to behave as disciplinarians with different perspectives. Their relationship may well be mutual and cumulative, but it is not interactive because there is no apparent connection or real cooperation.[4]

Genuine interdisciplinarity is described differently. Piaget[5] believed it meant reciprocal assimilation among the participating disciplines, Alpert[6] considered the fundamental ground for interaction to be "a problem," and Gusdorf[7] was convinced that teamwork is the essential element. One way, then, to portray the idea of interdisciplinarity is intense cooperation centered on a common problem-solving purpose. This provides a logical bridge of understanding for today's occupational therapist who is expected to be a project team member. Day[8] observed that several disciplines gathered around a patient ought to have sufficient opportunity to analyze the problem and plan a treatment program. However, "a truly functional and successful interdisciplinary team is never the byproduct of a series of serendipitous events."

STEPS AND TECHNIQUES FOR AN INTERDISCIPLINARY APPROACH

For the occupational therapist newly assigned to a team project requiring an interdisciplinary approach, the following steps are the integrative process common to most interdisciplinary activities:

1. Define the problem or topic
   - Determine all knowledge needs including appropriate disciplinary representatives and consultants, relevant models, traditions, and literatures
   - Develop a framework and questions to be investigated
2. Identify specific studies to be undertaken
   - Join in role negotiation with team members
   - Collect all current information on the subjects and initiate a search for new information
   - Work toward a common vocabulary in order to resolve disciplinary conflicts, and concentrate on reciprocal learning among team members
   - Use integrative techniques to build and maintain communication
3. Compile all contributions and assess their relevance and adaptability
   - Put together the individual pieces of information to find the common thread of relevance and relatedness
   - Weigh all aspects of the proposed solution, or answer, in relation to their support of your conclusions
   - Make decisions about the future management or disposition of the project

To assist in putting these steps into practice, the occupational therapist may use a number of integrative techniques. These procedures aid in assuring success for a team project:

1. Regular meetings with periodic reports and reviews
2. Internal and external presentations: joint presentations, papers, and publications
3. Joint organizing and planning
4. Internal and external seminars and continuing education
5. Joint legislative and patent work
6. Common data and equipment
7. Common data gathering and analysis using facilities and objectives in common
8. Common data reporting forms
9. Common teaching rounds and staff meetings
10. Discussion of differences among team members to assess what is needed and expected from each other while clarifying differences in methodology and ideology and to act as filters for each other as well as consulting experts
11. Training in group interaction skills, such as reading each other's work with an eye to common assessments
12. Building interdependence in analysis of object or objective in common by using techniques such as scenarios or the Delphi technique
13. Focusing on a "common enemy" or target (a common concern that overrides individual differences) through informal gatherings or telecommunication[9]

Independence First

As the roles of allied health professionals have blurred into teams, the strength in complementarity and the benefits of others' expertise have become apparent. First, though, entry-level occupational therapists are strongly urged to build a strong identity in their own profession to acquire a firm grasp on its unique values and orientation. Covey[10] advised, "Interdependence is a choice only independent people can make. . . . As we become independent—proactive, centered in correct principles, value driven and able to organize and execute around the priorities in our life with integrity—we then can choose to become interdependent—capable of building rich, enduring, highly productive relationships with other people." For most entry-level occupational therapists, a year or 2 of practice in a more structured job or in a job with access to an experienced therapist as a role model for emulation and guidance is advisable.

Collaboration allows professionals to market their own uniqueness by letting others see and know what they do well. This thought may perhaps be used to advantage in today's "team blurring," for cooperation and collaboration as a team member has a secondary benefit: a widening of individual competence.

When Teams Replace Hospital Departments

Patient-focused care (PFC) is a management concept that restructures a hospital's resources, including personnel, around patients. Placing the needs of patients over those of providers leads to decentralization, redeployment of staff, and multidisciplinary teams. Patients are assigned to treatment units according to diagnosis and are treated by team members (who also may be known as *care associates, care pairs, care partners,* or *clinical associates*). The concept evolved from Deming's total quality management process, a central aim of which is to reduce variation services or products by using critical pathways or protocols.

The advent of PFC has led to steadily growing numbers of multidisciplinary teams in place in hospitals today. Member makeup of these teams often includes occupational therapists, physical therapists, speech-language pathologists, psychologists, social workers, floor nurses, discharge planners, and rehabilitation nurse evaluators. Many occupational therapists are on teams with leaders from other disciplines. One advantage of the team configuration is that members can concentrate on what they do best and start doing it much earlier in a patient's rehabilitation process, which is important because clients usually remain in the acute care setting for only 5 to 7 days.

Each team member has specific functions as well as general responsibilities that complement the work of others. For example, in one hospital the occupational therapist may be generally responsible for upper extremity training, neuromuscular training, activities of daily living, cognition related to function, and perception. The physical therapist is commonly responsible for mobility, ambulation, transfer training, and lower extremity function. The speech-language pathologist looks at communication, the client's ability to follow directions, and swallowing problems. The psychologist usually holds responsibility for the client's problem-solving skills, cognition, and premorbid history, and the social worker helps with discharge planning and evaluation of the amount of support needed after discharge. Throughout the treatment process the occupational therapist, as a team member, is part of a system that is client-oriented, not discipline-oriented.[11] At the same time, the uniqueness that is occupational therapy can shine brightly when specific treatment is performed on a case-by-case basis.

The occupational therapist may also have a role in a rehabilitation facility. In this instance the occupational therapist contributes a unique perspective: the focus on clients' ability to perform daily living tasks that they want and need to do. As part of the discharge planning team, the value of occupational therapy is further evidenced in the capability to make housing recommendations, to match client skills with environmental demands, and to assess the impact on the client of many variables, such as social support.[12]

PROBLEMS DO ARISE

It takes patience, mutual understanding, and adaptation to succeed as part of a team. At the outset the overlap among team members' responsibilities can be disconcerting. Differences in documentation habits as well as ethical issues related to billing procedures require careful resolution. Mutual respect for strengths and expertise is requisite. Personality differences may easily interfere with smooth team functioning. Team decision making itself holds unique problems, such as *decision polarization,* in which group decisions tend to polarize toward an extreme point of view, and *groupthink,* a situation whereby cohesive groups fail to evaluate their decisions adequately because they are so focused on group solidarity.

Too-authoritarian leaders and too-diffuse responsibility for carrying out decisions are additional potential pitfalls. Although steering and coordination are necessary, particularly in a large-scale project, the more steering done by project leaders, the less opportunity there is for participants' innovation. By honing marketing and leadership skills, the occupational therapist can do much to address and ameliorate many of these problems and to demonstrate her or his inherent unique capabilities.

■ The Effective Healthcare Team

It is obviously not easy to build and sustain a good healthcare delivery team over a period of time. Most begin with enthusiasm and good intentions, and as they evolve any of these problems may become evident. Koepp-Baker[13] pictured a team as similar to "a polygamous marriage." The association is launched by the announcement of intentions, an engagement, considerable publicity, a honeymoon, and finally the long haul, which is inevitably threatened by the onset of ennui. Making it through that long haul depends on identifying key issues: where the difficulties lie, where and by whom goals are clarified and roles defined, what levels of communication exist inside and outside the team, how the team builds and maintains its identity and purpose, how much change the members can endure, and how and by whom points are assessed and achievements measured.[14] Many problems can be foreseen and avoided if, during a team's planning phase, six key ingredients are given attention:

1. Program philosophy
   - ☐ The program's mission statement defining your business
   - ☐ Written criteria for admission, continued service, and discharge

2. Client focus: all decisions including staffing, scheduling, and referral procedures designed around the client's best interests, not staff convenience

3. Role clarification: responsibilities of each team member made clear in writing and communicated with all concerned

4. Collaboration and information sharing

   □ Close teamwork to identify patient-care problems and possible solutions

   □ Open communication channels for continuous transmission among team members

   □ Functional, efficient meetings and charting methods

   □ Attention to physical arrangement of clinical areas and offices for most efficient coordination of services

5. Policies and procedures

   □ Effective operating systems

   □ Procedures in place for such events as scheduling team conferences, orienting clients and families to programs, and referring clients to outpatient services

6. Supportive staff

   □ Mutual respect and support among team members

   □ During recruitment interviews discussing applicants' attitudes toward program philosophy and thus identifying potential team participants[15]

Characteristics of a Team Member

Open-mindedness—a willingness to try new things, hear new ideas, tolerate change—is essential. You *can* be critical. In fact, you should question and at the same time be adventurous and innovative. Vision and creativity are to be encouraged and nourished. For an employer, fostering creative employees can be problematic, but the results make it well worth the effort.

LEARNING TEAM SKILLS

Punwar[16] recognized that entry-level occupational therapists must bring a high level of personal competence to the interdisciplinary team and went on to identify additional skills needed for successful participation. Communication abilities that facilitate group process are critically important, as is a capacity to support the group's ability to set team goals and to develop superior team programs. All members of a healthcare team tailor their own involvement according to that contributed by every other member. Each specializes in a segment of the person's total care, with the totality of the effect depending on each professional's individual contribution. The quality of each person's contribution directly affects the overall efficacy of the service delivery.

By communication skills is meant the ability to speak, listen, write, and read effectively. The spoken word in formal and informal situations is central to team functioning. Expression of findings, recommendations, and questions need to be brief, concise, and objective. Also critical is *active listening,* asking questions for clarification, not only hearing what is said but analyzing it in relation to other information available on the case. Accurate writing skills are needed to document assessments, interventions, and recommendations, as the written word has powerful legal significance and far-reaching potential effects today. Paralleling the responsibility to actively listen, the team professional is obligated to read other team members' documentation with understanding so as to know what each person is doing.

Given and Simmons[17] offered eight personal and team characteristics that support effective healthcare team function:

1. Open-mindedness or the willingness to accept differences and the perspectives of others

2. Independence to function interdependently

3. Negotiation skills

4. Willingness to accept new values, attitudes, and perceptions as appropriate

5. Tolerance of review and challenges of other team members

6. Risk-taking ability

7. Personal identity and integrity

8. Ability to accept and assume a team's philosophy of care after it is established by consensus

These eight characteristics help to summarize the preceding discussion in this chapter. For example, Covey's admonition to first gain independence in order to be interdependent is given support and corroboration by Given and Simmons in their second characteristic, and the essential role of communications, noted by Punwar, is a major factor needed to fulfill the fifth of Given and Simmons' attributes. Team members need to know that at times there will be a blurring of traditional roles and an obligation to accept shared responsibility. Such sharing of responsibilities requires a high level of trust among team members as well as willingness to accept appropriate guidance from those more expert in a specific area. As leadership roles shift, a spirit of cooperation, rather than competition, must be present. Resolution of issues should come about as a result of consensus instead of coercion or compromise. In addition, occupational therapy practitioners can draw on information and experience from their background in group process.

TEAMWORK IN ACTION

With managed care generally dictating how many visits a client can receive for a specific problem, occupational therapists must rely more and more on home programs and client compliance. Not only the occupational therapist but also the client, the caregiver, discharge planners, and other peer professionals may be construed as comprising a team in this instance.

An example of a team structure in place is the Good Samaritan Hospital, Center for Continuing Rehabilitation (CCR), in Puyallup, Washington, a postacute community-reintegration program for adults with head injuries. As part of the interdisciplinary team, the occupational therapists facilitate the clients' life-care planning, including access to mental health services, referrals to hand clinics, ADL training, and other hospital services. The community living program provides apartments for patients and families who are receiving services from Good Samaritan CCR and require continued 24-hour care. Fieldwork students who have the experience of working with these teams in action receive a good introduction to the concept.[18]

Zejdlik[19] illustrated from a nurse's standpoint how essential teamwork is with spinal cord–injured (SCI) clients, as she described how progressive intervention strategies initiated by interdisciplinary teams of professionals have begun to alleviate some of the major physical, social, and economic consequences of SCI. Her experience suggests that successful management requires a skilled, interdisciplinary approach that recognizes both individual and collective expertise. Commenting on the changing roles of rehabilitation professionals, she noted a transition toward stressing partnerships, with listening skills and shared exploration of problem areas critical. For an individual, being heard and having opinions respected during the rehabilitation process enhances self-esteem and increase the chances to do well in general, for all team members should realize that no one profession or professional can offer all the help available or needed.

Zejdlik urged that professionals should increasingly and actively seek input from consumers, such as the movement within rehabilitation research toward participatory action research that stresses consumer and interdisciplinary participation in research design and formulation of questions. Because the ultimate success or failure of rehabilitation of SCI individuals is determined by their ability to enjoy productive lives, Zejdlik suggested that rehabilitation professionals join SCI consumers to together overcome barriers to independence. Such a continuum of teamwork is not only ideal but also possible.

Across the country the many examples of fine teamwork conducted with SCI clients includes the Institute of Research and Rehabilitation in Houston, which has demonstrated teamwork in action for many years. The Craig Hospital in Englewood, Colorado; St. David's Rehabilitation Center in Austin; Shepherd Center in Atlanta; and St. Rita's Rehabilitation Hospital in Lima, Ohio, all take pride in their high-quality, team-oriented rehabilitation. With the SCI client as a focal point, team members represent occupational and physical therapy, recreational therapy, social work, nursing, and physiatry. At St. Rita's Rehabilitation Hospital cotreatment is in place for all clients, with any two of the following regularly working together: occupational therapy, physical therapy, speech-language pathology, and recreational therapy.

What the Team Leader Does

There is no single list of rules or directions for the would-be team leader to follow. The possibilities are as varied as the number of teams in existence. One general approach to analyzing the role of team leader is to compare four functional positions of team leaders according to their amount of involvement in the process of making final team decisions.

1. As team *leader* this individual initiates, manages, and continually exerts influence on the activities and productivity of the group and usually has excellent interpersonal skills.

2. As team *coordinator* the direct management aspect is smaller as other team members assume specific leadership roles. The team coordinator manages the group by coordinating members' skills and productivity and meanwhile developing liaisons with other groups and projects outside the team.

3. As team *leader-on-call* the individual is accountable for the group's productivity but reenters the group only if a problem arises, as there is no close contact with team members on a regular basis.

4. As team *consultant* this person usually has a great deal of high-level technical skill and remains available to the team to help if needed. The self-directed team is itself accountable for its own work accomplished through leadership within the team.

WHAT TEAM MEMBERS EXPECT

Disney, General Motors, Kellogg's, and Kodak recently sponsored a study to determine what expectations are held by team members and how to make teams work better. Headed by cultural anthropologist Clotaire Rapaille, the study showed that powerful forces within the American culture conflict with some of the requirements of teams as configured in businesses today. American employees are quite willing to work for the benefit of the company or the good of the team as a whole. At the same time, the study determined, Americans join teams with expectations of personal benefit as well and have strong needs for personal growth, new challenges, and individual recognition. Therefore, both group and individual goals must be met for the team to be successful.[20]

In Drucker's[1] apt comparison to a jazz ensemble in the opening paragraph of this chapter, he observed that each member has a turn to stand out and then blends back into the ensemble in a collaborative role. There is a lesson here for the team leader in any location.

BECOMING A TEAM LEADER

Becoming a team leader may not be one of your own natural inclinations; however, most occupational therapists can learn the skills needed to become one. Administrators underestimate the extent of shift in mindset and skills that are needed to shift from a traditional middle management role to that of a team leader in a new organizational structure. Conversion into a team leader who is ready to coach, motivate, resolve conflicts, and empower, especially if this has not been one's primary style of management, requires attention, effort, and adaptation.

Numerous stories of how men and women in the corporate world made the transition to team leader roles were crystallized in one author's set of tips for would-be team leaders. Based on leaders' experiences on the job, Caminiti[21] assured that people can learn such skills if they aren't afraid to admit ignorance, know when to intervene, learn to truly share power, worry about what they take on and not what they give up, and get used to learning on the job.

Such leaders are not expected to know everyone's job but rather to coordinate the individual expertise of all, to gather whatever information the team members need, and to "own" the project together. Learning when to intervene means that it is as important to know when to step in as it is to maintain hands off. One team leader asserted that this aspect of being a team leader is more art than science.

Supporting the team concept in today's healthcare organization is important but so are the rewards for members who fit this commitment. Encouraging the wonderfulness of teamwork while still rewarding me-first rather than team behavior soon scuttles a manager's efforts to introduce the team concept.

Mastering how to share power is still another lesson: planning, setting goals, and transferring responsibility. Becoming secure in handing over responsibility to other team members may be the most difficult step. Finally, keep in mind that you do not need to know everything, only where to find the answers.

■ An Example of the Team Approach at Work

Work hardening is one area of practice that customarily uses a team approach. *Work hardening* may be defined as an individualized work-oriented activity regimen performed by an interdisciplinary team and involving simulated or actual work tasks. The aim is to rehabilitate injured workers and return them to productive work as soon as possible with minimal functional restrictions. These programs address not only the physical elements of disabilities or injuries but also the psychological and emotional aspects. Clients progress through strengthening, conditioning, education, and simulated work tasks guided by an interdisciplinary team made up of, as required, occupational therapists, physical therapists, rehabilitation and vocational specialists, social workers, and psychologists.

In most cases a physical therapist evaluates the client for the purpose of planning an exercise program, while the occupational therapist develops a work-simulation routine based on her or his evaluation. Education is provided through a back school or in classes about body mechanics or cumulative trauma. The social worker leads support groups, and vocational classes are conducted by a counselor.

With the advent of managed care, a therapist must now sometimes begin a work-hardening program during the acute-care phase of client recovery. Therefore, more now than ever, injured workers must become proactive team members in their own treatment process and employers must assume roles as part of the teams. The employer as team member is increasingly evident in prevention of workplace injury in the first place. For instance, companies today are making ergonomic modifications, giving workers stretch breaks, and providing other means of reducing potential injuries.

AND IN THE NURSING HOME

Another site for growth in effective team performance is nursing homes. At Morris Hills Multicare Center, a 300-bed skilled nursing facility with 60 Medicare-approved beds in Morristown, New Jersey, the focus is on "realistic goals." Its multidisciplinary approach produces the outcome that about one-third of the clients return home, one-third go to residential facilities, and one-third remain in the nursing home. The geriatric rehabilitation team consists of a physiatrist, physical therapist, occupational therapist, speech-language pathologist, rehabilitation nurse, recreational therapist, psychologist, and social worker, all of whom meet for weekly conferences. Certified occupational therapy assistants and physical therapy assistants serve as part of the team as well.[22]

▓ Teamwork at the Association Level

Not only occupational therapists are affected by the changing boundaries of healthcare professions. Team demands affect everyone. All healthcare professionals must view changes in healthcare delivery as either encroachments or opportunities. It is incumbent on members of each profession to examine who they are and continually redefine what they can and cannot do. Those professions that feel diffuse and unstable are in more danger of being taken over than are professions with strong identities and an awareness of the limits of their expertise. Teamwork and mutual understanding at the professional association level is one recognized approach to this concern.

On local, state, and national levels of professional associations there are increasing numbers of team models, the Tri-Alliance of Health and Rehabilitation Professionals, for example. The American Occupational Therapy Association, American Physical Therapy Association, and American Speech-Language-Hearing Association formed this coalition for mutual support and promotion of projects; for use as a forum, resource, and advocate for public policy issues; to provide an arena for interprofessional communication on issues; and to promote joint educational opportunities.

▨ Teaching an Interdisciplinary Approach in Health Sciences Education

Although interdisciplinarity has great potential for widening vision among healthcare professionals, the effectiveness of integrative education will depend heavily on more thorough education at both the preprofessional and professional levels. If educational programs were better structured to reveal and explore differences among disciplines, alternative treatment approaches for similar problems could be compared and evaluated.[23]

Various methods are used to teach integrative care. These range from traditional lectures and conferences to innovative curricula. There are programs in place with an ethical focus as well as those that train in teamwork, group dynamics, conflict resolution, problem solving, decision making, interpersonal relations, and interpersonal, group, and organizational communications.

Aspects of all these have been incorporated into four major models of integrative education in the health sciences. The *traditional model* is found in some form in almost all health science teaching centers, usually a "multidisciplinary" content course. The *common-interest model,* described as a "nondisciplinary" topical approach, focuses on various aspects of healthcare delivery, healthcare financing, moral and ethical problems, and anatomy. The *case presentation model* is a passive patient-centered activity that relates some element of academic study to an actual patient. Based on the clinical case conference, this model focuses on topics related to disease, social history, and rehabilitation of the patient. Cases are used to demonstrate principles of comprehensive care. The *health team model* features students from several disciplines who take joint responsibility for a task in either research teams or client care teams. As research teams, the members study a particular problem through independent or guided study of research methods. Client care teams are responsible for comprehensive care in clinical work. Clinical conferences may have a professional orientation in a setting where the focus is on cooperation among designated disciplines, or a client orientation in a setting where a client's needs determine the disciplines to be involved. Usual topics include role definition, interdisciplinary communication, integrated client care, and noninstitutional client care.[24]

▓ Summary

This chapter described the nature of organizational teams today from the corporate perspective and specifically in occupational therapy–related sites of employment. What happens when teams replace traditional hospital departments and the composition of these teams were discussed, as were methods for organizing effective teams and the attributes necessary for their continued growth and efficacy. Examples were given of teamwork in diverse sites, including work-hardening programs, nursing homes, acute-care hospitals, and rehabilitation centers. The varying roles of team leaders as well as expectations for their performance were considered. Teamwork at the professional association level was recognized, and suggestions for integration of interdisciplinarity into health sciences curricula were made. Part Four summarizes the preceding chapters by illustrating how marketing and leadership can be synthesized with occupational therapy practice today.

REFERENCES

1. Drucker, PF: Post-Capitalist Society. HarperCollins, New York, 1993.
2. Dumaine, B: Who needs a boss? Fortune, May 7, 1990, p 52.
3. McEvoy, W, and McEvoy, J: Multi- and interdisciplinary research: Problems of initiation, control, integration, and reward. Policy Sciences 3(2):201, 1972.
4. Cluck, NA: Interdisciplinary approaches to the humanities. Liberal Education 66(1), 1980.
5. Piaget, J: The epistemology of interdisciplinary relationships. In Apostel, L (ed): Interdisciplinarity: Problems of Teaching and Research in Universities. Organization for Economic Cooperation and Development, Paris, 1972, p 130.
6. Alpert, D: The role and structure of interdisciplinary and multidisciplinary research centers. Address at Ninth Annual Meeting of Council of Graduate Schools, Washington, DC, Dec, 1969, p 2, ERIC ED 035 363.
7. Gusdorf, G: Project for interdisciplinary research. Diogenes 42:119, 1963.
8. Day, DW: Perspectives on care: The interdisciplinary team approach. Otolaryngol Clin North Am 14(4):769, 1981.
9. Birnbaum, PH: Academic contexts of interdisciplinary research. Educational Administration Quarterly 14:80, 1978.
10. Covey, SR: The Seven Habits of Highly Successful People. Simon & Schuster, New York, 1989, p 186.
11. Stancliff, S: Preserving OT's role when teams replace departments. OT Practice, Premiere Issue, Nov 1995, p 30.
12. Unsworth, CA: The role of occupational therapy in team discharge planning. OT Practice, Premiere Issue, Nov 1995, p 32.
13. Koepp-Baker, H: The craniofacial team. In Bzosch, KR (ed): Communicative Disorders Related to Cleft Lip and Palate. Little, Brown, Boston, 1979, p 54.
14. Logan, R, and McKendry, M: The multi-disciplinary team: A different approach to patient management. N Z Med J 95:722, 1982.
15. Reed, SM: Teamwork: A survival skill of the Eighties. Course of Action 2(12):1, 1984.
16. Punwar, AJ: Occupational Therapy: Principles & Practice. Williams & Wilkins, Baltimore, 1988.
17. Given, B, and Simmons, S: Interdisciplinary health care team: Fact or fiction? Nurse Forum 2:167, 1977.

18. Rogers, C: News from the fieldwork corner. OT Week 9(27):11, July 6, 1995.
19. Zejdlik, CP: Managing SCI. Rehab Management, Apr/May 1992, p 59.
20. Fortune, Sept 18, 1995, p S11.
21. Caminiti, S: What team leaders need to know. Fortune 131(3):93, Feb 20, 1995.
22. Pedinoff, S: Nursing homes: Team roles make rehab work. Advance for Occupational Therapists, June 20, 1994, p 13.
23. Greden, J: Interdisciplinary differences on a general hospital psychiatry unit. Gen Hosp Psychiatry 1(1):91, 1979.
24. Connelly, T Jr: Appendix 6: Interdisciplinary references III: A reference document for those contemplating interdisciplinary educational programs in the health sciences. Proceedings of the Workshop on Interdisciplinary Education, Kentucky January Prototype. Lexington College of Allied Health Professions, Lexington, Ky, Apr, 1975, p 6, ERIC ED 129 134.

PART FOUR

PARALLELS IN CONCEPTS AND PROCESSES

*If you want to feel secure, do what you
already know how to do. If you want to be
a true professional and continue to grow . . .
go to the cutting edge of your competence,
which means a temporary loss of security.
So whenever you don't know what you're
doing, know you're growing.*

Madeline Hunter, 1987

CHAPTER 9

The Therapeutic Relationship in Occupational Therapy

CHAPTER OBJECTIVES

- To note how definitions of occupational therapy have evolved.
- To acknowledge the essential nature of client choice in the occupational therapy process.
- To recognize the fundamental role of the therapist-client relationship in effective occupational therapy treatment.
- To appreciate the intrinsic part played by clinical reasoning in collaborative treatment.
- To realize where marketing fits into the parallel roles occupied by the maturing occupational therapist.

The aim of Part Four is to bring together the information that has been given in the previous chapters and to develop the idea that there are parallels and a sameness among the processes discussed. Not only a logical progression of thought but also overlapping and convergence are apparent as these parallel processes are analyzed. A major premise of occupational therapy is that it is a collaborative process between therapist and client. Some occupational therapy practitioners today may fail to remember that clients' self-identities, social worlds, histories, and personal goals are the primary components of their motivation to pursue daily tasks. After all, what matters most to people in their daily lives is ability to engage in their personal work, play, and self-care agendas. The natural conclusion on the part of the occupational therapist, then, should be to prioritize treatment time with clients to help them with health or performance problems that interfere with their life engagement.

Chapter 9 reviews the meaning of the collaborative process in occupational therapy and reiterates its fundamental role for effective treatment. The parallels among the processes of occupational therapy, management, marketing, and leadership are developed in Chapter 10, and the student is shown how to approach this way of thinking. Chapter 11 demonstrates with current examples successes and failures in all aspects of corporate business as well as in occupational therapy practice.

▨ Everything Old Is New Again

The theme of the 1996 conference of the AOTA was that everything old is new again. Royeen[1] had a similar thought, that "by pulling from the past we can go into the future taking with us the tried and true fundamentals of occupational therapy and applying them in current and future environments." The fundamentals of occupational therapy never change, even if appearances do. How the fundamentals are managed and handled does change. Heeding history and maintaining continuity are required of all occupational therapists if the profession is to grow and adapt successfully to monumental change, for fundamentals are the foundation of all practice. Look at the past year, the current year, and the upcoming year as part of the continuum of growth that began in 1917 and moves forward, regardless of obstacles along the way.

All occupational therapists should have a clear understanding of the origin and development of their chosen profession as well as determination to add to its richness and variety. The history of occupational therapy has been recounted in many publications and countries over the years and from various perspectives.[2-5] These references are representative rather than an exhaustive list, but a survey of the history of occupational therapy is not part of this text.

THE EVOLVING DEFINITION

Definitions of *occupational therapy* have evolved from the earliest formal one in 1922 by H. A. Pattison, who determined it to be "any activity, mental or physical, definitely prescribed and guided for the distinct purpose of contributing to, and hastening recovery from, disease or injury." That definition has been revised over the years to reflect changing circumstances. Beginning in the 1930s practice was influenced by techniques and components of function. This continued until the late 1970s, when a growing number of occupational therapy leaders wrote eloquently about the need to look, at the same time, more closely at the nature and realities of current practice compared to the origins of the profession. The reader is encouraged to review this progression of thought in Chapter 1 of Christiansen and Baum's text.[2]

From 1972 until 1981 the definition of *occupational therapy* was:

> the art and science of directing man's participation in selected tasks to restore, reinforce, and enhance performance, facilitate learning of those skills and functions essential for adaptation and productivity, diminish or correct pathology, and to promote and maintain health. Its fundamental concern is the development and maintenance of the capacity, throughout the life span, to perform with satisfaction to self and others those tasks and roles essential to productive living and to the mastery of self and the environment.[6]

An ongoing discussion in the literature about the definition of occupational therapy revolves around a comparison of this definition and the 1981 definition. Peloquin,[7] for example, asserted that eliminating the opening phrase of the 1972 definition does not serve the profession well.

At least four common propositions have characterized the profession throughout its history:

1. The use of occupation or purposeful activity can influence the state of health of an individual.

2. Individuals and their adaptation and total functioning must be viewed with respect to their own environment, and remediation must take into consideration all the physical, psychological, and social factors.

3. Interpersonal relationships are an important factor in the occupational therapy process.

4. Occupational therapy is an adjunct to, and has its roots in, medicine and must work in cooperation with medical professionals and other persons involved as health-care providers to ensure maximum benefits for clients.[8]

Note that the second and third statements introduce the notion of components parallel to those found in the marketing process. This idea is expanded further in Chapter 10.

▨ Client Choice and Client-Therapist Collaboration

When tracing definitions, assumptions, beliefs, values, and principles underlying the profession since 1922, the elements of client choice and client-therapist collaboration in the treatment process have grown in prominence. In the 1922 definition, prescription and guidance were stressed, in contrast to the six important beliefs and values continuing to influence occupational therapy practice in 1991. Two of these six are:

4. Autonomy implies choice and control over environmental circumstances, thus opportunities for exerting self-determination should be reflected in intervention strategies.

5. An individual's choice and control extend to decisions about intervention, thus occupational therapy is identified as a collaborative process between therapist and recipient of care, whose values are respected.[9]

MacDonald et al.,[4] viewing the development and status of occupational therapy in England in 1977, believed that much of the success of occupational therapy treatment depends on the occupational therapist, on the rapport developed with the client, and on the all-important therapeutic relationship. They further stated that the occupational therapist must be perceptive and in no way impose her or his will or intention on the client. They firmly believed that the occupational therapist must first identify the needs of the client, then help the client select the most valuable treatment activity, and, if necessary, offer suitable incentives to gain cooperation. The therapist was to see that interest, effort, and satisfaction were maintained during treatment. In this way, the client not only finds satisfaction in attaining the goal but also has justifiable opportunity for zest and pleasure in the process.

In 1980 Reed and Sanderson,[5] in their major criteria for a modern definition of occupational therapy for today's world, included as third on their list of seven "the population served."

Mosey began her 1981 book, *Occupational Therapy: Configuration of a Profession,* with the following definition: "Occupational therapy is defined as the art and science of using selected theories from a variety of disciplines and professions as a guide for *collaborating* [emphasis added] with a client in order to assess that individual's ability to perform life tasks and, if necessary, to assist the individual in acquiring the knowledge, skills, and attitudes necessary to perform required life tasks."[10] At the same time she asserted that the therapist is required to show skillful use of personal interactions.

Mosey expanded on her beliefs about the therapist-client relationship by saying that the intimate nature of this interaction requires reaffirmation of the client's individuality if the treatment is to be successful. As further evidence of the essential nature of this interpersonal association, Mosey noted therapists' need for rapport, empathy, and the capacity to guide others to understand and make use of their potential as participants in a community of others. This, she stated, was an illustration of the art of occupational therapy.

Mosey reiterated that occupational therapy is to be considered a collaborative process between therapist and client, a shared responsibility. She visualized this sharing as "truly a mutual process" and noted that instances of collaboration on the part of the occupational therapist are not limited to client relationships. Exchanges with others, such as the clients' family members, close friends, employers, teachers, and members of the healthcare team must also be kept in mind as part of the job. This assertion again parallels the marketing process described in Chapter 4, in that attention must be paid to both internal and external constituencies.

Peloquin[7] noted that a basic textbook available to occupational therapy students, Willard and Spackman's *Occupational Therapy*,[3] covered the patient-therapist relationship in only a fragmented fashion. Her contention was that occupational therapists needed to recommit to the patient as a vital partner in a collaborative relationship and return to concern about the client as a person essential to effective practice.

Viewing the client in context goes hand in hand with client-centered treatment and with the philosophical base of the profession. People influence their own development and health within their environments as they cope with change in themselves, their context, and the tasks to be done. Of greatest importance is that persons can choose what they need and want to do—and according to their own needs and preferences, not those of a professional. Purposeful activity, then, is the tool occupational therapists use to accomplish these goals.

▓ Need for Client-Centered Occupational Therapy Reaffirmed

Among healthcare professionals, occupational therapists should most readily understand the central importance of clients' needs. Clients' needs can be best met by conscientious listening to what clients are saying and thus full awareness of what clients perceive their needs to be. Trombly, in her 1995 Slagle lecture, declared that "meaningfulness is individual," that patients must determine which tasks and activities are meaningful to them, and that therapists themselves are not always good judges of what is important to their patients. She further said that meaningfulness in occupation comes from a person's culture and that a therapist "should not substitute his or her own values when selecting goals for the patient."[11]

In spite of the fact that occupational therapists' failure to first listen for expressed needs means less than effective, high-quality treatment, some troubling comments have been appearing lately. Spencer, Young, Rintala, and Bates[12] noted that "staff members seemed so intent on teaching the patient new skills that they often discounted the significance of his past experience and failed to engage in helping the patient connect his future life story to his past." Neistadt[13] found that "therapists are setting treatment goals without specific input from clients about their valued activities," and Breines[14] concluded a letter to the editor with a plea to "let patients' needs and interests dictate therapy, not therapists' and providers' biases."

Dijkers[15] stated that rehabilitation professionals have discussed and then failed to implement empowerment (or whatever synonym you wish to substitute, e.g., *consumer control, independence*) for years now and that decisions continue to be made for, about, and without the clients involved. To emphasize his point, he cited what he felt were examples of good plans for empowerment that had not materialized.[16,17]

Csikszentmihalyi[18] offered proof of the value of empowerment from still another perspective, flow, and stated that when individuals feel in control of their actions they experience a sense of exhilaration and of deep enjoyment. He said the optimal experience is when a person's body or mind is stretched to its limits in a voluntary effort to accomplish something difficult and worthwhile. The person is "making it happen" and has a strong sense of mastery. The author said that this theory of optimal experience is based on the concept of *flow*, a state in which a person is so involved in an activity that nothing else seems to matter. The experience is so enjoyable that the individual does it even at great cost.

▓ Clinical Reasoning and Collaborative Treatment

Clinical reasoning is an essential part of the therapeutic relationship in occupational therapy. An extensive amount of excellent research, explanation, and analysis of the concept is available. (See the reading list related to the clinical reasoning process at the end of this chapter.)

"The therapist with the three-track mind" is an apt and intriguing description of the clinical reasoning process. The three tracks—procedural, interactive, and conditional—have continually evolved as a concept following extensive study. The procedural track focuses on the disability and on treatment as a means of remediation. The interactive track centers on the client as a human being by engaging the client in the occupational therapy process. The interpersonal skills of new therapists are a critical factor in this track. The conditional track integrates the two other tracks and expands to view the client in the context of his or her past and probable future.[19]

Clinical reasoning provides the framework within which information is processed, and elements of the transactions with clients or consumers complete the integration of art and science so essential to all aspects of successful therapeutic performance. Proficiency in all these areas grows as experience accumulates. The centrality of the client and the collaborative process can be clearly seen in the clinical reasoning process.

■ The Helping Relationship and the Marketing Process

At the point of entry to practice, professional education has prepared the occupational therapy student conceptually and elementally with the tools required to evaluate and treat. Approaches to patient-therapist interaction have been introduced in a manner that can be identified as parallel to a marketing approach. For example, to have an exchange in any helping relationship, the professional needs to receive more than money. The therapist needs the satisfaction of seeing his or her professional help *used*. Listening must go both ways in the therapist-client interchange. Regarding mutually satisfying exchanges at the therapist-client level of interaction, authors such as Purtilo[20] offer beneficial heuristic observations that enable the therapist to achieve satisfaction and fruitful exchanges through successful treatment outcomes.

■ Continuing to Grow by Applying the Marketing Process

As the entry-level occupational therapy practitioner progresses to staff level, the need for marketing skills becomes apparent, for the number of daily interactions and transactions grows: professional colleagues, supervisors, aides, clients' families, insurance representatives, staff, and more. Moving up the professional ladder, recognition of all potential constituencies and mutual satisfaction of needs are important if personal and professional objectives are to be realized.

As the occupational therapy practitioner's career develops, the integration of art and science should continue. The increasing responsibilities deal more and more with supervision, management, teaching, business, government, funding, and consultation. Knowledge of these additional competencies in varying degrees is required. All this is accomplished by using marketing skills, consciously or unconsciously, if each progressive stage of professional development is to be attained. For that reason, marketing literature offers a perspective rich in potential value to occupational therapists. By developing a conscious awareness of the marketing process in all daily interactions, every occupational therapist can use marketing techniques to improve daily practice.

Interestingly, a "marketing" approach with a consumer-oriented focus originally helped to form the occupational therapy profession. Adolf Meyer, in his presentation to the fifth annual meeting of the National Society for the Promotion of Occupational Therapy (today known as the American Occupational Therapy Association) held in Baltimore in 1921, explained to his audience that the personal abilities and interests of patients should be considered. He also stated that the job of an occupational therapist was to provide opportunities, not prescriptions. We can see once more that history should be heeded.

Such ideas demonstrate how occupational therapy can be visualized in tandem with marketing and leadership. Marketing is a social process that *is*, and occupational therapy is also a process that *is*. Marketing techniques are tools used to implement the marketing process; occupational therapy media and techniques are tools used to implement the occupational therapy process.

▩ Authentic Occupational Therapy

A well-known and respected leader in occupational therapy, Elizabeth J. Yerxa, PhD, OTR, FAOTA, in her 1966 Eleanor Clarke Slagle Lecture, shared a description of the therapeutic occupational therapy process that is as appropriate today as it was in 1966.[21] The inclusion of mutual exchange can be noted. Her view was that authentic occupational therapy is based on a commitment to helping clients make their own choices, not forcing the therapist's value system on clients. Clients are the only ones who can discover their own particular meanings and the only ones who are intellectually and emotionally involved in realizing what is purposeful to them. The occupational therapist engages in a *mutual* relationship with the client by involvement in the process of caring. Occupational therapy practitioners cannot really help clients unless they take time to truly listen and feel and care. Yerxa declared that "our service to the client is unique in its application of choice, self-initiated, purposeful activity and its emphasis upon the goal of function with self-actualization. Our media have been identified as those activities which are at the very source of human motivation."

▩ Summary

This chapter has traced the evolution of definitions of occupational therapy and its elements of therapeutic interaction. The meaning of client choice is recognized as being of central importance throughout the development of the occupational therapy profession. Client-therapist interaction is described, and the essential part it plays in successful treatment outcomes is discussed. The idea was introduced that a marketing approach can be identified as being present in the client-therapist relationship beginning with the origin of occupational therapy as a profession, in occupational therapy education, and in the roles of student, staff therapist, manager, and consultant.

REFERENCES

1. Royeen, CB: Editor's note. In AOTA Self-Study Series: The Practice of the Future: Putting Occupation Back into Therapy (Lesson 1, ps). American Occupational Therapy Association, Rockville, Md, 1994.
2. Christiansen, C: Occupational therapy: Intervention for life performance. In Christiansen, C, and Baum, C (eds): Occupational Therapy: Overcoming Human Performance Deficits. Slack, Thorofare, NJ, 1991.
3. Hopkins, H, and Smith, H: Willard and Spackman's Occupational Therapy, ed 6. JB Lippincott, Philadelphia, 1983.
4. MacDonald, EM, MacCaul, G, and Mirrey, L (eds): Occupational Therapy in Rehabilitation, ed 3. Bailliere, Tindall and Cassell, London, 1970.
5. Reed, K, and Sanderson, SR: Concepts of Occupational Therapy. Williams & Wilkins, Baltimore, 1980.
6. AOTA: Occupational therapy: Its definition and function. Am J Occup Ther 26:204, 1972.
7. Peloquin, SM: The issue is: Occupational therapy as art and science: Should the older definition be reclaimed: Am J Occup Ther 48(11):1093, Nov/Dec, 1994.
8. Hopkins, H, and Smith, H: Willard and Spackman's Occupational Therapy, ed 6. JB Lippincott, Philadelphia, 1983, p 20.
9. Christiansen, C, and Baum, C (eds): Occupational Therapy: Overcoming Human Performance Deficits. Slack, Thorofare, NJ, 1991, p 9.
10. Mosey, AC: Occupational Therapy: Configuration of a Profession. Raven Press, New York, 1981, p 3.
11. Trombly, C: Eleanor Clarke Slagle lecture: Occupation: Purposefulness and meaningfulness as therapeutic mechanisms. Am J Occup Ther 49:960, 1995.
12. Spencer, J, Young, ME, Rintala, D, and Bates, S: Socialization to the culture of a rehabilitation hospital: An ethnographic study. Am J Occup Ther 49:53, 1995.
13. Neistadt, ME: Methods of assessing clients' priorities: A survey of adult physical dysfunction settings. Am J Occup Ther 49:428, 1995.
14. Breines, EB: Let patients, not bias guide therapy. Advance for Occupational Therapists 11(23):3, June 12, 1995.
15. Breske, S: Should rehab patients be recipients or participants of care? Advance for Occupational Therapists, Jan 18, 1993, p 14.
16. Kutner, S: Milieu therapy in rehabilitation. Journal of Rehabilitation 34:14, 1968.
17. Wright, M: Client as Co-Manager in Rehabilitation. Harper & Row, New York, 1983.
18. Csikszentmihalyi, M: Flow: The Psychology of Optimal Experience. Harper & Row, New York, 1990.
19. Fleming, M: The therapist with the three-track mind. The AOTA Practice Symposium 1989: Program Guide. AOTA, Rockville, Md, 1989, p 70.
20. Purtilo, R: Health Professional and Patient Interaction, ed 4. WB Saunders, Philadelphia, 1990.
21. Yerxa, EJ: 1966 Eleanor Clarke Slagle lecture. Am J Occup Ther 21:1, 1967.

RELATED READINGS ON CLINICAL REASONING

Burke, JP: Selecting evaluation tools I. In Royeen, CB, (ed): AOTA Self-Study Series: Assessing Function (vol 3). AOTA, Rockville, Md, 1989.

Cohn, ES: Fieldwork education: Shaping a foundation for clinical reasoning. Am J Occup Ther 43:240, 1989.

Fleming, M: The therapist with the three-track mind. The AOTA Practice Symposium 1989: Program Guide. AOTA, Rockville, Md, 1989, p 70.

Mattingly, C: Clinical reasoning in occupational therapy. The AOTA Practice Symposium 1989: Program Guide. AOTA, Rockville, Md, 1989, p 67.

Mattingly, C, and Fleming, M: Clinical Reasoning: Forms of Inquiry in a Therapeutic Practice. FA Davis, Philadelphia, 1994.

Parham, D: Toward professionalism: The reflective therapist. Am J Occup Ther 41:555, 1987.

Rogers, JC: Eleanor Clarke Slagle lectureship: Clinical reasoning: The ethics, science, and art. Am J Occup Ther 37:601, 1983.

Rogers, JC, and Holm, MB: The therapist's thinking behind functional assessment II. In Royeen, CB (ed): AOTA Self-Study Series: Assessing Function, vol 2. AOTA, Rockville, Md, 1989.

Rogers, JC, and Masagatani, G: Clinical reasoning of occupational therapists during the initial assessment of physically disabled patients. OTJR 2(4):195, Oct, 1982.

Royeen, CB: AOTA Self-Study Series: Assessing Function. AOTA, Rockville, Md, 1989.

CHAPTER 10

The Convergence of Marketing, Management, and Occupational Therapy

CHAPTER OBJECTIVES

- To see what occupational therapy, marketing, and management have in common.
- To understand how the same approach can be used to teach marketing, management, and occupational therapy treatment processes.
- To realize that a marketing attitude helps to build self-confidence in the developing occupational therapy practitioner.
- To detect the presence of potential exchanges in all areas of daily practice.
- To acknowledge the critical need to have ethics as part of every transaction.
- To recognize consultation as still another process that can be taught in tandem.
- To once more realize how client-centered occupational therapy treatment has always been a professional essential.
- To conclude that the marketing process is part of effective occupational therapy treatment and management.

For any who even momentarily might doubt the fundamental simplicity, common sense, and wisdom underlying occupational therapy—of using occupation to empower and heal—there are daily reminders of its value. The powerful fact is "discovered" over and over and reported in sometimes surprising places and circumstances. Chuck Colson, special counsel to President Nixon from 1969 to 1973, and Jack Eckerd,[1] founder and former CEO of the Eckerd Drug chain, traveled to the Soviet Union in 1990 as part of an American delegation to visit the most notorious Soviet prisons. Their purposes were to share expertise about prisons with Soviet officials and to press for release of political prisoners. In visiting these depressing, gray institutions, they were amazed to find efficient production lines there, with each inmate employed in a job 6 days a week, 8 hours a day, and high morale despite the brutality of the Soviet prison system. They were impressed by the effect of purposeful work on the prisoners. This chapter continues to explore the art of occupational therapy but with an added perspective.

This chapter describes how the processes of occupational therapy, management, marketing, consultation, and helping itself are parallel and complementary. The concept of mutually satisfying exchanges is identified throughout. This idea of mutual needs satisfaction can be used to teach the processes of occupational therapy treatment, management, and marketing. Chapter 11 continues with examples of successes and failures in the achievement of mutual needs satisfaction and a consumer orientation.

■ Client-Centered Care Is the Answer

In 1910 Susan Tracy identified interpersonal relationships between teacher or nurse and patient as a vital factor in successful occupation treatment. She further valued recognition of patient needs when she advocated a great variety of activity choices to meet individual patient preferences, with occupations chosen to provide tangible associations with those preferences. Eleanor Clarke Slagle developed a treatment model used in occupational therapy with mentally ill patients until the 1950s. Her method was rooted in heeding and responding to patients' needs, providing tasks of increasing interest, and requiring increasing degrees of concentration.

From the extensive body of literature that has contributed to development of the philosophical assumptions underlying occupational therapy, Mosey[2] offered a distillation in the form of five assumptions, one of which is that "each individual has the right to seek his or her potential through personal choice within the context of some social constraints." Mosey's contention was that ultimately clients have the right and privilege to choose how they wish to live. This thought offers further evidence that the components of mutual exchange lie at the foundation of the art and science of occupational therapy.

Before an occupational therapist can plan and implement any treatment program, the feelings and expressed needs of the client must be of primary concern. Should the client be unable to express or perform this function, the family or responsible caregiver, of course, is to be consulted. Because the definition of *assumption* is "a fact or statement taken for granted"[3] and there is agreement that clients have the ultimate right to make their own life choices, logically there should be no disagreement whatsoever among occupational therapists that collaborative treatment is a cornerstone of practice.

Mutual Satisfaction of Therapist and Client

Because collaboration is fundamental to the frame of reference used throughout this book, the words *client* or *consumer* are used in most cases rather than *patient*, which connotes the state of being a passive recipient of services instead of an active participant in satisfying exchanges. In 1974 Mosey[4] proposed to occupational therapists an alternative to the medical and health model, the "biopsychosocial model." Through this model she suggested that attention be directed to the body, mind, and environment of the client.

In 1981 Mosey[2] went on to state that "collaboration has the connotation of sharing; of doing with, not doing for or doing to. It is truly a mutual process." She observed that occupational therapy is a collaborative process between therapist and client, with the client having the right to be treated as a unique individual and to benefit from the therapist's skill and knowledge. Conversely, the client has a responsibility to participate in planning and carrying out the treatment program, for the therapist has a right and a need for respect and remuneration for having applied skills and knowledge, acting ethically, and participating in mutual planning and implementation of the client's program of treatment. Here we see Mosey's mutual process, as described in Chapter 9, expanded.

EXCHANGE IN CRITICAL THINKING

One conceptual example of the mutual process at work could be taken from today's recognition of critical thinking in occupational therapy. Parham[5] stated that critical thinking and analytic ability have a direct relationship to the profession's autonomy and recognition as a legitimate profession. Here a transaction is taking place. It is similar to that recognized in marketing: Clients need efficient and accurate assessment and treatment in exchange for their attribution of autonomy and respect to occupational therapists individually and to the profession.

THE ART OF HELPING

Carkhuff,[6] looking at the art of helping from a developmental standpoint, offered a model: "Responding prepares us for initiating." His definition of *re-*

sponding was that the helper saw the world through the eyes of others; *initiating* meant seeing that world through the helper's eyes. Regardless of the nature of the help being given—as teacher, parent, therapist, or counselor—the helper must first listen well to the experiences and feelings of the person to be helped to be able to initiate assistance that is accepted and effective. The helping relationship can end successfully only if a mutually satisfying transaction takes place, with each participant heeding and appreciating what is being given in the exchange.

Becoming a helper is a time-consuming process if done correctly. It is a deeply personal process of self-discovery to learn how to use oneself most effectively to help others. The mature healing therapist must listen carefully, evaluate, assist, support, help develop alternatives that lead to healing, apply therapeutic measures aimed at alleviating pain and dysfunction, teach, and help others discover how to adapt to the world, do their own problem solving, and function as independently as possible.[7] This is no small assignment, but the rewards are infinite, beginning with the helper's gratification in watching the client adapt and grow in independence and self-esteem.

THE COMMON DENOMINATOR

In this discussion a common denominator has begun to emerge: To have a successful outcome, both parties in a transaction or exchange must expend attention and effort so as to emerge with feelings of satisfaction that each has received something of value. Quite often the thing of value received by the therapist or helper is not of a monetary nature. It may be recognition, as mentioned by Parham, or respect, as suggested by Mosey, or the feeling of gratification for having managed a successful encounter as proposed by Carkhuff. In all cases, there is the obvious presence of a mutually satisfying exchange or transaction having taken place.

In occupational therapy the therapist-client relationship is usually the first level of interest and experience of an entry-level therapist. Nevertheless, already the marketing process—the need for mutual needs satisfaction, that common denominator—can be recognized.

The Graduating Student

Occupational therapy students have learned many things during their academic education, including the theoretical underpinnings of the profession; the beliefs, ethics, and values of occupational therapy; occupational therapy practice issues; fundamentals of activity; service models; tools and techniques; management of services; and the basic sciences needed for practice. Excellent educational programs provide students with the content needed for preparation to practice; however, both faculty and emerging students often feel that all the elements of occupational therapy practice have been taught but in a fragmented, unconnected fashion. For instance, students often tolerate the management course primarily because it is required, not because its role and value are appreciated at that point in their education.

In students' final evaluations of their academic educational preparation, in my experience, they frequently express concern that there seems to be an indistinct relationship, or even a gap, between the theoretical and practical. A bridge between the learned occupational therapy process and the student's first interpersonal encounter with a client as a therapist can be built through a marketing approach. The occupational therapy treatment process and the marketing process both consist of mutually satisfying exchanges. I suggest that the marketing process be taught and used as the bridge across that first gap for entry-level therapists.

HOW MUCH DOES THE EMERGING STUDENT KNOW?

Armed with a professional education and certification, the entry-level therapist arrives on the scene to begin practice. Not surprisingly, many new occupational therapy practitioners feel uncertainty, although it is not often admitted or communicated. Consciously or unconsciously, many graduates have aspirations for careers that will progress through stages of becoming proficient therapists, efficient supervisors, effective managers, to respected professionals and leaders. Achievement of these milestones is overtly or covertly desired, but how to proceed is seldom clear, and burnout often intervenes.

This feeling of unreadiness is not new among occupational therapy graduates. Fike[8] conducted a study in response to complaints over the years from both graduates and their employers that new therapists felt unprepared for management roles, that they were educated along narrow professional lines, and that their conceptual thinking was limited. Fiscal planning and marketing skills were also often found lacking. Because, on one hand, most management texts emphasize that the guidance of human resources is the primary and most important task of management and, on the other hand, occupational therapy has within its concept helping individuals become productive and independent, it would seem to be a logical maturation from effective therapist to effective supervisor. However, according to Fike's findings, this transition did not appear to be taking place.

THE MANAGEMENT PARALLEL

The purpose of Fike's study was to demonstrate that parallels exist between the conventional theories and practice of human resource management (supervision) and of occupational therapy theories and practice. To illustrate this hypothesis, she developed a model to assist students in understanding how to acquire basic supervisory skills while they learn occupational therapy skills and thus demonstrated that supervisory skills could be derived from coursework already included in occupational therapy curricula and that there is a relationship between the principles and practice of occupational therapy and the primary roles and tasks required of managers (Fig. 10–1).

ADD MARKETING

A marketing exchange viewpoint can be added here to the management transaction idea, as the occupational therapy supervisor or manager must first seek

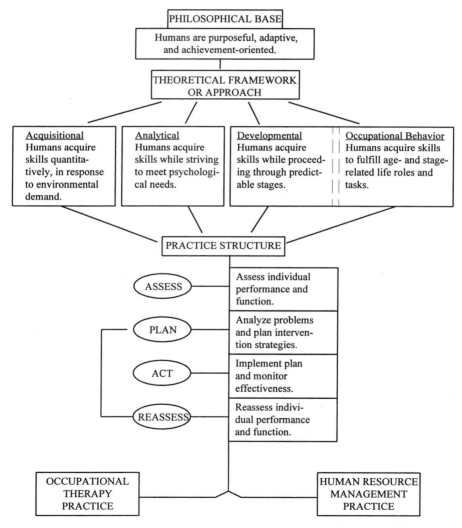

FIGURE 10–1. Professional practice model shared by occupational therapy and human resource management. (Fike,[8] p 34, with permission.)

to understand an employee's needs and then, in collaboration with that individual, assess how well those needs can be met in the organization. With this information in hand, the manager can develop a plan to meet the employee's needs. In exchange, of course, the manager expects to receive the needed professional services of the employee and to thus achieve the productivity goals of the organization. How well this transaction is managed determines the success or failure of the manager's marketing plan developed for that employee.

Exchanges All Around You: Four Illustrations

Regardless of a person's place of employment, every day is made up of a series of mutual exchanges. All aspects of the daily employer-employee relationship contain potential transactions whose successful resolution has a direct bearing on the mutual satisfaction sought by both parties in the equation. As reengineering invades places of employment, the number of potential confrontations at all levels will continue to grow. Everyday facts, such as the weight to be placed on seniority of employees when downsizing, consolidation, or reorganization takes place, grow into understandably major concerns to the individuals involved. As the economic pressure of managed care significantly cut reimbursements to hospitals and reduce inpatient days by emphasizing subacute care and other alternatives, hospitals must cut costs and restructure services. In every case there are examples of mutual needs to be satisfied.

With the idea of marketing exchanges in mind, think of your job security as depending on how valuable you are to your on-the-job "customers." Picture those "customers" as your personal target markets by reviewing Figure 4–4 and considering coworkers or bosses as your publics. Are you taking those "customers" for granted and not providing the best possible service at the best possible price? Are you inviting the decision makers to replace you with a better service provider?

Resolution of these and other dilemmas varies from one institution to another, from one state to another. In California, where many hospital employees are union members, most contracts detail specific "bumping procedures" enabling many senior workers to be given preference for rehire or reassignment. In Texas, a right-to-work state, employers are not legally obligated to recognize seniority when reorganizing. There are a variety of possible applications of marketing and related negotiations here.

PHYSICIAN-THERAPIST EXCHANGES IN HOSPITAL SETTINGS

Potential exchanges in hospitals occur daily today between occupational therapists and referring physicians. Helen Mierzwa, OTR,[9] a director of occupational therapy with 15 years' experience, shared some of the ways in which she has maintained mutually satisfactory exchanges with referring physicians. For example, she suggested that this sometimes might simply be through attitude and manner when communicating with the physician. Observations may be phrased in the form of a question such as "I noticed the patient is dragging his foot. Do you think he needs a drop-foot brace?" rather than voicing the same concern in a more demanding, directive manner. For all involved the result is more satisfactory: The therapist gets the referral, the physician retains control, and the patient gets the most effective care.

Leah Winkler, OTR, and Charity Gleeson, OTR,[10] followed an approach to improve physician-therapist communications that begins with presenting an overall professional image and attitude. In addition, by sending written acknowledgment of referrals and progress updates and networking with physicians in grand rounds, they take advantage of those opportunities to present information on unique occupational therapy treatment outcomes and methodologies. Physicians are included in team meetings, and occupational therapists join community associations with strong physician bases as further networking strategies. In reporting, they have found that brevity is essential, as is user-friendly documentation.

EXCHANGES BETWEEN AOTA AND THE VOLUNTEER SECTOR

The same principles of mutual exchange satisfaction can be applied to service in local, state, and national professional associations. The goals of the associations are achieved in great part because responsible professionals donate time, effort, and money. Being part of the reason one's profession grows in visibility, respect, and strength brings satisfaction to both paid and unpaid participants. Formal recognition of voluntary service in the form of special awards professional associations give to volunteers is an added satisfaction for the volunteer. It takes awareness and hard work on the part of each participant in these transactions to bring successful conclusions to all those ongoing interactions.

With AOTA as an example, constant attention must be paid to the quality of interactions between national office staff and the volunteer sector of the organization. Often a small misunderstanding can effectively erase months of work on a joint project. Careful listening and perceptive observation are critical to keeping a balance of mutual satisfaction and thus are a never-ending responsibility for both.

EXCHANGES IN ACADEME

Throughout academic programs, for both occupational therapists and occupational therapy assistants, there is marketing. Beginning in the classroom, instructors have needs for satisfaction in seeing their students become enlightened and develop knowledge through having their full attention and appreciation. On their part, students need patience and perception as they try to synthesize much information. Faculty members try to design the best method to assist students to problem-solve and to acquire adaptive skills. Another exchange takes place when faculty develop clinical reasoning skills through instruction that fosters critical thinking and, as a result, students emerge to join the faculty members' ranks as independent and resourceful therapists.

Faculty members have mutual needs to fill through collaborative research with peers inside and outside their own educational programs. Faculty members' needs for being appreciated and for rewards such as salary increases are balanced against the university's need for a high quality of teaching and publication.

Across the country the needs of working students on all levels of education from associate degree programs through doctoral programs are increasingly met through weekend instruction, one-day-a-week formats, evening offerings, and other curriculum configurations. The institutions receive the satisfaction of increased numbers of enrolled students and accompanying revenues, and the students are gratified by educational opportunities at convenient times and places. The simplicity of the marketing process is obvious.

Treatment planning is one of the basic and required courses included in occupational therapy educational programs. In her textbook on this subject, Trombly[11] presented treatment planning as problem solving applied to patient care, noting that the methodology is similar to that used by scientists and businessmen to solve problems in their operations. She used diagrams to illustrate the treatment planning process. This, too, parallels the marketing process, as the therapist collaborates with the client to gather all pertinent data, interprets the data, identifies the problems, sets priorities and goals, plans the treatment approach, treats the client, then reevaluates results to determine progress, and subsequently adjusts priorities and goals to maintain progress.

In the manner similar to that proposed by Fike, why not, during the same academic semester in which treatment planning is taught, provide instruction about the nontreatment aspects of practice by applying this same treatment planning process? Rather than management being "still another thing added on" to be studied, the common sense of it all can be recognized and simultaneously absorbed.

EDUCATION, RESEARCH, AND MARKETING

Every treatment plan holds potential as a research topic. A marketing approach can be easily applied to development of collaborative research ventures between academicians and clinicians. Begin by finding out how each can help the other to achieve their individual and organizational goals; the practice setting can provide the subjects and treatment goals while the academician supplies the methodology and the personnel to conduct studies. The time and efforts of both faculty and students can be planned so that all participants satisfy their personal professional needs.

▓ Occupational Therapy Consultation and the Marketing Process

As mentioned previously, an increasingly common form of occupational therapy practice is consultation. Consultation is included in this book because of its present and future role in occupational therapy practice and its singular affinity for the marketing process. *Occupational Therapy Consultation* by Jaffe and Epstein[12] comprehensively explains consultation and the variety of models in which it is found. Consultation does not culminate in a favorable outcome without assimilation of the marketing process, so a mutuality of purpose and process is clearly discernible here. Figure 10–2 illustrates the role of marketing in consultation.

Diligent listening is an essential component throughout the consultation process, regardless of the location and the client or consultee involved. The most valued skills of a successful consultant include a willingness to learn, respect for divergent points of view, effective communication, active listening and responding, and conflict and confrontation management, all aimed at maintaining that critical collaborative relationship and resulting in a mutually satisfying transaction.

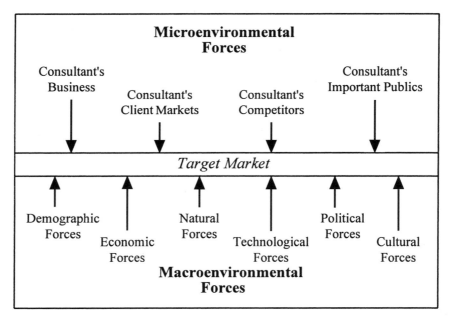

FIGURE 10–2. Analyzing the consultation market. (From Jaffe and Epstein,[12] p 659, with permission.)

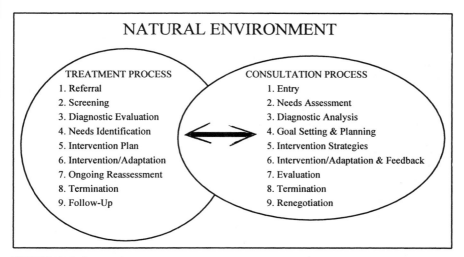

FIGURE 10–3. Occupational therapy treatment and consultation: a comparative process. (From Jaffe and Epstein,[12] p 684, with permission.)

Jaffe and Epstein[12] asserted that comparative processes are at work in consultation and in occupational therapy treatment. Figure 10–3 demonstrates their conceptual approach to this comparison and provides an understanding of the logic and commonalities present. Thus, still another perspective, that of consultation, suggests that students who master the fundamental occupational therapy treatment process can carry forward their knowledge and use it to understand another parallel process.

Marketing, Management, and Ethics

Marketing intersects daily with ethics and management in occupational therapy practice. All healthcare marketing is value-laden for all participants in daily transactions: clients, families, caregivers, occupational therapy personnel, reimbursers, professional colleagues, and all others who appear in one's own "circles of constituents."

Gardner[13] proposed one way to distinguish the "moral" person from the transgressor, the manipulator from the motivator, among managers and leaders. He suggested that all be judged on the basis of generally accepted American values. According to Gardner, "bad" leaders:

- Are cruel to their followers
- Encourage their followers to do immoral or illegal things
- Motivate by appealing to bigotry, hate, revenge, fear, and/or superstitions

- Render their followers dependent and childlike by diminishing them
- Destroy or lessen the processes established to protect freedom, justice, and/or human dignity
- Lust for power in and of itself
- Betray the trust of others in their judgment

Morally acceptable leadership:

- Accepts power, but not as the sole purpose of the position
- Serves the common good in addition to that of special interests
- Prefers to use persuasion rather than coercion
- Is "first among equals," not just "first"
- Treats followers as persons, not objects for manipulation
- Fosters individual development and tries to release human potential for the common good
- Seeks to balance the reciprocal needs of the group and the individual for the common benefit of both
- Respects and works within the law, custom, and traditional values
- Encourages individual initiative while pushing personal responsibility and involvement to the lowest levels of the organization

Regardless of specific circumstances, employees who are provided with considerate leadership forgo their own separate goals and ambitions, at least temporarily, and cooperate to achieve a common objective. This kind of efficient group action reflects sound ethical management and a marketing attitude. It is remarkable how quickly and intuitively subordinates can sense a leader's ethics. Leadership today is being judged on attitude and action rather than on authority, for executives reveal much of their character in the attitude exhibited toward associates and particularly toward subordinates. Actions in the leadership role are even more significant.

How to Begin

One way to summarize the foregoing discussion is a simple pictorial approach. With the mutually satisfying exchanges of the marketing approach applied, the processes of occupational therapy treatment and of management can be facilitated and goals achieved. Figure 10–4 illustrates these parallel processes.

Summary

This chapter asserted that because occupational therapy, marketing, and management can be viewed as both parallel and convergent processes, stu-

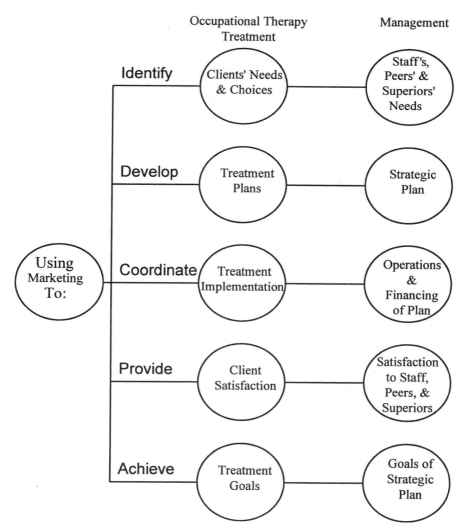

FIGURE 10–4. The marketing process at work in occupational therapy treatment and in management.

dents can be taught in a way that helps them progress logically from one to the other. Exchanges in critical thinking, therapist-client collaboration, and the helping relationship were presented as having a common denominator: the social process of marketing. The synthesizing nature of the marketing process as the entry-level occupational therapy practitioner matures was explained. The ubiquitous exchange process was shown in all practice settings, in the volunteer sector, and in academe. Ethical concerns should be inseparable throughout all these exchanges. How occupational therapy students are already learning supervisory skills in existing coursework was discussed. Finally, the topic of consultation was used as a further example of how similar processes could be taught.

REFERENCES

1. Colson, C, and Eckerd, J: Why America Doesn't Work. Work Publishing, Dallas, 1991.
2. Mosey, AC: Occupational Therapy: Configuration of a Profession. Raven Press, New York, 1981, pp 5, 61.
3. Webster's Ninth New Collegiate Dictionary. Merriam-Webster, Springfield, Mass, 1983, p 110.
4. Mosey, AC: An alternative: The biopsychosocial model. Am J Occup Ther 28:140, 1974.
5. Parham, D: Toward professionalism: The reflective therapist. Am J Occup Ther 41:555, 1987.
6. Carkhuff, R Jr: The Art of Helping. Human Resource Development Press, Amherst, Mass, 1977, p 3.
7. Davis, CM: Patient Practitioner Interaction. Slack, Thorofare, NJ, 1989.
8. Fike, ML: Professional Occupational Therapy Education as a Basis for Supervisory Skills: A Conceptual Model. Unpublished master's thesis, Texas Woman's University, 1983.
9. Stahl, C: The success of deinstitutionalization in DD. Advance for Occupational Therapists 11(20):15, May 29, 1995.
10. Stahl, C: Dealing with doctors. Advance for Occupational Therapists 11(45):12, Nov 13, 1995.
11. Trombly, CA (ed): Occupational Therapy for Physical Dysfunction, ed 2. Williams & Wilkins, Baltimore, 1983.
12. Jaffe, EG, and Epstein, CF: Occupational Therapy Consultation. Mosby–Year Book, St. Louis, 1992.
13. Gardner, J: On Leadership. Free Press, New York, 1990, p 29.

CHAPTER 11

Successes, Failures, and
Occupational Therapy

- To share examples of successes that evolved out of failures.
- To emphasize the importance of translating client-therapist collaboration into formal practice procedures.
- To recognize the move toward empowerment of clients as consumers throughout rehabilitation today.
- To realize the effects and challenges of deinstitutionalization.
- To be encouraged by a growing consumer orientation in CARF and ACSD.
- To appreciate the use of outcome-based performance measures applied to services for people with disabilities.
- To identify positive examples of a marketing orientation in adult day care.
- To emphasize the critical importance of COTA-OTR teamwork.
- To acknowledge the role of academic programs in promotion of OTR-COTA partnerships.
- To understand why occupational therapy practitioners can and must build successes out of today's problems.

Occupational therapy today has something in common with Life Savers and Swatches. Each has at times experienced a lack of appreciation, and each has emerged to be recognized as a successful idea. This chapter describes problems, failures, and successes in healthcare delivery today.

▓ Successes in the Business World

Rarely, if ever, does success just "happen." Behind a story of success there is usually a tale of conviction, hard work, and perseverance. This chapter begins with the stories behind two products that illustrate that point.

LIFE SAVERS

In 1913, Clarence Crane, a candy manufacturer in Ohio, could get no orders for his chocolate candy during the hot summer months and decided to develop a line of hard mints. Because his factory was set up to manufacture only chocolates, he resorted to having a pill manufacturer make his mints. Because the pill manufacturer's machine was malfunctioning, it kept punching holes in the center of the mints. The manufacturer promised to try to fix the machine, but Crane looked at them and decided they looked like little lifesavers, and the name was born. Because he considered them just a summer sideline, nothing happened until he sold the Life Saver brand to Edward Noble in New York. After a series of packaging and marketing failures, Noble introduced the idea of moving the now tinfoil-wrapped Life Savers out of candy stores and into drug stores, tobacco shops, barber shops, restaurants, and saloons. A new promotional technique was used: counter displays for impulse sales. By taking a commonsense, high-quality product and introducing it in new ways and places, Life Savers flourished.[1]

SWATCHES

Swiss manufacturers were recognized worldwide for centuries for their watches, which were famous for reliability and craftsmanship. Relying on their certainty that most consumers would continue to demand genuine Swiss watches because of their style and high quality, the watchmakers ceded the low end of the watch market to upstart companies in Japan and Hong Kong. However, Seiko, Casio, and other Asian companies continued to perfect their products and expand their lines out of the low end and into the middle. By 1980 the Swiss had lost all of the low end (under $75) and all but 3 percent of the middle ($75 to $400). Tradition, once a strength, became a liability. Simply waiting for watch customers to come to their senses and begin buying Swiss watches again did not work at all. Hundreds of Swiss companies went out of business. In 1978 Ernst Thomke, 20 years earlier an apprentice watchmaker-mechanic and by then an industrial managing director, responded to a request from his old boss at the parts-making arm of the country's biggest watch manufacturer, SMH, to come back and take over. Based on his experience in marketing and research, he went to work. At this point, Japanese innovation had begun moving into even the high end of the watch market with an ultrathin analog watch that made Swiss models look chunky and ungainly.

Thomke challenged his engineers to design a high-priced analog watch, thinner than 2 millimeters, in 6 months. Thomke's rationale was to make the engineers rethink their whole approach, find new solutions, and develop new modules. The result was a 1-millimeter-thick watch with a revolutionary design; instead of placing separately manufactured moving parts into the watch housing, the mechanism was built directly into the case. Five thousand were sold at $4700 each.

Thomke next demanded an analog watch that cost less than $6.65 to produce. The engineers pronounced the idea impossible until two of them took on the challenge. With no loss of traditional Swiss quality but with a totally new perspective, they found a way to produce a watch under $6.65 that was waterproof and designed to withstand abuse. Contracting the words *Swiss watch,* the new product was called the Swatch. The first Swatch came out for $40 in 1983, and the price has remained constant. Every year Swatch releases 140 strikingly different designs, while collectors sell and trade unusual and early editions.

The CEO of SMH, Nicholas Hayek, says that the Swatch story has two lessons: (1) "It is possible to build high-quality, high-value, mass-market consumer products in a high-wage country at low cost. . . . We must build where we live. . . . [We] must say to [our] people 'We will build this product in our country at a lower cost and with higher quality than anywhere else in the world.' And they have to figure out how to do it." (2) "The second lesson is related to the first. You can build mass-market products in countries like Switzerland or the United States only if you embrace the fantasy and imagination of your childhood and youth. People may laugh . . . but that's the real secret behind what we have done. . . . We kill too many good ideas by rejecting them without thinking about them, by laughing at them."[1]

▨ Occupational Therapy: The Success, the Responsibility

Like Life Savers and Swatches, occupational therapy has experienced periods of challenge. Because of adaptability, resourcefulness, risk taking, and common sense, there has been rapidly growing recognition of the high quality and soundness of occupational therapy. It is now the responsibility of current and future occupational therapy practitioners to ensure that occupational therapy continues to be "one of the great ideas of 20th century medicine."[2] Remembering that the therapeutic value of an activity is dependent on its meaning to the person performing it is one way to assure that occupational therapy will continue to evolve.

Recent clinical reasoning literature has added support for the fact that a collaborative model of treatment—one that responds to *clients'* perceptions of their illness and disability experiences—is central to occupational therapy practice. However, occupational therapists must do more to strengthen that collaborative treatment model. Neistadt[3] conducted a study to determine what methods occupational therapists were currently using to assess clients' priorities in adult physical disability settings. Results indicated that the majority of occupational therapists were using informal interviews to ascertain clients' priorities on admission. Resulting data were vague and did not identify meaningful occupations. Her conclusion was that occupational therapists need to work harder to translate their core professional and personal values about client-therapist collaboration into a formal set of procedures for practice. Following are illustrations of how some professionals are proceeding.

▨ Problems and Failures in Rehabilitation Services

No matter how thin you slice it, there are two sides to everything, including a slice of bread, my grandmother often told me. Evidently the field of rehabilitation is no exception, as evidenced by two presentations given during a recent conference of the American Congress of Rehabilitation Medicine (ACRM) and American Academy of Physical Medicine and Rehabilitation (AAPM&R). On the one hand, Marcel Dijkers, director of research at the Rehabilitative Institute of Michigan and associate professor at Wayne State University, declared that "empowerment is just the latest catch-phrase for concepts that the field of rehabilitation has discussed and failed to implement or fully implement for years," a dead-end ideology.[4] On the other hand, Mildred Matlock, assistant vice president of clinical services at the Rehabilitative Institute of Michigan, contested that a power shift is already in progress to replace the medical model with a partnership or empowerment model.

Dijkers stated that rehabilitation professionals fail miserably when it comes to empowering patients as decision makers and participants in treatment programs; instead, decisions are made for them, about them, and without them. He cited numerous indicators of this premise as he reminded listeners that patients do not set daily routines, are not addressed as Mr. or Mrs., are subjected to staff jargon, and are not held responsible for their own behavior. Such indicators he termed "proposals for empowerment that went nowhere,"[4] as professionals are loathe to give up authority and have no need to do so in that they have the power base, the prestige, the status, the precision, and expertise. Dijkers continued that "providing the patient with information, [having] discussions and making decisions with the patient takes time, and we don't have time. Even if we had the time, making decisions the democratic way is messy. . . . Autocratic systems are much more efficient."[4] Matlock noted that some may see empowerment as an aggressive challenge to professional expertise, but it should instead be understood as a reciprocal sharing of power.

INITIAL SUCCESS

Matlock described ways in which she had observed that the idea of patients as consumers was gaining in momentum as a model, with the rehabilitation team itself benefiting by finding out the clients' needs and sharing responsibilities, power, and control of the rehabilitation process. She detected movement in this direction in such changes as informing patients of their rights and how to voice concerns about care deficiencies, providing alternatives to restrictions for patients who tend to wander, learning about patients' individual values and beliefs, involving patients and families at team conferences, teaching patients to manage their medication and diets while using professionals as consultants, and training staff in empowerment techniques such as coaching, delegating, and mentoring. Matlock strongly urged continuation of this positive and successful movement by *replacing* the medical model with the empowerment model, not merely adding it on. She concluded with the admonition that all rehabilitation professionals should establish contacts with clients based on a mutual understanding of the clients' priorities and the professionals' expertise.[4]

▨ Failure and Success Following Deinstitutionalization

Often counted among failures in practice today, deinstitutionalization in mental health has created obvious problems; however, many professionals have worked diligently on solutions with varying degrees of success. The "revolving door syndrome" sends 50 percent of chronic schizophrenia patients on drug therapy back to hospitals at least once a year, according to William M. Glazer, associate clinical professor of psychiatry at the Yale University School of Medicine.[5] Among suggestions he has made toward amelioration of such problems are giving more incentives to help some mentally ill keep up with outpatient care, balancing entitlements with responsibility for follow-up care, and having clinicians negotiate with patients to work on treatment alliances, a mutual process.

David Braddock, director of the Institute on Disability and Human Development in the College of Associated Health Professions at the University of Illinois at Chicago, stated that more proactive approaches, such as one in which case managers take the clinic out into the community, do a better job of meeting the needs of people with mental disabilities. This mutually satisfying process has been successful in many parts of the United States, as teams of professionals provide for the needs of the clients in their environments and work regularly with their consumers to develop trust.

Braddock, making his presidential address to the American Association on Mental Retardation, also expressed the view that even severely retarded individuals can live in the community with little help.[6] Gary Blumenthal, executive director of the President's Committee on Mental Retardation, credits much of this success to focusing on the abilities of this population rather than on their disabilities.

Accreditation Bodies Work Toward Successful Outcomes

Among healthcare services accreditors, redefining *quality* in terms of outcomes for those people who are served rather than compliance with program processes reflects trends such as those described by Matlock. The expressed needs and priorities of the disabled are heeded and subsequent actions required to be taken. Across the entire service industry the definition of *quality* should rest with the perception of those receiving the services. Authors such as Peppers and Rogers[7] stress dialogue with and feedback from consumers, with the central question being "What does this customer really want?" Listening to the consumer is not germane only to those in health services delivery. Across the country *all* businesses are acutely aware that if you want your customers to remain your customers you must find out what specific factors—faster delivery? electronic billing and payment? better-trained personnel?—make the most difference in your retention rate and how much that difference is worth. To do this means that measuring and managing customer satisfaction cannot be left to a market research department. It is the responsibility of everyone in the business; it is the whole business.[8]

In the healthcare services delivery world, a heartening response to these increasing market pressures for consumer orientation can be seen in such regulatory agencies as the Commission for Accreditation of Rehabilitation Facilities (CARF). This agency now requires therapists to document clients' goals for treatment and client-therapist collaboration on treatment plans.[9]

THE ACCREDITATION COUNCIL ON SERVICES FOR PEOPLE WITH DISABILITIES: A SUCCESS

Proof that disabled individuals can live successfully in the community can also be found in the diligent work of The Accreditation Council on Services for People With Disabilities (ACSD). This accreditation body evolved from the work of the American Association on Mental Deficiency (AAMD), which published its *Standards for State Residential Institutions for the Mentally Retarded* in 1964.[10] Through a series of organizational changes, beginning in 1996, the name of the ACSD evolved into today's designation. During the 1980s the Accreditation

Council published standards (in 1984 and 1987) and operated a national accreditation program for organizations that provided services to people with developmental disabilities. The 1988 Intermediate Care Facility for the Mentally Retarded regulation of the Health Care Financing Administration (HCFA) was based on the 1984 standards of ACSD. During the 1990s the ACSD reexamined the role of accreditation and developed a new system for quality improvement and measurement that emphasizes responsiveness to individual needs rather than compliance with organizational processes. This system, now in place and implemented across the country with increasing success, is called *Outcome Based Performance Measures.*[11]

Evidence of the marketing approach used by the ACSD interviewers, who provide the baseline data for making decisions that determine the futures of those persons being served, can be readily seen in the 30 outcome-based performance measures around which the interview questions are devised (Table 11–1). Four principles are embedded throughout the measures: individual differences, choice and decision making, rights and responsibilities, and organizational process and personal outcomes.

In addition to the 30 performance measures for people being served, the council administers a series of measures related to organizational performance. Six of the 16 organizational performance measures, those relating to the personal health, safety, and welfare of the people being served, are given in Table 11–2.

Successes in Adult Day Care

Scarcely a day goes by that one does not see reference to "the graying of America" or to the statistics indicating steady growth in the proportion of citizens over age 65 in United States. Daily news contains encouraging examples of the ways in which a marketing approach has been applied to the growing need for enjoyable, satisfying solutions to the questions posed by adult day care. The Spring 1995 issue of *Advances,* the newsletter of the Robert Wood Johnson Foundation, described scenarios representative of the marketing approach used for the mutual benefit of organizations and their clients.[12]

At Elderly Services in Middlebury, Vermont, the sponsoring facility acquired an income surplus to create building and reserve funds while the persons being served received what they wanted and needed without disclosing personal financial information, an aspect of special importance to them. The mutual exchange at work here is clearly evident. Joanne Corbett, project director, credits improved "customer service" as one strategy that has boosted Elderly Services' appeal, as the staff looked at what people said they wanted, not only what they, the staff, decided was needed.

The source of support for this initiative is Partners in Caregiving: The Dementia Services Program funded by the Robert Wood Johnson Foundation. Created in 1992, the national program has three main objectives: "(1) test the via-

TABLE 11–1

Outcome-Based Performance Measures for People

Personal goals	1. People choose personal goals. 2. People realize personal goals.
Choice	3. People choose where and with whom they live. 4. People choose where they work. 5. People decide how to use their free time. 6. People choose services. 7. People choose their daily routine.
Social inclusion	8. People participate in the life of the community. 9. People interact with other members of the community. 10. People perform different social roles.
Relationships	11. People have friends. 12. People remain connected to natural support networks. 13. People have intimate relationships.
Rights	14. People exercise rights. 15. People are afforded due process if rights are limited. 16. People are free from abuse and neglect.
Dignity and Respect	17. People are respected. 18. People have time, space, and opportunity for privacy. 19. People have and keep personal possessions. 20. People decide when to share personal information.
Health	21. People have healthcare services. 22. People have the best possible health.
Environment	23. People are safe. 24. People use their environments. 25. People live in integrated environments.
Security	26. People have economic resources. 27. People have insurance to protect their resources. 28. People experience continuity and security.
Satisfaction	29. People are satisfied with services. 30. People are satisfied with their personal life situations.

From The Accreditation Council on Services for People With Disabilities,[11] p 15, with permission.

bility of adult day centers as alternatives to nursing home care for the elderly, (2) determine if consumers would be willing to pay out-of-pocket for the full cost of the services if those services were designed to respond to their needs, and (3) see if with proper training, relatively small grants and limited technical assistance, day centers could become financially self-sufficient."[12] In Middlebury, since 1993 daily attendance climbed from 13 to 34, while total enrollment jumped from 39 to 82, due to what Corbett called "a real revolution in our minds of what customer service means. We learned how to treat every family member as a customer from the first phone call."[12]

TABLE 11–2

Performance Measures for Organizations: Personal Health, Safety, Welfare

1. The organization protects the rights of people.

2. The organization demonstrates a commitment to using positive approaches in all service and support activities.

3. The organization's service practices and staff demonstrate sensitivity and concern for personal dignity and respect.

4. The organization implements procedures for investigation and intervention in all instances of alleged abuse and neglect.

5. The organization owns, operates, or leases buildings that comply with all applicable fire and sanitation codes.

6. The organization implements procedures for meeting all emergencies, such as fire, severe weather, and health.

From The Accreditation Council on Services for People With Disabilities,[11] p 137, with permission.

Other marketing constituencies mentioned by Corbett were referral agencies and a family member support group. Part of the strategy of Elderly Services is to spend time with prospective clients or their family members, solidifying its family member support group for caregivers who have not yet enrolled relatives but may in the future. A concerted effort has been launched to strengthen and nurture relationships with referral agencies.

Partners in Caregiving has also given technical assistance to the Jewish Community Centers Association (JCCA) adult day care program in St. Louis, with similar successes. Sylvia Nissenboim, project director, credited lessons in marketing as the key to the newfound prosperity of the program. She observed that marketing is not a skill customarily encouraged in nurses, social workers, or therapist: "We're not marketing people. . . . The weakness in [our] training is a mindset that says, 'if you can't sell it, you give it away.'"[12] She has since learned that giving away a program is the same as reducing its value. Today Nissenboim and her colleagues, instead of telling clients about their frailties or impairments, show them how the center could enrich their lives; they promote the center as a place for people to socialize and enjoy themselves despite physical limitations. As a result, JCCA enrollment increased from 26 to 40 daily participants, which is capacity. Hours have been expanded to 7:30 A.M. to 6 P.M. rather than from 10 A.M. to 3 P.M. to appeal to more working caregivers. Also, daily operating cost is now set based on 90 percent of full enrollment to account for people who do not show up and who were costing hundreds of dollars daily.

Further mutual exchanges can be detected with a closer look at the processes at work in these two cases. The growing numbers of elderly or chronically ill adults who are living longer, many with disabilities such as Alzheimer's, mental retardation, developmental disabilities, or chronic mental illness, find that the adult day programs provide them with companionship, activity, and caring. Simultaneously, the burden felt by the growing number of caregivers unable to spend as much time as they feel they should with loved ones is eased.

These examples may be more fully understood in a graphic representation similar to that found in Figures 4–3 and 4–5. Visualizing in this way the potential constituencies or publics surrounding the daily operations of an organization enables the systematic process that is marketing to be set in motion, leading to positive results. The role of occupational therapists as essential members of the teams in adult day care is evident; however, these potential roles have not been universally recognized and occupied by occupational therapists. Thus future roles in this practice area have been greatly threatened.

■ Occupational Therapy Successes in the Community

Growing numbers of occupational therapy practitioners have recognized the necessity and reality of moving practice into the community as psychiatric clients leave hospitals. The essence of the marketing process is evident as these therapists advocate that the secret is to alter and adapt attitudes toward the community environment. The advice is similar from those who have already successfully made the transition, now working in partial hospital programs, mobile treatment teams, day treatment centers, homeless shelters, and clubhouse model programs.

It is up to occupational therapists to create their own markets, fill unfamiliar roles, justify occupational therapy in new configurations, take risks, and work in programs with no clear boundaries. The creative registered occupational therapists (OTR) and certified occupational therapy assistants (COTA) who have pioneered their own new roles are working with people where they need help, using community service systems, and finding community practice to be practical and rewarding. They are demonstrating to others how much occupational therapy services are needed in new settings every day.[13]

■ Mutual Understanding of COTA, OTR, and OT Aide Roles

For successes such as these to continue and to increase, a problem within the profession must be addressed: mutual unfamiliarity and misunderstanding of the comparative roles and responsibilities of the OTR, COTA, and OT aide. Standards for the training of occupational therapy assistants were adopted by AOTA in 1958 and implemented in 1960. Since then, the profession has been justly proud of the effective work that certified occupational therapy assistants have accomplished. However, uncertainty often exists when the comparative roles of the registered occupational therapist (OTR) and certified occupational therapy assistant (COTA) are not made clear. The complementarity of OTRs and COTAs in practice is inhibited at times in spite of the AOTA publication of specifics regarding comparative roles and responsibilities. When boundaries within a profession are not made clear, there is less agreement about purpose, goals, and direction, which makes difficult the promotion of professionalism.

Role-modeling for these two levels of occupational therapy practitioners must begin in their academic programs. Educating students in isolation affects future teaming with members of their own profession and with other disciplines as well. This has been amply documented in occupational therapy literature for the past decade. Both OTR and COTA educational programs must provide more and better information and experiences for students about the depth and variety of education and expertise possessed by graduates of both types of programs.

When work was begun in 1989 on the entry-level role delineation document, the first fact to be recognized was that the OTR and COTA both have important and distinct roles in practice settings. Moreover, both the OTR and the COTA have responsibilities to each other as service provision is carried out. Where better to lay the foundation for such collaborative practice than in academic classrooms?

The 1991 *Essentials and Guidelines for an Accredited Educational Program for the Occupational Therapy Therapist* and for the *Occupational Therapy Assistant* reiterated and reemphasized this responsibility. The *Essentials* for the occupational therapist programs are explicit in their requirements for content concerning COTAs. Curriculum content must include increased attention to the COTA role, such as the appropriate part played by the COTA in the screening and assessment process, in collaboration with patients, caregivers, and other professionals, and in collaboration with the OTR in treatment implementation.

The OT aide, as another level of practitioner, does not at this time have the same uniformity and regulation of preparation as the OTR and COTA. A further dilemma derives from the changes resulting from increased interest in multi-skilled practitioners and from separating skilled and unskilled responsibilities of healthcare workers. Occupational therapy practitioners are advised to remain continuously informed about current decisions being made concerning the role of OT aides by reading state and national publications from professional associations and from state regulatory boards.

SUCCESSES IN ACADEMIC PARTNERSHIPS

Educational programs have implemented *Essentials* requirements in many ways. For example, the University of New England's senior class in occupational therapy hosted COTA students from Kennebec Valley Technical College for the purpose of giving students of both programs opportunity to explore the meaning of collaborative OTR-COTA relationships prior to the fieldwork phase of education. A forum emphasized the recognition of individualism, levels of competence, advocacy, respect, and open communication as ways to facilitate collaboration. One session used small groups to experience critical thinking, role delineation, and collaborative teamwork and give the students opportunity for mutual exploration of therapeutic issues. Four pairs of working COTA-OTR teams described partnerships in psychosocial, school system, subacute rehabilitation, and general hospital settings, including types of supervision needed, levels of responsibility, and tasks shared. The result was a shared understanding among all the students that collaborative relationships are rewarding and that everyone is working toward the same goal: providing high-quality, holistic client care.[14]

In 1988 the School of Occupational Therapy at Texas Woman's University (TWU) and Cooke County College (CCC) in Texas, after conducting a needs survey, began working together to develop an occupational therapy assistant program at CCC. Space and equipment at TWU were leased by CCC, and scheduling of TWU labs was adapted to accommodate the occupational therapy assistant program until separate facilities could be located. Plans were made to have OTA and OT students meet together for some classes. Today CCC has its own buildings nearby, and accreditation was awarded to CCC for the first time in 1992.

At Loma Linda University in California, the OT and OTA students participate in a patient management course together, team-taught by an OTR and a COTA. Among the course objectives are facilitation of communications between the two levels of professionals, encouragement of collaborative problem solving and decision making, and opportunities for mutual discussion of roles and supervision issues. Joint fieldwork assignments of OTA and OT students add to the experiential education of both.[15]

After concerns voiced by both COTAs and OTRs during the first annual COTA forum held in 1994 during the Occupational Therapy Association of California's (OTAC) annual state conference, the first COTA-OTR partnership seminar was conducted in California in 1995. It was followed by several new joint OTR-COTA educational programs, including a seminar hosted by Mount Saint Mary's College for its own students and for students from the University of Southern California.[16]

OTR AND COTA TEAMWORK IN PRACTICE

There are many examples of success as OTRs and COTAs form new partnerships while developing mutual appreciation for each other's skills and expertise. The annual award given by AOTA for the most exemplary OTR-COTA teamwork is a continual illustration of fruitful collaboration in daily practice. Such partnerships not only serve the clients who benefit but also can decrease burnout and increase job satisfaction among the OTRs and COTAs. When there is a shortage of occupational therapy personnel, it is advantageous to have a greater number of persons with skills and expertise among whom to choose to fill positions.

A recent example demonstrated how successful COTA-OTR teams can provide home healthcare clients with optimum care and skill in a cost-effective way, no small consideration in a managed-care climate. According to Rebecca Robinson-Brown, OTR/L, owner of an allied healthcare company that specializes in home care hospice, the future of occupational therapy lies in "developing strong working teams in home care, meaning the OTR-COTA relationships."[17] Robinson-Brown made the statement from her multiple personal perspectives of clinical OTR, business owner, and manager.

A marketing approach is obvious in Robinson-Brown's assertion that, from a management standpoint, communication between COTA and OTR, between the team and the client, and between the team and other members of the home care agency is the biggest and most essential element of success. She meets these challenges through such means as pagers, voice mail, mobile phones, and FAX. Robinson-Brown asserts that the OTR-COTA partnerships have been a positive addition to her practice from every perspective. By drawing on each other's strengths, sharing ideas, and problem-solving together, the OTR-COTA teams provide the best care for their clients.

From the clients' point of view, this optimum care is provided within the mandates set by the managed care and healthcare reimbursement systems. Robinson-Brown's opinion is that this team approach serves the elderly population very well, especially those who have limiting problems in the home environment. The client and family work with the OTR-COTA team on specific goals of choice to ensure that the client's needs and values are addressed. "It is imperative that the goals be established in partnership with the client and the family. We have the client sign off on the goals," says Robinson-Brown.[17] Because clients are now released from hospitals sooner and need additional care at home, the focus is not just on physical treatment but also on educating the family and providing emotional support, a primary function of the occupational therapy partnership. This is no small aspect of healthcare delivery, for how illnesses impact families and their lifestyles on a long-term basis will be of growing importance in the future.

Contemporary Problems

Failure to acknowledge the presence of the many dilemmas in contemporary practice would be foolish; however, having identified a problem the fault would lie in not then analyzing and working toward its solution. Following are but two examples of challenges identified in healthcare settings today and to which occupational therapists need to respond.

CARDIAC REHABILITATION

According to data released by the federal Agency for Health Care Policy and Research (AHCPR), more than 13.5 million people with coronary heart disease could benefit from cardiac rehabilitation, yet only 11 to 38 percent of those people participate in cardiac rehabilitation programs. Because those in need of cardiac rehabilitation have many different needs that can be met through the combined expertise of a group of professionals, a team approach is the most effective solution.

Occupational therapists serve as team members in many facilities; however, the occupational therapist is frequently left out as a provider, despite the valuable potential role that occupational therapy could play on the team: to determine activity guidelines using monitored task evaluation in ADL, leisure activities, and work; to modify activity for high-risk patients by reducing cardiac work and teaching principles of energy conservation; and to provide education for clients and their caregivers regarding risk factors. No occupational therapists were included on the panel that wrote the ACHCPR guidelines, and there is not presently any special interest section in cardiac rehabilitation through AOTA.[18]

CULTURAL AND LANGUAGE DIFFERENCES

Mary Taugher, MS, OTR, FAOTA, director of rehabilitation services at the Milwaukee County Mental Health Complex in Wauwatosa, Wisconsin, observed that cultural and language differences between therapist and client can lead to incorrect diagnoses and misinterpretation of symptoms as well as ineffective treatment. An estimated 10 percent of clients seen in public and teaching hospitals speak a primary language other than English. Taugher asserted that therapists need at least to become educated about the various cultures represented in their communities. For example, in treating psychiatric diagnoses, therapists need to be able to distinguish between a commonly shared superstition and a personal delusion, between culture and illness. A therapist who is not fluent in a client's language should rely on the services of a professional interpreter.[19]

More Occupational Therapy Successes

There is not enough space here to describe all the tales of success achieved by resourceful occupational therapy practitioners. Throughout this book I have shared examples and have referred readers to information sources such as *OT Week* and *Advance* to learn about more. Each day there is evidence of the infinite variety of opportunities open to occupational therapy practitioners and new chances to demonstrate what can be done. For example, occupational therapists are recognized as members of many oral motor teams, with occupational therapists responsible for assessing and planning dysphagia interventions. Education in evaluating muscle tone and sensory system impairments combined with knowledge of facilitative neuromuscular techniques, wheelchair seating design, and adaptive eating equipment, make the occupational therapist a well-qualified member of the dysphagia team. Several problems that may be handled by the occupational therapist include poor lip closure, decreased tongue movement, delayed or absent gag reflex, decreased or absent sensation, choking, and decreased motor skills.[20]

Along with other diagnostic categories, acute care of the spinal cord–injured (SCI) client is being compressed by shorter hospital stays that result in clients heading back to the community more quickly. Occupational therapists have risen to the occasion. In addition to those noted in previous chapters, Claire Yanoshak, MS, OTR, at Thomas Jefferson University Hospital in Philadelphia, reported that shorter stays in acute care have caused occupational therapists to concentrate on gathering information and establishing rapport with clients to enable them to regain control of their own care and lives. To do this, she says that occupational therapists must tailor acute and long-term rehabilitation of SCI clients by first ascertaining who they were before their injuries, what they liked to do, and what they most wished to work on first. In that way, the clients are more fully involved in their own care. In short, Yanoshak believes that a big part of the therapist's job is to educate both client and family and that the most prominent aspect of acute care is psychosocial.[21]

Summary

This chapter discussed the problems, failures, and successes in healthcare service delivery today. The movement throughout rehabilitation to incorporate a consumer orientation was noted and its positive results shown through examples. Effects of deinstitutionalization were acknowledged with an expanded role for the occupational therapy practitioner in community treatment of this problem suggested. It was shown how the Commission for Accreditation of Rehabilitation Facilities (CARF) and the Accreditation Council on Services for People with Disabilities (ACSD) have provided support for the supposition that disabled individuals can live successfully in the community when their needs and goals are determined collaboratively with those responsible for their care. Examples of successes in adult day care settings were described. The importance of OTR-COTA partnerships was stressed, beginning with role-modeling in occupational therapy educational programs at both levels. Change as a dominant factor in the work world in which success must be achieved is discussed in Chapter 12.

REFERENCES

1. Mingo, J: How the Cadillac Got Its Fins. HarperCollins, New York, 1994.
2. Reilly, M: Occupational therapy can be one of the great ideas of 20th century medicine. Am J Occup Ther 16(1), 1962.
3. Neistadt, ME: Methods of assessing clients' priorities: A survey of adult physical dysfunction settings. Am J Occup Ther 49(5):428, 1995.

4. Breske, S: Should rehab patients be recipients or participants of care? Advance for Occupational Therapists, Jan 18, 1993, pp 17, 19.

5. Kerr, T: Revolving door syndrome in MH sends 50% back to hospital. Advance for Occupational Therapists 11(20):14, May 29, 1995.

6. Stahl, C: The success of deinstitutionalization in DD. Advance for Occupational Therapists 11(20):15, May 29, 1995.

7. Peppers, D, and Rogers, M: The One to One Future: Building Relationships One Customer at a Time. Doubleday, New York, 1993, p 16.

8. Stewart, TA: After all you've done for your customers, why are they still not happy? Fortune, Dec 11, 1995, p 178.

9. Commission on Accreditation of Rehabilitation Facilities: Standards Manual and Interpretive Guidelines for Organizations Serving People with Disabilities. The Commission, Tucson, 1994.

10. Gardner, JF, and Campanella, T: Beyond compliance to responsiveness: New measures of quality for accreditation. Work 5:105, 1995.

11. The Accreditation Council on Services for People With Disabilities: A Guide to Using Outcomes Based Performance Measures in Employment Services, The Council, Towson, Md, 1993.

12. Robert Wood Johnson Foundation: Partners in caregiving: Lessons in customer service. Advances 8(2):9, Spring 1995.

13. Hettinger, J: Leap of faith. OT Week 9(47):11, Nov 23, 1995.

14. York, CD, and Gitlow-Archer, L: UNE exposes students to the OTR-COTA relationship. OT Week 8(39):2, Sept 29, 1994.

15. Hewitt, L: Loma Linda's inspiring approach. Advance for Occupational Therapists 12(36):11, Sept 11, 1996.

16. Olivas-De La O, T: What the partnership really means. Advance for Occupational Therapists 11(36):12, Sept 11, 1995.

17. Woodard, K: A team approach to recovery. OT Week 9(32):18, Aug 10, 1995.

18. Federwisch, A: Guide says teams should lead cardiac rehab. Nursing and Allied Healthweek 2(26):1, 1995.

19. Joe, BE: Breaking barriers in psychosocial OT. OT Week 9(29):20, July 20, 1995.

20. Posner, T, and Eckford, C: Dysphagia Resource Manual: Training for Caregivers of Patients with Swallowing Problems. AOTA, Bethesda, Md, 1991.

21. Hettinger, J: Acute care of SCI gets aggressive. OT Week 9(29):18, July 20, 1995.

PART FIVE

CHANGE AS THREAT
AND OPPORTUNITY

He not busy being born is busy dying.

Bob Dylan

CHAPTER 12

The Nature of Change and How It Is Adopted

CHAPTER OBJECTIVES

- To comprehend the nature of change.
- To realize why the habit of lifelong learning is inextricably bound to the reality of change today.
- To know how to recognize and deal with change and innovation.
- To identify the reasons for resistance to change.
- To recognize the role of motivation in acceptance of change.
- To realize how an organization's culture is central to adaptation to change.
- To recognize conflict: its sources, levels, management, and consequences.
- To visualize the diffusion of innovation.
- To value negotiation and the part it plays in marketing.
- To know how public opinion works.
- To acknowledge the inherent value of one's attitude toward change.

Designing the future of occupational therapy requires an attitude often not encouraged among those employed in the healthcare industry. Change is inevitable, but how you handle it makes all the difference between success and failure, satisfaction and disappointment. The idea of change is closely akin to *crisis,* a word the Chinese write in two characters, one meaning danger and the other opportunity. Occupational therapists can approach change in much the same way—as a threat or as an opportunity. To explain any action with "I've always done it that way" simply doesn't work any more. The big picture must be seen and in new ways, with new niches where none existed before.

Even though Bennis,[1] in his book *Why Leaders Can't Lead,* painted an overall pessimistic picture of American leadership today, he did conclude with the observation, "I do think change is possible—even for the better. Change begins slowly, however, as, one by one, individuals make the conscious choice to live up to their potential." The potential of individual occupational therapists is awesome, but even more so is the collective future they represent.

Part Five looks at change and at how occupational therapy practitioners have continuously adapted. Chapter 12 examines the nature of change itself, and Chapter 13 offers heartening evidence of how occupational therapists historically and currently have anticipated and successfully adapted to change.

▨ Understanding Change

Change is inherently neither good nor bad. It is dynamic and possesses several special characteristics. Change affects your organization, disrupts the balance, and causes forces within the organization to work to restore equilibrium. Both internal and external forces influence change. Because organizations today must change in order to survive, understanding the process of change is essential. So important has the management of change become, as upheaval has become endemic to corporate America, that professional consultants who specialize in "change management" have appeared on the scene to assist in transitions.

Because everyone exists and acts in two time periods—today and tomorrow—and because no one can assume that tomorrow will be an extension of today, openness and adaptability to change are the keys to occupational therapists' personal and professional transitions. Understanding how to manage change is a key element in the final production of an effective marketing plan.

Students are advised to take seriously the advice to assume the habit of lifelong learning because anyone with any kind of knowledge has to acquire *new* knowledge every 4 or 5 years or else become obsolete. Purposeful innovation, both technical and social, has become an organized discipline in the last 40 years. Fortunately, it can be both taught and learned.

Management of change must be built into every organization today, with carefully planned abandonment instead of attempted prolongation of policies, practices, or products that have previously been successful. Added to this planned abandonment must be a way to systematically welcome and create the new. Drucker[2] suggested building into the organization three practices: (1) continual improvement of everything you do (called *kaizen* by the Japanese, whose aim is to improve every service or product until within 2 or 3 years it becomes truly different), (2) exploitation or development of new applications for already successful services or products, and (3) systematic innovation. Following these three practices brings the manager back to abandonment and beginning the process again.

FORMS THAT CHANGE WILL TAKE

Alexander Graham Bell has been credited with saying that "when one door closes, another opens; but we often look so long and so regretfully upon the closed door that we do not see the one that has opened for us," for change is not a one-time event that occurs and is over. It is instead a constantly evolving process requiring vigilant management.

An organization is confronted with change in various ways; however, most changes fall into one of three categories: technological, structural, or people. Technological changes involve equipment or procedures used on the job, with more complex equipment causing more anxiety. Structural changes can include everything from hierarchical organization to policies or procedures. The organization's human resources constitute the people category, a major factor to be kept in mind.

RESISTANCE TO CHANGE

It is not the *change* people resist so much as *being changed*. Drucker advised, "What creates resistance to technological or structural change is fear: fear of the unknown, fear of being lost, of being alone, of being an outcast. . . . And it is precisely because the real problem is fear of the unknown, fear of being abandoned in a world the worker does not know or understand, that . . . organized planning is so badly needed."[3]

Resistance to change is natural and inevitable, for with change comes uncertainty, whether conscious or unconscious, and uncertainty produces a disruption of the status quo. Human beings exist in a homeostatic condition; when this balance is disrupted, an individual resists change to retain that state of equilibrium. Many reasons are given for this innate resistance to change, any one of which begins with Drucker's analysis. People may have an inaccurate perception or understanding of the nature and implications of the change, and when job security or status is threatened or any sort of personal loss put in jeopardy, resistance to the change is to be expected. Resisting change is usually attributable to not knowing, understanding, or appreciating all of the implications of the change.

Resistance to change can be kept to a minimum through careful preparation, genuine interest in those with whom you work, an understanding of the causes of resistance to change and innovation, and attention to ways to support those who have been affected by the change. Although human beings are amazingly adaptable, you have to make it logical for them to want to change in some way.

ATTITUDE AND MOTIVATION FOR CHANGE

The success of any change within the organization depends primarily on the employees' attitudes and motivations. Building on early motivational work of E. C. Tolman in 1932 and Kurt Lewin in 1938, later theorists developed several theories of expectancy or instrumentality. One of the most popular versions was that of Victor Vroom,[4] who attempted to explain individual motivation in a process theory that used an effort-outcome framework. He was primarily concerned with answering the question of *how* individual behavior is energized, directed, maintained, and stopped, and he based his theory on three concepts: expectancy, valence, and instrumentality.

Expectancy refers to the perceived probability that a given level of effort will result in a given outcome. For example, a person wonders how likely it is that extra effort will result in a promotion. This leads to the second concept: *valence,* or the value (to the worker) of the possible outcome. It reflects the strength of the individual's desire for, or attraction toward, the outcomes of different courses of action. Vroom described performance as a *first-level outcome* and its valence or strength as the individual's probability estimate that it will lead to *second-level outcomes* (e.g., promotion, raise) and the strengths or valences of these outcomes.

The degree to which an individual believes that a first-level outcome leads to a second-level outcome (e.g., that high performance leads to a promotion) is what Vroom labels as *instrumentality.* The combination of the valences of second-level outcomes and instrumentality (that performance will result in the second-level outcome) determines the importance, or valence, of the first-level outcome.

In essence, Vroom pictured people going through a three-step thought process: How badly do they want the ultimate, second-level outcome, the promotion (valence)? Will a higher performance level—working harder—really lead to that promotion? Will exerting effort, in fact, result in high performance? By understanding the components of this and other theories of motivation, a manager may be helped to successfully introduce and establish change.[4]

THE IMPORTANCE OF CULTURE
WHEN ADAPTING TO CHANGE

One way to analyze change and its role in your professional life is first to determine the culture of your organization. *Culture* is defined here as the shared beliefs, behaviors, and assumptions that have developed over time in your particular organization. Self-assessment and analysis should be the first step in identifying and articulating your corporate culture. This in turn will go far in helping you understand and deal with resistance to change as it occurs.

Expanding this thought to your own practice specialty and to the occupational therapy profession as a whole, you can see that when change occurs in one part it can and will affect others, much like the ripples created when a stone is thrown into the water. Occupational therapists will do well to ask of themselves, "What was our 'practice culture' 10 years ago? Five years ago? What beliefs, behaviors, and assumptions characterize occupational therapy today? Is it not changed—and changing? What must I do to be an effective part of it?" Strategies must change, and when that happens, cultures must change. "It is the nature of the task that determines the culture of an organization, rather than the community in which that task is being performed.[5]

These sobering facts give further credence to the need for all occupational therapists to be aware of what is going on locally, statewide, nationally, and globally. Changes must be at best anticipated and at least understood in a world where the rules change daily.

▦ Change and Conflict

It is highly unlikely that the word *change* can be uttered without the word *conflict* being at least implied and expected. Conflict is an element of life with which each person must cope, an inevitable part of personal growth and development. Conflict is always found in the work environment because it is an unavoidable part of human relationships. In itself, conflict has no value; even though it is usually viewed as negative, however, conflict can also be beneficial to organizations and a powerful motivator for positive change.

SOURCES OF CONFLICT

Schmidt and Tannenbaum[6] offered a categorization of conflict that is of potential benefit to occupational therapists on the job. The four categories progress from simple to complex, and the resolutions of those conflicts follow a similar progression in complexity. The simplest kind of conflict involves *facts*, information that is inadequate or inaccurate. Easy resolution of this type of conflict requires only seeking information from reliable sources. The second type of conflict is associated with *methods,* when no one standard way of doing things is in place. Differences in methods can be resolved by setting guidelines for creating procedures.

The third kind of conflict involves *goals*. Differing goals are not uncommon within the most compatible of organizations. Long-range and short-term organizational goals are in conflict with individual personal goals for career and family. Identifying and understanding goal commonalities is a first step toward managing goal-related conflict.

By far the most difficult type of conflict involves *values*. Differences in belief systems, their personal importance, and their subjective nature make these conflicts at the same time the most crucial to organizational stasis. The goal in managing these values conflicts is to develop an understanding and acceptance of the beliefs of others.

LEVELS OF CONFLICT

In the workplace the potential for daily conflict is evident. One way to view it systematically is to begin with the identification of your marketing constituencies and publics, as directed in Part Two. With that configuration in mind, conflict can occur within yourself (under stress and making decisions with no clear choices available), interpersonally (one on one, competing or cooperating), intragroup (being expected by the other group members to behave in a certain way), or intergroup (often due to threats to group survival and differentiation).

CONSEQUENCES OF CONFLICT

Consequences of conflict in the work environment can be positive or negative. Douglas[7] suggested that conflicts can have positive results: *recognition of issues* through fostering open and honest communication; *improved group cohesion* when group members face the conflict, erase former disagreements, and present a united front; *changes in performance* to increased productivity when the worker feels respected or to lower productivity if the worker chooses to accept the status quo; *leadership changes* if the conflict brought out a new leader who might not have been otherwise recognized; and *understanding* if the conflict was successful in promoting a deeper understanding of other people's beliefs, values, attitudes, and viewpoints.

Among the ways of dealing with organizational conflict, five are most commonly used: denial or withdrawal, suppression or smoothing over, power or dominance strategies, compromise or negotiation, and integration or collaboration. Having completed the preceding chapters, by this time you should have a growing understanding of the comparative merits and detrimental qualities of each choice. The related readings at the end of this chapter contain more in-depth information on conflict and its resolution.

Diffusion of Innovation

Even though openness and adaptability to change are acknowledged to be keys to successful transitions, the fact remains that all managers have problems when changes are introduced because not everyone who is affected responds in the same way or at the same time. Rogers[8] effectively described this phenomenon as *diffusion of innovation*, asserting that a consumer goes through the following stages of acceptance of a new idea or product: awareness, interest, evaluation, trial, and adoption. His definition of *innovation* was "an idea, practice, or object that is perceived as new by a unit of adoption."[8] He went on to graphically categorize how a group of people adopt an innovation according to the amount of time they take to do so. He defined *innovators* as the first 2.5 percent to adopt a new idea; *early adopters* are the next 13.5 percent to accept it; the *early majority* group comprise 34 percent of the total, and the *late majority* 34 percent, with 16 percent of the individuals labeled as *laggards,* the last of the group to adopt an innovation.

It is interesting to look at this categorization in light of an organization's having first assessed its individual "corporate culture," for Rogers went on to characterize the individuals who make up the five groups in terms of their personal values. The overriding value held by innovators is venturesomeness, a liking for new ideas and cosmopolitanism. Early adopters value respect, are considered to be opinion leaders, and adopt new ideas early but with discretion. Deliberateness is the dominant value of the early majority, as they like to adopt new ideas before the general public; however, they are rarely considered to be leaders. The primary value held by the late majority is skepticism, not adopting an innovation until most people have authenticated its value. Finally, the ruling value of the laggard is tradition, suspicious of any changes until the innovation has become nearly a tradition itself.

Judson[9] presented a similar, yet interestingly different, way of looking at how people respond to change. His spectrum of possible behavior toward change ranged from a response of acceptance, through states of indifference and passive resistance to active resistance. Specific reactions of those who exhibited acceptance (a similarity to Rogers's innovators) were enthusiastic cooperation and support, cooperation, and passive resignation. Those classified as indifferent showed apathy, loss of interest in job, or doing only what was ordered. The passively resistant showed regression behavior or nonlearning, while those who actively resisted engaged in protests, slowing down, spoilage, or personal withdrawal.

The important point here for occupational therapists to associate with marketing is that changes and innovations—ideas, practices, or objects—that must be introduced to constituencies can be physical or behavioral entities. Some innovations are substantially hardware: computers, videos, curriculum materials, heart monitors. Others are process or practice: diet, aerobic exercise, stress management methodology. In the case of each innovation, its adoption presents a myriad of related considerations for occupational therapists to ponder as they select a plan of action. Logic suggests that a manager intending to introduce a new idea should aim the message at those in the organization considered to be in Rogers's innovator or early adopter categories or in Judson's acceptance category. The road ahead may well be smoother.

▦ Innovation and Resistance Personified

Cook[10] chronicled an occupational therapist's successful introduction of an innovative outpatient service of multidisciplinary team case management within a general community hospital. With the purpose in mind of meeting the needs of discharged clients with severe mental illnesses trying to live satisfactorily in the community, Cook persevered for 3 years to overcome resistance to change by confronting power, politics, and differing cultural visions as she introduced a new service within a bureaucratic organization. The lessons she learned personify innovation and its introduction as previously described:

> Nothing changes quickly
> Have a clear and consistent vision. . .
> Maintain the vision with new language . . . In order to change a culture (both the values and the practices) new . . . terminology must be developed . . . and used consistently . . .
> Put in writing . . . writing memos and proposals
> Build coalitions . . . supported by other professionals . . . for success in both the initiation and the maintenance of the innovation once implemented
> Recognize stakeholders' interests . . . everyone involved in institutional change has "turf" or professional concerns that can hinder or help the process of change . . . [so] adjustments can be made . . . to encourage support
> Be flexible
> Don't give up or give in . . . initiating change often requires a long term commitment of energy.[10]

▦ Managing Conflict

Regardless of the source or level of the conflict, there is a general way to approach it. First, the conflict should be recognized and put into words. Understanding that each party in the conflict feels that his or her side is reasonable, discussion should focus on the future and not the past. Clear up misperceptions by using techniques such as role reversal or any means to raise the level of trust and openness. Develop objectives or goals both have in common. Outline what must be done, who is responsible for doing it, and deadlines for completion.

NEGOTIATION

Understanding the rationale and techniques of negotiation is one more valuable asset in the conduct of a successful marketing approach. Negotiation is, of course, at the core of the conflict resolution.

As early as 1941 Mary Parker Follet[11] pointed out that problems or disagreements can be resolved in three ways:

1. Authority, as the person in command makes a decision that those under his or her supervision are to follow

2. Compromise, with each party surrendering part of its wishes and some, often most, not entirely satisfied with the solution

3. Problem-solving by integration, with the wishes of everyone concerned integrated into the solution. Such solutions are not easily achieved and require a high degree of management competence

Admittedly, elements of the marketing concept can be found in the process of negotiation; however, for the intent of this book it is presupposed that the process of negotiation is more often initially begun for the purpose of gaining or winning points in an agreement. Metzger's *The Health Care Supervisor's Guidebook* (in the list of related readings at the end of this chapter) is a source that can help you develop familiarity with the process of negotiation. To become an effective, productive leader-manager, it is essential to be a proficient negotiator.

ASSERTIVENESS

As observed previously, there are often differences between men and women in communication patterns and goals that may have a direct effect on the outcome of not only a conversation but also an important project. Similarly, a lack of understanding or attention to assertiveness holds the potential for disappointing results. With that in mind, a brief introduction to the subject is included here.

Nonassertive behavior, failing to get your point across by remaining quiet or passive, is perceived by others to be weak and conveys the message that your feelings are not important. At the other extreme is aggressive behavior, through which you get your point across but are perceived by others to be hostile, angry, offensive, sarcastic, or humiliating. The message given to others is that what you want is most important and what they want, feel, or think does not matter to you.

Through assertive behavior you get your point across by direct, congruent expression of your thoughts, feelings, beliefs, and opinions in an inoffensive way. Alberti and Emmons[12] listed 10 key elements that characterize assertive behavior:

1. Self-expressive

2. Respectful of the rights of others

3. Honest

4. Direct and firm

5. Equalizing; benefiting both self and relationship

6. Verbally appropriate, including the content of the message (feelings, rights, facts, opinions, requests, limits)

7. Nonverbally appropriate, including the style of the message (eye con-

tact, voice, posture, facial expression, gestures, distance, timing, fluency, listening)

8. Appropriate for the person and the situation; not universal
9. Socially responsible
10. Learned, not inborn

One explanation for difficulty in acting assertively in appropriate situations may lie in feeling a real or perceived threat of rejection, anger, or disapproval. Assertiveness helps people realize that they can stand up for themselves and hold onto their power in difficult situations. Assertive behavior is not inborn; it is a skill that can be developed by learning four new behaviors, according to Alberti and Emmons[12]:

1. Recognize situations in which you are tempted to become passive or aggressive. Observe yourself. Be conscious of situations in which you automatically give up your power, have unreasonable thoughts unrelated to the present moment, or feel it is necessary to put down the other person.

2. Confront these ingrown habits with different thoughts. Mentally interrupt the old thought patterns such as "You're right, I'm no good" or "How dare you correct me, you arrogant fool?" By yourself or with a good friend,

   □ Outline the environment of the situation that caused the emotion

   □ Face the tendency to respond passively or aggressively

   □ Determine what belief underlies your reaaction

   □ Challenge the inaccurate belief with a counteracting right

3. Practice thinking new thoughts as a first step toward changing the feelings that accompanied the old thoughts.

4. Practice the new behavior that goes along with ownership of the right. Be assertive.

One aspect of assertive communication is the use of "I" statements, essentially telling the other person the effect that his or her behavior has on you. Negative thoughts must be challenged with more affirming, positive thoughts that confirm your rights as a human being. Then you are ready to express your honest thoughts, feelings, and beliefs in the situation.

Bower and Bower[13] expanded on the "I" statements idea by applying it to a more detailed interaction designed to draw the other person's attention to your point of view. They used DESC as an acronym for:

D—Describe the situation
E—Express your feelings about the situation
S—Specify the change you want
C—Consequences (identify the results that will occur)

When confronting a person who will not care how or what you feel, eliminate the expression of feeling and substitute *I* for *Indicate*, indicating the problem the behavior is causing. Both DESC and DISC are amplifications of the "I" statement that can be practiced and used in a disciplined ways to replace an old, ineffective method with an assertive response.

How Public Opinion Works

Understanding another concept may be of help when you wish to introduce certain changes. That is the phenomenon of public opinion. Its formation has been described by Yankelovich[14] as a seven-step process. For an especially complex issue, public opinion may take as long as 10 years to evolve from multiple individual opinions into a generalized, considered, thoughtful public judgment.

When visualized in association with Rogers's and Judson's observations about the diffusion of innovation, there is an interesting progression of thought. Yankelovich used the topic of the rising cost of health care to illustrate the seven stages by which public opinion moves into a state of public judgment:

1. Dawning awareness—but largely unaware of specifics
2. Greater urgency—global and diffuse—free-floating concern
3. Discovering the choices—beginning focus on alternatives—proposals for action
4. Wishful thinking—resistance to facing trade-offs
5. Weighing the choices—pondering the pros and cons of the options—resisting hard choices—struggling with change
6. Taking a stand intellectually—recognition but not yet commitment
7. Making a responsible judgment morally and emotionally—wholehearted acceptance—unwelcome realities accommodated—doing the right thing[14]

This interpretation of how public opinion forms has special value to the occupational therapist who is attempting to introduce change into an organization. It is especially apt when the prospective change requires wrestling with moral and emotional components. An understanding of the possible stages of resolution through which individuals' opinions are progressing may help an occupational therapist whose patience is tested. Knowing the stage of a person's opinion may help you reach a successful mutual exchange with that particular constituency in your marketing plan.

Managing Change

Based on the assumption that a participative or consultative approach is the best way to accomplish things through employees and that the best means to reduce fear of the unknown is to use communication and involvement in decision making, the following steps are suggested for introduction and management of change within an organization:

- Plan carefully and completely the full potential impact of the change throughout the organization.
- Begin early to avoid any surprises, fully communicate with everyone who will be affected, and request their comments and suggestions.
- Convince employees of the values and benefits to them and to the organization.
- When possible, involve employees as a source of job knowledge, for acceptance of change as well as for their improvements on the idea.
- Conscientiously follow up and monitor implementation until the change has become established, as new habits are not formed easily.

To summarize the foregoing discussion, a manager who is introducing a change has three ways to approach employees: (1) issuing specific orders or commands, an approach most likely to generate resistance and one that should be used rarely, when it is the only way possible; (2) making each employee at least aware of the reasons and necessity for the change by using explanations and persuasion to convince them; and (3) involving them in planning for the change because they are far more likely to understand and comply when they have helped to determine the form and substance of the change.[15]

Conflict and Marketing

Not only is conflict usually present in the healthcare service delivery environment but also there usually are several types of conflicts existing at any one time and with a number of the marketing constituencies. Conflicts may involve staff members, administrators, clients, or families. These conflicts, however, do not have to be negative. They can instead stimulate creativity, innovation, and progress for, after all, a static organization offers little challenge or progress. When participants are able to consider various alternative solutions to a conflict scenario and arrive at a mutually acceptable decision for action, that conflict has been constructive.

Once again the marketing concept is discernible in that needs of both constituencies have been satisfied through a negotiated resolution of the conflict that was interfering with that mutual exchange. The status of that particular exchange can then be changed to satisfactory when the next marketing audit is conducted.

Why Develop a Positive Attitude Toward Change?

Embracing change is crucial and life enhancing. Change can herald growth, and without growth there is only the absence of life. Those individuals who continually evolve, develop, and mature—personally and professionally—have more hope and a positive belief in the future and in their own capacity to make a difference in the world. The ability to cope with the process of change determines, in large part, a person's adjustment to all of life.

Occupational therapists must remember that their core competencies have not changed; what they do with them should change. Don't discard your skills; take them where no one before has imagined going as you open up those new windows of opportunity. In the past, to find security, a worker forged a successful career through being inflexible and unchanging in his or her pattern of living and by having a lifelong commitment and loyalty to one employer. Stability today is too often equated with security, and unfortunately security now lies in being flexible and adaptable to change.

Summary

This chapter has addressed the nature of change and its relevance for occupational therapists. The role of lifelong learning in association with change was discussed. Resistance to change was analyzed, as well as ways to recognize and overcome it. Conflict as one potential aspect of change was discussed, specifically its sources, levels, and consequences. How to go about dealing with conflict was introduced, and sources for further information on the subject suggested. Levels of acceptance among individuals following introduction of innovation were outlined, as well as the stages through which members of the community progress toward formation of final public opinion. Negotiation was recognized as an element of adjustment to change and of the marketing process. Chapter 13 continues discussion of change, with more specific attention to occupational therapists.

REFERENCES

1. Bennis, W: Why Leaders Can't Lead. Jossey-Bass, San Francisco, 1989, p xiii.
2. Drucker, PF: Post-Capitalist Society. HarperCollins, New York, 1993, p 58.
3. Drucker, PF: Managing in Turbulent Times. Harper & Row, New York, 1980, p 146.
4. Vroom, VH: Work and Motivation. John Wiley, New York, 1964.
5. Drucker, PF: Post-Capitalist Society. HarperCollins, New York 1993, p 62.
6. Schmidt, WH, and Tannenbaum, RM: Management of differences. Harvard Business Review 38(6):107, Nov/Dec, 1960.
7. Douglas, LM: The Effective Nurse Leader and Manager. Mosby, St. Louis, 1992.
8. Rogers, EM: Diffusion of Innovation. Free Press, New York, 1962, p 11.
9. Judson, AJ: A Manager's Guide to Making Changes. John Wiley, New York, 1966.
10. Cook, JV: Innovation and leadership in a mental health facility. Am J Occup Ther 49:604, 1995.
11. Metcalf, HC, and Urwich, L (eds): Dynamic Administration: The Collected Papers of Mary Parker Follett. Harper and Brothers, New York, 1942.
12. Alberti, RE, and Emmons, ML: Your Perfect Right, ed 5. Impact Publishers, San Luis Obispo, Calif, 1986, p 34.
13. Bower, SA, and Bower, GH: Asserting Yourself. Addison Wesley, Reading, Mass, 1976.
14. Yankelovich, D: How public opinion really works. Fortune 132:102, Oct 5, 1995.
15. McConnell, CR: The Effective Health Care Supervisor. Aspen, Rockville, Md, 1982, p 191.

RELATED READINGS ON CONFLICT RESOLUTION AND NEGOTIATION

Ducanis, AJ, and Golin, AK: The Interdisciplinary Health Care Team. Aspen, Germantown, Md, 1979.

Haimann, T: Supervisor Management for Healthcare Organizations. The Catholic Health Association of the United States, St. Louis, 1989.

Liebler, JG, Levine, RE, and Rothman, J: Management Principles for Health Professionals, ed 2. Aspen, Rockville, Md, 1992.

Lyles, RI, and Joiner, C: Supervision in Health Care Organizations. John Wiley, New York, 1986.

Metzger, N: The Health Care Supervisor's Guidebook, ed 3. Aspen, Rockville, Md, 1988.

CHAPTER 13

Occupational Therapy Professionals Adapt

CHAPTER OBJECTIVES

- To realize that change, adaptation, and growth are a continuous process.
- To discover the variety of models of adaptation developed by occupational therapists.
- To study adaptation to change from the multiple perspectives of corporate executives, rehabilitation managers, occupational therapy practitioners, and fieldwork and classroom educators.
- To review changing models of occupational therapy practice.
- To remember that occupational therapy is highly effective when practiced in the home.
- To understand the critical need for intraprofessional occupational therapy collaboration.
- To recognize the attributes of a change leader.

Change is here, whether you like it or not. The world does not care about our opinions or our feelings and instead rewards only those who catch on to what is happening and find those opportunities that were brought on by change. Advice to occupational therapists today to be resilient, resourceful, and adaptive is not new. Leaders in the profession have been urging this for years. The very characteristics of those who choose to become occupational therapists should make this a natural and logical move. Chapter 13 demonstrates how members of the occupational therapy profession have continuously adapted to change, beginning at the inception of occupational therapy and continuing until today. Tomorrow is your responsibility.

Entrepreneurship in Occupational Therapy Is a Continuing Story

The history of occupational therapy is itself a tale of adaptation and entrepreneurship, of resourcefulness in response to changing times and needs. Eleanor Clarke Slagle, with a background in social work, organized the first professional school for occupational therapists after recognizing the need for a balanced program of work, play, and rest for mentally ill patients.[1] The National Society for the Promotion of Occupational Therapy was formed, incorporated, and chartered in 1917 by a group who recognized a need to provide care for the sick and disabled through a technique called occupational therapy.[2] William Rush Dunton, elected president of the society in 1917, saw a need to have local organizations for exchange of ideas and concepts and established the model for state-affiliated organizations that continues today.[3] In 1919 the Boston School of Occupational Therapy, which had been closed after training reconstruction aides, responded to a need for trained occupational therapists in civilian hospitals by reopening, followed shortly by the opening of the Philadelphia and St. Louis Schools of Occupational Therapy.

After World War II the type of patients to be treated changed and increased in number, putting new demands on occupational therapists and requiring new treatment procedures.[4] This in turn required extensive adaptation and reorganization of curricula of the accredited schools of occupational therapy. Global issues became more apparent, and Clare S. Spackman represented the United States when the World Federation of Occupational Therapists was founded in 1954. Her recognition of the importance of a world view facilitated good relationships with member countries and expansion of the profession into many underdeveloped countries.[5]

In 1966 Wilma West[6] brought to the profession the observation that the shift from medical to health concerns had implications for occupational therapy and urged therapists to become involved in this new emphasis. She recommended that occupational therapists take on new roles as evaluators, consultants, supervisors, and researchers and move into the community to work in positions associated with prevention of disease. Also in 1966, Reilly[7] reminded occupational therapists that the future depended on them and what they were doing right then; through the efforts of occupational therapists themselves, their personal history would take a new and unprecedented turn. In 1974 Mosey[8] proposed an alternative to the medical and health model, the biopsychosocial model, to bring attention to the body, mind, and environment of the client.

In 1978 the representative assembly authorized a special session to examine the status of the American Occupational Therapy Association (AOTA) and the field. During this landmark meeting, issues and concerns about the changes and needs of healthcare delivery were identified and discussed.[9] Many of these concerns and needs have since been addressed by diligent, resourceful occupational therapists: a growing amount of research is being conducted to verify practice, theoretical positions are being brought forward, practice in new settings and with new categories of clients has developed, and a philosophical base was adopted.

With these and other foresighted individuals over the years pressing occupational therapy practitioners to continue widening their horizons, and with continual examples of entrepreneurship in successful responses since 1917, why is anyone hesitating now?

▨ Ongoing Change, Growth, and Innovation

Growth and development can happen only when change is considered to be both natural and acceptable. Adaptation follows, and the next step is innovation—providing different, better and new services and products, new conveniences, new responses. The best innovation is one that is different and creates a new potential for satisfaction, whether it is totally new or is a new use for an old product. Like change and marketing, innovation must be built in and extended throughout an organization if it is to grow and prosper. The need for occupational therapists to adopt this way of thinking is obvious during this time of healthcare services transformation. Managing innovation is a challenge and an excellent test of competence for all managers.[10]

CHANGES IN HEALTHCARE DELIVERY

Lessons can be learned by heeding managers from industries outside health care, leaders of high-tech corporations, for example. Advice from one such manager was to adapt or die.[11] His view was that everyone is operating in a new environment shaped by globalization and the information revolution, with everything happening faster. The resulting changes have created a less kind, less gentle, and less predictable workplace. He saw a need for managers to develop a higher tolerance for disorder, to be mentally and emotionally ready for turbulence, and to anticipate the unexpected. His motto: Let chaos reign, then rein in chaos. The kind of planning he advocated was the way a fire department plans: not able to predict fires, the firefighters shape a flexible organization capable of responding to unpredictable events. He concluded with the observation that nobody owes you a career; instead, continuously look for ways to make things better, increase your output, "plug in" to what is going on around you, and try new ideas.[11]

Within the healthcare delivery system, professionals other than occupational therapists are also having to adapt to changes. Physiatrists are acting as case managers for patients with chronic conditions and disabilities, providing primary care services to their patients, collaborating with a variety of other medical specialists, joining other specialty groups to provide a wider spectrum of care, joining HMOs, and providing industrial and occupational medicine services.[12] Physical therapists with private practices that manage to survive have done so by analyzing the marketplace and using strategic planning to ensure that their practices grow. They have reacted to change by negotiating contracts with HMOs, joining provider networks, merging with other independent practices, and introducing new services and packages. Occupational and physical therapists have found that multidisciplinary networking and banding together of practices has been the answer in some cases, contracting with insurers and other payers to market healthcare services, and sharing knowledge instead of engaging in competitiveness.

As previously noted in and from a *philosophical* perspective, too many are watching for too long the doors that are closing and missing those that are opening. Looking at that same concern from a *practical* viewpoint, the same forces that close the doors and reduce one's income also bring about once-in-a-lifetime opportunities to grow and prosper. You must be open, aware, and ready to direct fundamental occupational therapy skills in new directions, perhaps to where no one has yet imagined going. Why not? "In the New Economy there are no tracks to guide careers, only stars—skills, habits of mind."[13]

REHABILITATION MANAGERS ADAPT

A recent survey of rehabilitation services managers in the Chicago area[14] found that they have used a variety of strategies to cope effectively with changes in organization and service delivery and with the industry's goal to "do more with less." Ways they have discovered to be effective include increasing staff productivity through larger caseloads and work redesign, expanding hours, flexing staff, using more part-time staff, developing new patient care programs, expanding outpatient services, and supporting and educating staff to maintain morale, prevent burnout, and aid retention.

SOME ADAPTED TO COMMUNITY MENTAL HEALTH CARE, SOME DIDN'T

Nielson[15] provided an appropriate example of those closing and opening doors in her opinion of community health and occupational therapy in 1994. Her belief was that occupational therapists in the United States failed to respond successfully to deinstitutionalization in the 1960s. Because of that, she observed, they did not progress to their full potential as a rehabilitation presence in community mental health programs.

There were other earlier warnings, such as Ethridge's[16] in 1984. At that time he declared that the ongoing shift of mental health services from state administrations and facilities to community and local administrations dramatically affected the traditional occupational therapy service delivery pattern. He warned that, in response, occupational therapists should move into a different model of service, one that is consultative, community oriented, and independent, or they would be replaced entirely by other professions.

According to Nielson,[15] some occupational therapists did meet the challenge proactively to position themselves as dynamic rehabilitation professionals in community mental health. They are employed in services that include crisis intervention and management, day and partial hospitalization, group homes, and addiction programs as agency employees, consultants, or administrators. It was her further contention that any healthcare practitioner, to be successful, must either gain autonomous power or work with existing power sources.

One example of a successful outcome in community mental health is an innovative project, headed by an occupational therapist, that is teaching high-cost utilizers of mental health services how to live independently in the community. Cynthia McCoy, OTR, heads a multidisciplinary team of 24 workers in a nonprofit organization that stresses self-sufficiency and productivity. Since initiating the program, there has been an average savings to her California county of $8800 per person served. The 110 people in the program receive preemployment training, are helped to obtain employment at local businesses, and are provided opportunities for paid work experience. Teamwork among peers and self-help rather than dependence on staff are encouraged. For McCoy this type of position demonstrates successful adaptation, as she came into it following 23 years of working in a traditional medical model. She now considers it to be the way that psychiatric occupational therapy is best practiced.[17]

Nielson agreed with Ethridge that a key premise underlying working within the community mental health system is a shift in occupational therapy emphasis from direct involvement with clients to more indirect roles. Nielson said that indirect roles such as those of consultant, case manager, or program administrator do not lessen the impact of occupational therapy. To work in other than a clearly defined role is an idea that does not come easily and naturally to many experienced occupational therapists. Adams,[18] too, described community mental health occupational therapists as those who bridge gaps in service provision, coordinate discharge plans, serve as liaisons to family members, and interact with the public.

Nielson found a number of occupational therapists practicing in community mental health who had successfully re-formed and integrated their identities as occupational therapists into community health positions, contributing a unique perspective clearly focused on client needs and outcomes. Here again can be detected the basic marketing process at work in new mutual exchanges, as she noted that these occupational therapists "know their consumers and their needs, and they speak the language of each group." More evidence of the marketing process at work can be found in her comment that "community mental health occupational therapists have succeeded because they *understood the barriers* and faced them as challenges. [They] share a strong belief in and understanding of intervention programs that are functionally oriented and *meaningful to their consumers, to agencies, and to people who pay the bills*" [emphasis added].[15]

▦ Continuous Adaptations in Education

Two Pew Health Professions Commission reports in 1991 and 1993 made suggestions relevant to potential additions to occupational therapy educational programs. From among those suggestions, only two are mentioned here. Shugars, O'Neil, and Bader[19] encouraged professional training in multicultural, community-based service delivery, and O'Neil[20] charged healthcare professional schools to provide clinical education programs in emerging settings and to foster environments that promote innovation and leadership.

EDUCATIONAL CHANGE AND ADAPTATION

Different knowledge and skills will be required to meet the responsibilities accompanying these new roles and environments. Occupational therapy educational programs and professional associations are obligated to make their own adaptations in order to continue responding with new continuing education topics and updated academic course content.

The AOTA was cognizant of the short amount of time and limited space available in already crowded professional education curricula. For example, in response to the *Essentials* requirement for increased education related to the COTA-OTR relationship, AOTA formed a task force in 1995 to address this issue. A combined group of certified occupational therapy assistants and registered occupational therapists developed an educational unit to send to academic programs around the country, having recognized that this is a content issue as well as one of quality. (See Chapter 11 for more detailed coverage of this topic.)

FIELDWORK INNOVATION

Occupational therapy educational programs have begun to respond to some of the statements of the Pew publications. Locating fieldwork placements has become a challenge that grows at an alarming rate, and educational program fieldwork placement staff are using creativity and innovation to locate alternative types of training sites that reflect current trends in healthcare delivery. As practice settings have expanded beyond traditional medical facilities into schools, employment settings, day care centers for both children and the elderly, technology centers, residential care facilities, and independent living centers, proactive educational program directors have directed their attention to these same sites. Opacich[21] suggested that matches be made among students' needs and aptitudes, the philosophies of the educational programs, and the potential fieldwork sites. The result should be highly invested, independent clinicians who are able to address a wide range of human performance problems.

Now that public school systems are becoming the largest employers of occupational therapy practitioners, training students to work in schools has become a critical challenge for educators. Rural school-based occupational therapists are particularly beset with on-the-job pressures for large daily caseloads, travel, school scheduling, educational duties, and bureaucratic regulations. Providing level 2 fieldwork opportunities for students is a major problem. The Division of Occupational Therapy at the University of Washington in Seattle responded by developing a model training program to improve the training and distribution of occupational therapists specializing in pediatrics in rural areas of the northwestern United States. Specialized courses provided occupational therapy students with the specific skills they needed in their level 2 placements in pediatric rural settings. A fieldwork 2 training manual furnished guidelines and examples of training components so that other therapists could implement similar programs.[22]*

Further progress toward addressing the fieldwork challenge was made when the Representative Assembly passed Resolution D in 1996. Authored by Penny Moyers, EdD, OTR, and Sharan Schwartzberg, EdD, OTR, the resolution called for continuous marketing for clinical facility administrators, cost-effective research studies, and academic fieldwork coordinator training in obtaining and developing new fieldwork level 2 sites. Amendments provided funding for market research, cost-benefit analysis, and a plan based on research findings.[23]

▨ Transformations in Practice

New "rules" are changing the location and kind of care that most clients receive today. Occupational therapy clinics respond daily to new insurance mandates, outcomes measures requirements, niche marketing, cost containment, and consumer demands. In addition to these changing incentives, the settings and the client populations have themselves changed in many instances and have caused expansion in the scope of occupational therapy practice. For instance,

---

Occupational Therapy Fieldwork II Training Manual: School-Based Practice in Rural Settings can be purchased for $18 from the Health Sciences Center for Educational Resources, University of Washington, Mail Stop SB-56, Seattle, WA 98195.

not too many years ago neither traumatic brain-injured (TBI) nor high-level spinal cord–injured (SCI) patients usually survived, and today they form a growing percentage of those benefiting from the services of occupational therapists, as do pulmonary patients. Many pediatric clients previously seen as inpatients are now treated by occupational therapists in school-based and early intervention programs.

In Virginia, occupational therapists Jean Hearst and Sherry Johnson responded to a demand for pediatric services in their community by expanding their private company to respond to the need. Heeding parents' comments and local therapists' observations and using their innovative and determined staff, they provide therapeutic summer groups for children with developmental needs. A sensorimotor group, therapeutic aquatics program, and a loops and groups handwriting program were developed and offered in summer when these services were most needed. In addition to that venture, their organization is working to make housing more accessible to the elderly and to other persons with disabilities.[24]

In Texas, occupational therapists Jean Polichino and Jaclyn Low helped shape the state's policy on managed care and the provision of Medicaid services to children with disabilities. They were selected by the Texas Department of Health to serve as vice chair and member, respectively, on a Medicaid panel, along with two physical therapists, two speech-language pathologists, a pediatric neurologist, orthopedic surgeon, a parent of a child with a disability, and an adult who received services as a child.[25]

▨ New Opportunities for Intraprofessional Collaboration

One of the most promising "opening doors" is the burgeoning opportunity for expanding collaboration among all levels of occupational therapy personnel. Potential gains for everyone concerned are immeasurable, whether these persons are occupational therapy aides, certified occupational therapy assistants, occupational therapists educated at the bachelor's, master's, or doctoral level, or occupational therapists with specialized advanced clinical certifications. Registered occupational therapists are and will be moving into the more indirect service roles of consultation, supervision, research, and management, while growing responsibilities for direct therapy relationships are assumed by certified occupational therapy assistants and by aides.[26] Graduate-level occupational therapists, especially those with doctorates, will continue to be expected to serve their profession through research that develops the theoretical base and validates practice. Maximum use of budgeted funds in practice settings can be made with wise division of work among personnel who share complementary occupational therapy educational backgrounds and professional organizational memberships.

▦ Occupational Therapy Shines on the Home Front

Under managed care, less time is spent with patients than previously, thus requiring extensive adaptations in approach and regimen; however, many occupational therapists have found the more goal-oriented model of treatment to be an improvement, once they have become accustomed to this service delivery transformation. Rather than seeing an acute care client in a series of treatment sessions complete as much functional independence as can be accomplished on site in the occupational therapy clinic, as previously, the occupational therapist has become part of an interdisciplinary team during this early phase of care.

The even greater strength of occupational therapy lies in the postdischarge phase of care. Where clients actually live is where occupational therapists shine, for they understand the critical need for every person to be helped to adapt as fully as possible to his or her living environment after discharge. Universal outcome measures seldom address those needs that have subjective, personal, individualized meaning and priority for clients. Discharged clients face complex challenges that are best perceived, understood, and resolved together with occupational therapists.

So far, changes in the healthcare system have been aimed primarily at efficiency measures to improve productivity. Occupational therapists must pay attention to what they do and why they do it and join together the business of saving money *and* improving clients' health. Occupational therapists must assume the responsibility for the part they played—through action or inaction—in bringing about the current state of affairs. Furthermore, changes made must have built-in evaluation components that provide the data needed to prove assertions that occupational therapy services are important and valuable and truly make a measurable difference.

▦ The Change Leader

Those who are successfully leading change in today's workplace have a nice balance of abilities: They are technically skillful and also very capable in personal relationships, are tough decision-makers who know how to energize people and align them in the same direction, can operate with more than one leadership style, and can shift easily from a team approach to command and control, if necessary. It's an attitude. It can be learned and developed!

▦ Summary

This chapter highlighted the development and growth of occupational therapy and showed that the very history of occupational therapy is a tale of adaptation, innovation, and entrepreneurship. With this precedent, tales of the continuation of adaptation to change in practice and education today reveal that occupational therapy practitioners have continued to make the role of change leaders natural and evident. Examples were given of change that has been successfully accommodated and enhanced by corporate executives, by health professional peers, and by occupational therapy colleagues, with lessons to be learned from all of them. It was strongly urged once again that more attention be paid and effort given to building intraprofessional collaboration among all levels of occupational therapy personnel. The potential strength and powerful role to be played by occupational therapy in home-based care was reiterated, as was the inherent capacity of occupational therapy practitioners and educators to be change leaders in this domain as well. Part Six continues with a closer look at structural reorganization and changing management styles in today's business and its meaning for occupational therapy.

"The tiger who does not prowl is a potential rug." (Charles Farrell)

REFERENCES

1. Slagle, EC: Training Aides for Mental Patients: Papers on Occupational Therapy, State Hospital Press, Utica, NY, 1922.
2. Constitution of the National Society for the Promotion of Occupational Therapy. Sheppard Hospital Press, Baltimore, 1917.
3. Bing, R: William Rush Dunton, Jr.: American Psychiatrist, a Study in Self. Unpublished doctoral dissertation, University of Maryland, 1961.
4. Spackman, CS: A history of the practice of occupational therapy for restoration of physical function: 1917–1967. Am J Occup Ther 22:68, 1968.
5. Hopkins, HL, and Smith, HD: Willard and Spackman's Occupational Therapy, ed 6. JB Lippincott, Philadelphia, 1983.
6. West, W: The occupational therapist's changing responsibility to the community. Am J Occup Ther 21:312, 1967.
7. Reilly, M: The challenge of the future to an occupational therapist. Am J Occup Ther 20:221, 1966.
8. Mosey, AC: An alternative: The biopsychosocial model. Am J Occup Ther 23:140, 1974.
9. American Occupational Therapy Association: Occupational Therapy 2001. AOTA, Rockville, Md, 1979.
10. Drucker, PF: An Introductory View of Management. Harper's College Press, New York, 1977.
11. Grove, AS: A high-tech CEO updates his views on managing and careers. Fortune 132:229, Sept 18, 1995.
12. Christopher, RP: Physiatry adapts to change. Rehab Management 7(6):47, 1994.
13. Stewart, TA: Navigating by starlight: Career guidance from the class of 1970. Fortune 132:253, Aug 7, 1995.
14. Grace, IA: Charting changes in rehab. OT Week 9(7):15, Feb 7, 1995.
15. Nielson, C: Occupational therapy and community health: A new and unprecedented turn. WFOT Bulletin 30(13):11, Nov, 1994.
16. Ethridge, DA: Issues and trends in mental health practice. Occupational Therapy In Health Care 7(4):3, 1984.
17. Hettinger, J: The portals partners project. OT Week 9(34):18, Aug 24, 1995.
18. Adams, R: The role of occupational therapists in community mental health. Mental Health Special Interest Section Newsletter, Mar, 1990, p 1.

19. Shugars, DA, O'Neil, EH, and Bader, D (eds): Healthy America: Practitioners for 2005: An Agenda for Action for U.S. Health Professional Schools. The Pew Health Professions Commission, Durham, NC, 1991.
20. O'Neil, EH: Health Professions Education for the Future: Schools in Service to the Nation. The Pew Health Professions Commission, San Francisco, 1993.
21. Opacich, KJ: Is an educational philosophy missing from the fieldwork solution? Am J Occup Ther 49:160, 1995.
22. Amundson, SJ, and Kanny, E: Off the beaten path. OT Week 9(13):18, Mar 30, 1995.
23. Kerr, T: Implications of resolution D: Can we end the fieldwork crisis? Advance for Occupational Therapists 12(24):13, June 17, 1996.
24. Mraz-Geary, K: Filling the gaps. OT Week 9(13):11, Mar 30, 1995.
25. Hettinger, J: Texas OTs help shape Medicaid. OT Week 9(43):10, Oct 26, 1995.
26. Hettinger, J: A question of roles. OT Week 9(39):18, Sept 28, 1995.

PART SIX

THE CHANGING WORLD OF ORGANIZATION AND MANAGEMENT

In the middle of difficulty lies opportunity.

Albert Einstein

CHAPTER 14

The Flattened Pyramid and Managed Care

CHAPTER OBJECTIVES

- To realize that there is a new career paradigm for everyone, including occupational therapists.
- To follow the pattern of changes in organizational structure and management.
- To visualize the transitioning organizational structures.
- To understand the structure of the horizontal company.
- To become acquainted with the altered roles and approaches of most managers.
- To comprehend the nature of work redesign and the depths of transformation that result.
- To appreciate employee empowerment and the complexities of teamwork in action.
- To apply examples of corporate team-based management to healthcare services delivery.
- To see the role of competition related to team behavior.
- To recognize illustrations of reversals today in priorities of humanism and technology.

- To see variations in forms of managed care and how they have evolved.
- To realize that there are variations in the definitions and realities of utilization review.
- To understand how occupational therapists should approach their roles in managed care.

An occupational therapist is rarely, if ever, offered a lifetime career by an institution anymore. Occupational therapists today create their own career ladders through their own productivity and innovation. The business of earning a living and planning for the future requires a major attitude adjustment on the part of every new graduate emerging from an educational program of study with that hard-earned credential in hand. This is in no way a condemnation, for most Americans today share a feeling of confusion as they face new ways of earning their livings, feelings in many ways similar to 18th-century workers at the outset of the Industrial Age.

The new paradigm requires all workers to continuously reassess where they stand vis-à-vis their careers and financially and be ready to change direction if obligated or if a new opportunity sounds inviting. Often a challenge provides the incentive and perspective needed to dispel the confusion and find a secure new career direction. As Naisbett, Toffler, and other futurists have pointed out beginning 25 years ago, there has never in history been such a breathtaking acceleration in the rate of change. People must run to stay in place, let alone respond and innovate. Simply managing the accumulated knowledge of individual employees into a usable asset is an overwhelming task. Some large corporations are trying to make knowledge management a recognized discipline similar to human resources or fiscal affairs, as they have found their information systems are inadequate to collect useful management data and are not user friendly.

Part Six discusses how the structure, organization, and management of work and jobs has changed, how the role of manager has also been transformed and has evolved as a result of those changes, and some of the problems and issues faced by occupational therapy practitioners as a result of these evolving changes.

Changes in the Way a Manager Manages

The basic functions generally performed by a manager at any level continue to consist fundamentally of planning, organizing, directing, coordinating, and controlling. This book, however, does not include the study of management functions and processes. For those readers seeking information about the fundamentals of management, a list of selected references has been provided at the end of this chapter.

When Peter Drucker published his classic *The Practice of Management* in 1954, management had been seen mostly as the expression of rank and power. Today the quality of managerial leadership is being judged on attitude and action rather than authority. In 1983 Rosabeth Moss Kanter's[1] *The Change Masters: Innovation for Productivity in the American Corporation* created a stir in the business community as she asserted that business organizations were facing the most fundamental changes since the "modern" industrial system took shape between 1890 and 1920. She contended that these changes in the American business community came from several sources: the labor force, patterns of world trade, technology, and political forces. By 1995 Bridges[2] believed that the job had become a social artifact from the Industrial Revolution. In today's workplace the benchmark is no longer title or status but who gets the work done.

Compounding the gravity of the unusual situation is the fact that these changes were all profound and occurring simultaneously. Ubiquitous evidence demonstrates that the pace of change has accelerated since 1983 through every part of the corporate world, including healthcare service delivery. Indicative of this changing order, Peter Senge's[3] *The Fifth Discipline* in the 1990s stressed that people are more than cogs, that they are to be empowered, and their thoughts, feelings, and insights are to be heard and understood.

In the 1950s and 1960s, U.S. industry more or less pleased itself as to what products were manufactured, especially as far as autos were concerned. However, in the 1970s global competition began to expand, and American corporations began to realize that they needed to organize around the notion of serving the customer: the marketing concept.

It is the opinion of some that over the past 40 years only a few broad management principles have proved to have surviving power and are worthy of serious consideration today:[2]

1. Management is a practice.
2. People are a resource.
3. Marketing and innovation are the key functions of a business.
4. Discover what you do well.
5. Quality pays for itself.

▓ The Pyramid Falls

The new organization is like a symphony orchestra, Drucker suggested; Boyett and Conn[4] pictured it as a "flatter and leaner pancake organization." Others have dubbed it a transformation from hierarchical and bureaucratic to flat, flexible, and quality focused. Many have attempted to describe the posthierarchical organization in a more detailed fashion, but a clear, universal picture seems still out of reach. One thing is certain: Organizational structure is different today. Customer needs define business units, and the people and processes necessary

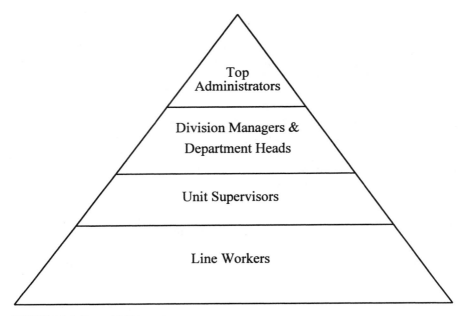

FIGURE 14–1. Pyramidal hierarchy.

to serve these needs are grouped into business units. Three characteristics appear in most: empowering employees, management of processes rather than functional departments, and rapid distribution of knowledge, accountability, and results. Companies put the three together in forms that are uniquely practical for each of them. The planned change that goes into such organizational transformations involves common sense, continuing hard work, an organizationwide goal-oriented approach, and solid knowledge about organizational dynamics. With the understanding that there are many configurations in place today, Figures 14–1 to 14–3 illustrate basic differences among a pyramidal hierarchy, a variation of the matrix type of organizational structure, and a version of the program management model.

BIG CORPORATIONS CAN SURVIVE IF . . .

Articles concerning organizational transformation appear in almost all recent American business publications, most centering on corporate culture, changing attitudes of American workers, greater employee participation in managerial decision making, and employees as an important asset of corporations. For years, companies' top executives worked on operating plans mostly centered around specific projects and based on "what we are going to do in the next year." Instead, they now begin with "where we want to be in the next 3, 4, and 5 years."

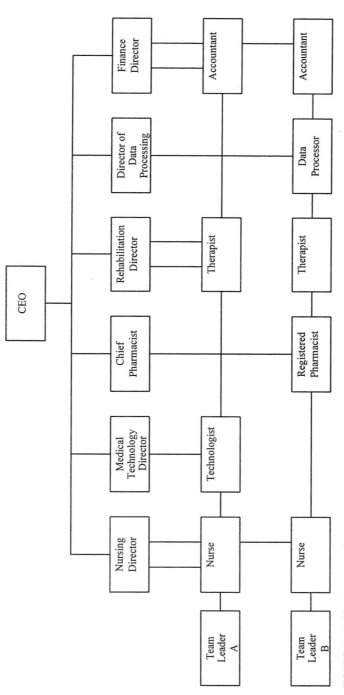

FIGURE 14–2. Matrix organizational structure.

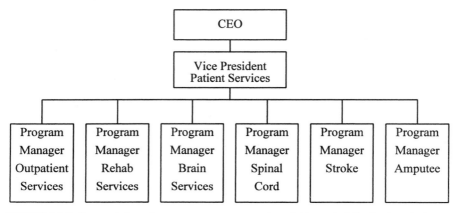

FIGURE 14–3. One variation of a program management model in a rehabilitation hospital.

A well-grounded, well-conceived vision of what the organization seeks to become is the cornerstone of a fast-tracking transformation effort. It is the master plan through which the transformation process can be assessed and modified.

Big corporations are not going to disappear, but to survive they must combine the benefits of size (money and talent) with the best features of small businesses: focus, flexibility, and speed. Drucker's opinion is that "they will slowly and painfully transform themselves into a new kind of creature that combines the clout of a giant with the nimbleness of an entrepreneurial elf,"[5] and Chuck Ames of Clayton, Dublier, and Rice of New York says, "Small is not better, focused is better."

GONE IS THE OLD CEO TYPE

Many alterations within major corporations have evolved out of changes in relationships among management, boards of directors, and shareholders. In 1992, 13 CEOs from the Fortune 500 were ousted from their positions. As the Alcoa chief said, "The imperial CEO is doomed."[6] The move was declared to be a reversal of the decades-old tendency of corporate power to be in the hands of executive officers rather than directors or owners, a reversal that was predicted to change corporate America for a long time. If not actually dethroned, many CEOs were reduced to far less than imperial powers.

In answer to a question about what the manager's role would be like in the future, many agreed that executive *leadership* is becoming more indispensable than ever. Only the executive can mediate among all the constituencies trying to influence every corporation: investors, lenders, communities, employees, and customers; however, that person is now more constrained by needing to stay in closer touch, to listen to the constituents, and to manage for the long term.[6]

Not all leaders of large corporations have worn blinders, however. At General Electric, Chairman John F. Welch seemed to be Drucker's "entrepreneurial elf." Few corporations are bigger and none more complex, for GE makes 65-cent light bulbs, 400,000-pound locomotives, and billion-dollar power plants. Its chairman, however, wants to run it like a small business, taking out the boss element. His opinion is that 21st-century managers will give up their old powers of planning, organizing, implementing, and measuring to assume new duties: counseling groups, providing resources for them, and helping them think for themselves. His statement was, "We're going to win on our ideas, not by whips and chains."[7] Welch maintained that there is no contradiction between his hardnosed reputation for demanding superior performance and soft concepts like employee involvement. He insisted on getting everyone in the organization involved and, by doing that, found that the best ideas rose to the top.

GONE ARE MANY MIDDLE MANAGERS

In addition to those at the top of the hierarchy who have, in many cases, found their jobs to be "redundant," many in middle management positions have found themselves victims of restructuring. Because of the great number who are seeking new positions, outplacement firms have found themselves doing booming business. The most successful unemployed managers are finding new niches born of change.

Displaced managers are being advised that if they expect to be hired they must expect to pursue some unfamiliar paths: transform themselves from being overseers into doers, from bosses into team leaders or maybe just team players. They are being informed that they will less often tell people what to do and more often take responsibility for the success or failure of the business. Skills will be measured on a global scale, and computer fluency will be required. They are also being told that the leadership challenge in the 21st century will be to recalibrate people to global standards. The leader who is multilingual, multicultural, and fluent in information technology will come out ahead, predict some who are advising new managers.[8]

▨ The Need to Expect Change

W. Edwards Deming, father of the quality-management movement, at 92 still commanded respect, admiration, and close attention for his wisdom, perception, and endless energy. One day when Deming was teaching about fear and anxiety in the workplace at General Motors, one of the employees there, who helped workers learn about quality-control techniques, was asked how the GM employees felt about all the changes they were having to make. His reply was, "For the most part, people accept that if we don't change no one's going to have a job. We can't continue to run with blinders on."[9] Occupational therapists would do well to think about this observation.

Organizational Responsiveness

One way to be better prepared and to make accommodations for change is to develop the habit of being open and responsive to others, listening carefully, and responding. Being responsive individually as well as on an organizational level is recognized as essential throughout the healthcare service delivery scene. Organizational responsiveness can be classified on four levels:

1. The unresponsive organization does not encourage customer inquiries, complaints, or suggestions; does not monitor whether customers are satisfied; and does not promote staff who are tuned in to customers.

2. The casually responsive organization listens to customer suggestions or opinions but does nothing about them.

3. The highly responsive organization conducts ongoing consumer satisfaction surveys, investigates unmet consumer needs and preferences, passes the information gathered on to employees to help them better serve consumers, and hires and trains staff to be attentive and polite as well as clinically competent.

4. The fully responsive organization expands the work of the highly responsive organization by thoughtfully accepting or rejecting consumer complaints and suggestions on the basis of established organizational priorities.[10]

WHERE TO BEGIN

One first step toward creating a fully responsive organization would be to ask yourself and everyone employed within the organization to complete the statement, "I could serve our clients better if. . . . " Beginning with each individual's personal commitment to accountability for his or her actions, the collective contributions of everyone will move the organization toward the goal of becoming a responsive institution.

The Horizontal Company

As pyramids flatten as a result of changes in structure, a more horizontally configured organizational shape emerges. A 10-point blueprint for a horizontal company was conceived by Frank Ostroff and Doug Smith[11] for McKinsey & Company. Following is an adaptation of those points:

1. Organize primarily around process, not task, with performance objectives based on customer needs, the processes identified that meet those needs, and these processes incorporated as the company's main components.

2. Flatten the hierarchy by minimizing the subdivision of processes, thus eliminating having a series of teams with each doing fewer steps.

3. Give a senior leader charge of processes and process performance.

4. Link performance objectives and evaluation of all activities to customer satisfaction.

5. Make teams, not individuals, the focus of organization performance and design.

6. Combine managerial and nonmanagerial activities as often as possible. For example, let teams take on hiring, evaluating, and scheduling.

7. Emphasize that each employee should develop several competencies. You need fewer specialists.

8. Inform and train people on a need-to-perform basis.

9. Maximize interpersonal contacts and joint problem-solving teams.

10. Reward both individual skill development and team performance instead of individual performance alone.[11]

WORK REDESIGN

Another consequence of organizational changes has, in many cases, been elimination of some jobs. Downsizing or reduction in numbers of staff in an organization became increasingly prevalent in the 1990s. How to proceed was a topic about which many had—and have—opinions. One study of more than 300 organizations, including 117 hospitals, compared the results of hospitals that used across-the-board cuts to reduce given numbers of positions and those that used data-driven work-redesign methods. *Work redesign* means using "a clinical model to collect data, diagnose organizational problems, and prescribe solutions which redesign individual work roles."[12] The skills mix in an organization was changed, and people with certain levels of training and pay were placed to perform work at corresponding levels. It was admitted that problems did arise when duties and tasks were not objectively assigned based on patients' needs and the essential functions of specific roles. Overall, the results of the study determined that there were sustained cost savings, no increases in mortality and morbidity rates, improved perceptions of quality of care by patients and physicians, and higher rates of leadership retention. The work-redesign method of change was found to be a client-focused restructuring methodology.

DEPTH OF TRANSFORMATION

While some reengineering requires minimal change within an organization, many companies are changed in ways beyond just a shifting of boxes on an organizational chart. Managers are expected to promote and nurture improvement and innovation; control is replaced as the fundamental management job. To be successful, the manager must be able to confer empowerment and account-ability simultaneously. (One can detect here the time-honored admonition that rights and responsibility must go hand in hand in delegated tasks.) New and serious recognition has been given to this particular managerial responsibility.

One variation of this can be found at AES Corporation in Montville, Connecticut, where members of an ad hoc team manage a $33 million plant investment fund; CEO Dennis W. Bakke claimed that the more individual responsibility is increased, the better the chances for improved operations. A member of the company's board, Robert H. Waterman Jr. (coauthor of *In Search of Excellence*), insisted that employees can get involved however they wish without being concerned about crossing boundaries.[13]

Another example would be Sam Walton and his Wal-Mart stores. He created the chain by giving customers what they wanted: low prices and a modicum of service administered by employees who care because they share the company's ideals as well as its profits. Regardless of personal opinions, the fact that the idea has been successful cannot be denied. It developed through total communication, constant awareness of all aspects of the operation, a push of responsibility—and thus authority—toward the "front lines" and toward those who are in daily contact with customers, ideas forced to percolate by encouraging store associates to share ideas for improvement, and avoidance of big egos.

Walton[14] shared his personal "rules":

1. Be committed to your business.
2. Share your profits with all your associates, and treat them as partners.
3. Motivate your partners constantly, setting high goals, encouraging, challenging, and rewarding them.
4. Communicate everything to your partners, as they will understand more and thus care more.
5. Appreciate everything your associates do for the business.
6. Celebrate your successes and find some humor in your failures. Loosen up and don't take yourself too seriously. Always be enthusiastic.
7. Listen to everyone in your company because the people on the front lines are the only ones who know what's going on. You *must* listen to what your associates are trying to tell you.

One final comment made by Walton regarding the main reason for his success was that for people to achieve success in business they must overcome one of the most powerful forces in human nature: resistance to change. To succeed in this world, you have to change all the time.[14]

ORGANIZATION AROUND PROCESSES

Using a structure that organizes around processes rather than functions permits (actually requires) greater self-management and allows organizations to dismantle unneeded supervisory positions. Law firms, having only three levels of hierarchy—associate, partner, and senior partner—might be considered as a model for one's career path, with the new graduate progressing through more and more complex work on the way to career goals. Titles would not change, but advancement would result from successful performance, with everyone recognizing those with the highest status. This is one more illustration of the fact that a major outcome of organizational restructuring is a renewed emphasis on the employee and a new recognition of individual responsibility.

The work-redesign issue is reminiscent of the dilemma, in healthcare delivery, of cross-trained personnel. The effects of some decisions about cross-training have already been felt among occupational therapy practitioners, and there are indications that this will continue. Chapter 18 discusses this decision and its ramifications.

Employee Empowerment

Employee empowerment is a broad term that can mean an employee suggestion box or, at the high end of the scale, self-directed work teams. Recent studies found that 83 percent of the companies surveyed had experimented with self-directed work teams and planned to increase their usage.[15] Employee empowerment gives workers four major responsibilities: authority, resources, information, and accountability. At the same time, quality assurance and continuous quality improvement must be addressed on the job. To accomplish such multiple assignments, self-directed teams have appeared in hospitals and other healthcare institutions.

Although relatively autonomous in many cases, teams do require guidance and boundaries. The manager's role has been modified but certainly not eliminated in organizations in which self-directed work teams are found. Employees on the teams still need management support and guidance. Generally in these situations managers concentrate on team development while keeping the vision and purpose of the organization before the members.

Teamwork Is Harder Than It Looks

In the 1990s the corporate world adopted team-based management as a miracle cure for what ailed organizations. In many cases this was a great success, such as the egalitarian teams introduced at Boeing, Volvo, Hewlett-Packard, and Federal Express; however, in some instances the difficulties associated with successfully integrating the notion of team-based management resulted in less than ideal situations. Managers who did not realize the amount of patience and perception required were disappointed. Human nature intervened, as team leaders refused to share authority and team members disagreed on who got credit for what.

One study looked at successful teamwork found outside of the corporate scene among such diverse groups as the U.S. Navy SEALs, the five Dallas Cowboys offensive linemen, the Tokyo String Quartet, and the University of North Carolina women's soccer team. The common thread throughout was that in each case the team members had created a collective ego, getting results different than those engendered by a group of people merely working side by side. A main ingredient was humility, a scarce thing, concluded the writer, in the business world. The four members of the string quartet did not think about who got to showcase a great sound or technique; instead, they projected as one and put forth the group's musical personality. The Cowboys' linemen reported that the anonymity of playing on the line did not bother them a bit and that they felt good whenever their work as a "family" in the background brought about a touchdown.[16]

Sabbagh[17] described successful teamwork at Boeing in a book about the construction of the 777 jetliner. The team-based management scheme came about when Boeing officials broke up the departments of engineers, designers, and manufacturing workers and re-formed them into 250 multidisciplinary groups. Each of the design-build teams, or DBTs, was totally responsible for its own part of the jet from conception to final assembly. The group dynamics were reportedly sometimes chaotic, and the problems of integrating the work as the project neared completion were many, but the 777 became the ultimate technical success.

▨ Teamwork in Health Care

The quest for ideal teamwork configurations and attitudes, whether it is the Cowboys' linemen or the Tokyo String Quartet or Wal-Mart or a healthcare team, will no doubt continue. Most human work is carried out in teams, and even the most solitary artists or painters depend on others for their work to become effective.[18] As described in Chapter 8, three kinds of teams can be envisioned. Those on a baseball team are similar to a surgical team: they are playing *on*, but not *as*, a team because each has a fixed position. A soccer team resembles the emergency room group that plays *on and as* a team. A symphony orchestra can be likened to doubles tennis, as all have preferred positions but *adjust, adapt, and cover* for each other's strengths and weaknesses. Only by choosing the appropriate team players and combinations can a manager improve the productivity of healthcare workers in program management models.

Another perspective on ideal teams among healthcare professionals was offered by Diane Komp,[19] a pediatric oncologist at Yale University School of Medicine, who suggested that healthcare reformers look at the hospice model for bringing professionals, clients, and the community together to solve other healthcare problems. Komp recognized the importance of not only treating the body but also providing comfort and help for the mind and spirit. Forming a team during the hospital phase of cancer treatment or when hospice care is needed, the goal is always to keep the client as the central figure on the team. With the central focus on the client, the team moves as a unit to provide the special care needed by client and family.

According to professionals in acute care settings in Texas, increased patient acuity, decreased reimbursement for services, and shorter lengths of stay affect all hospital clinicians. Initial reactions to recent changes in how critical care is provided have ranged from stoic to emphatically positive. However, critical care staff have learned that accepting new ways to perform work is not optional; to survive today with managed care means to work as teams. Actually, in many instances, the emphasis on teamwork has helped to smooth over old divisions among professionals. In most hospitals, intensive care unit (ICU) staff members expressed being pleased, for the most part, by the changes in the way they work. Elizabeth DeGuzman, nurse manager of the 30-bed ICU at Ben Taub General Hospital in Houston, summed it up by saying that "the more understanding we have, the more marketable we'll be."[20]

▓ Competition as It Relates to Team Behavior

There is most certainly a realistic and important place for competition in an infinite variety of situations, such as entrepreneurism itself. However, in keeping with the need for team approaches stressed in this chapter, it need not become a stumbling block to the kind of performance expected in healthcare teams. Competition is pervasive but at the same time has a destructive component. Kohn[21] conducted several studies on the subject that resulted in pinpointing four prevalent myths:

Myth 1: Competition is inevitable. Rather than attributing competition to "human nature," the studies determined that competitive behavior is a matter of social training and culture instead of a built-in feature. Competition is a learned behavior.

Myth 2: Competition keeps productivity high and is necessary for excellence. Kohn found that other researchers across the country agreed with his conclusion that many who claim that competition boosts achievement and brings out the best in us have simply confused success with competition. He cited one series of studies that found a significant negative correlation between competitiveness and achievement. Additional findings were that competition is often highly stressful and that competition makes it difficult to share skills, experiences, and resources, as can be done with cooperation.

Myth 3: Recreation requires competition. Results found that recreation does not have to involve activities in which each player is trying to make the other fail.

Myth 4: Competition builds character. Competing does nothing to strengthen the shaky self-esteem that gave rise to it because the potential for humiliation is present in every competitive encounter. Moreover, victory is never permanent, and empirical evidence shows that competition is anything but constructive.[21]

The conclusion is that competition has its value and place in certain human endeavors, but it does have destructive components. If successful teamwork is the goal, the presence or use of competition should be carefully evaluated. Managing competition and teamwork are but two of an infinite number of human resource problems associated with management today. Those responsible for the development of technology itself acknowledge the need to recognize human factors, as the following discussion shows.

Humanism and Technology

Frederick Taylor, in the 1880s, sought to increase productivity by making workers more like machines. Today, those responsible for computer development aim to increase the "humanness" of their "machines," an interesting thought for anyone wrestling with balancing humanism and technology in the workplace today. The computer has revolutionized work to a greater extent than any technology since Edison introduced electricity. A common feature touted by purveyors of computers and software is that they are "user-friendly," reminiscent of Naisbett's "high tech–high touch" deliberation in 1982.[22] Computers can be employed to perform the mechanical, repetitive elements of work, which leaves time for the essential human aspects: judging, creating, sensing, and developing human relationships. The 10 most common reengineering mistakes in Hammer and Stanton's *The Reengineering Revolution* all involved managers who ignored such human elements as leadership, courage, and the concerns of the people involved. The decision need not be made *between* technology and humanism but rather a complementary choice that maximizes the values of *both*.

Evolution of Managed Care

Disparate viewpoints of which values hold the highest priority characterize the whole topic of managed care decisions today. A brief explanation of managed care is offered here for clarification as part of the discussion of changes in organizational management in this chapter because the effect of managed care on healthcare delivery is of critical importance. A broad, general definition of *managed care* is management of all aspects of health care by employing both medical expertise and technology to improve the quality of care and to control and reduce the cost. An essential part is the management and processing of information concurrently during delivery of healthcare services.

Group practice prepayment was initiated in the United States in a small clinic in Elk City, Oklahoma, in 1932. It was first put into operation on a large scale by the Kaiser Foundation Health Plan on the West Coast. Since then, the groups who have organized plans, from medical schools to insurance companies, have been widely diverse, and those plans have taken equally diverse forms.[23]

Managed care has entered the healthcare delivery scene in the United States as a measure for providing cost-effective services. One of its elements is *case management*, first initiated to address major traumatic injuries, a model holding one person responsible for developing a plan that takes an individual from the point of injury through medical and rehabilitation interventions to functional independence.

Growth of HMOs precipitated emergence of the *preferred provider organization* (PPO), a managed care system formed by providers who joined forces to discount their fees and become HMO competitors. This competition resulted in the evolution of particular prices for per annum coverage that included most healthcare needs and usually encompassed 60 days of rehabilitation.

In the late 1980s another model of managed care appeared, the *competitive medical plan* (CMP), which covered seniors and allowed them to save some up-front costs on Medicare. Seniors sign over their Medicare rights to the managed care provider and allow the provider to deliver or not deliver in accordance with Medicare guidelines.

Finally, *independent practice associations* (IPA) are physician associations that charge on a capitated basis to maintain health and provide restoration from illness and injury. These associations can have a strong impact on rehabilitation utilization through testing of less expensive alternatives.

Physicians have been admonished in many cases that the manner in which they have previously done business must change and that developing or joining networks is a proactive way to make those changes. Giving up a little independence is suggested as a small price to pay for long-term financial security and increased medical collaboration.[24]

FORMS IN WHICH MANAGED CARE IS CURRENTLY FOUND

The forms managed care takes today cover a wide variety of configurations. As occupational therapy practitioners become increasingly involved, they must become fully familiar with the characteristics of all these structures. Following, in more detail, are explanations of the types of care existing today, with the understanding that new forms and additional approaches are no doubt about to appear. They are mentioned in order from the loosest integration (PPO) to the most complex integration (HMO).

1. Preferred provider organization (PPO): a group of providers who offer healthcare services to beneficiaries through a discounted fee-for-service

   arrangement, with the beneficiary able to choose within the network for a discounted fee, obligated for minimal copayment, and also allowed to seek care outside of the network.

2. Exclusive provider organization (EPO): similar to a PPO, but beneficiaries may seek health care only from participating providers, usually in a program implemented by employers.

3. Independent practice association (IPA): a group of distinct providers who together invest money to form a for-profit association with health care provided by the independent providers in private practice sites; admission rules are set for providers, with each provider choosing contracts for participation.

4. Clinic without walls (CWW) and group practice without walls (GPWW): multisite practices owned by private or public corporations.

5. Physician hospital organizations (PHO): a corporation or foundation formed of physicians and a hospital, usually hospital driven and, usually administered by a management service organization.

6. Health maintenance organization (HMO): a fully integrated system that provides a comprehensive range of health services to an enrolled population for a fixed sum of money paid in advance for a specific period of time.[24]

HMOS: DEFINITION AND CHARACTERISTICS

The term HMO has been used to identify many kinds of healthcare delivery systems. The most commonly adopted definition is a medical care delivery system that accepts responsibility for the organization, financing, and delivery of healthcare services for a specific population.[23] The HMO is characterized by the combination of a financing mechanism (prepayment) and a particular way of delivery (group practice) implemented through a managerial-administrative organization responsible for making sure that health services are available for the subscriber population. The HMO philosophy is that through working with all involved people, healthcare expenditures can be reduced by eliminating unnecessary steps, and money will be saved as compared with the fee-for-service model.

   There are six primary characteristics of HMO operations:

1. Responsibility for organizing and delivering health services: besides providing a financing mechanism, the HMO must secure contracts with providers in order to assure a source of health services for members.

2. Prepayment: fixed periodic payments from subscribers meet the costs of the organization, with some plans supplementing these payments with copayments charged at time of treatment.

3. Group practice: multispecialty groups of physicians maintain facilities capable of providing comprehensive, continuous care.

4. Comprehensive benefits: a complete range of medical services including some forms of preventive care, in most instances.

5. Compensation of physicians: usually the physicians are compensated through use of the capitation principle (payment of a sum equal to a fixed per capita amount for each subscriber multiplied by the number of subscribers enrolled). Also, in most cases, physician groups share in savings generated through effective management of the plan.

6. Voluntary enrollment: most HMOs enroll through a dual choice mechanism; that is, employees may choose between an indemnity plan or the HMO.[23]

NEW PARTNERS

Rehabilitation practices have changed with the continued growth of managed care. More services are delivered in subacute and home settings, and new designs for rehabilitation management have emerged. For example, in all types of settings more professionals are found as consultants and rehabilitation technicians as assistants.

Subacute rehabilitation was a little-known phenomenon a few years ago, but now there is estimated to be a $600 to $750 million subacute industry. For a variety of reasons, political and financial, acute rehabilitation providers have faced greater challenges in developing the subacute rehabilitation level of care. Establishing alliances with other providers has been one way to develop subacute services. Some forms of alliance structures have been leased bed arrangements, long-term contract management, and joint venture development.[25] Rehabilitation providers must develop regional networks, standardize care plans and outcomes standards, and prospectively contract for patients on a per-case basis with insurance companies, HMOs, and self-insured employers. Many small, independent providers have found it prudent to develop networks and consolidate into regional organizations.

▓ Utilization Review

An aspect of healthcare services delivery that affects occupational therapists is utilization review. By definition, *utilization review* is the process of evaluating the medical necessity and appropriateness of healthcare services, frequently by the application of review criteria. *Medically necessary* means that a service or treatment is consistent with the diagnosis and could not have been omitted without adversely affecting the client's condition or the quality of medical care rendered. *Appropriateness* is defined as the right service given to the right client at the right time in the right setting, including consideration of efficacy and efficiency.

Utilization review can be broken down into three basic areas: precertification or prospective review, concurrent review, and retrospective review. By *prospective review* is meant that the managed care organization must be notified before any nonemergency treatment or service is rendered; the insurer then determines if the therapy service or procedure is appropriate and medically necessary, the basis for determining payment. *Concurrent review* amounts to a running second opinion, as continued treatment is approved by the managed care organization at regular intervals. At this point the therapist may be required to furnish clinical information and patient progress reports before additional visits are approved. Throughout this time the therapist's treatment plan is measured against a particular protocol for that specific injury or diagnosis. The review organization collects these data over time to help determine future authorizations and payment decisions.

Retrospective review occurs after treatment has been rendered and is usually used to determine future policy. Claims that do not have prior authorization are reviewed restrospectively. Because most rehabilitation services are not of an emergency nature, payment for services that did not obtain proper authorization would generally be denied.[26]

U.S. Health Care in Flux

Ideally, at this point in the discussion, a typical example of a healthcare community would be offered. However, at this writing in 1996 there is no typical healthcare community in the United States, for the experience of each area has been understandably unique. Results of an initiative to address this situation were reported by the Robert Wood Johnson Foundation, through the Center for Studying Health System Change in 1996. Healthcare delivery was surveyed in 15 diverse communities across the country. Subjects were providers, purchasers, and consumers. Findings of the Community Snapshots project included:

- All markets saw increases in managed care and consolidation of healthcare providers such as hospitals.
- Primary care practitioners' power relative to specialists is rising dramatically.
- To cut costs, many employers switched to managed care or self-funded plans, negotiated aggressively with insurers, and changed plan options. Some contracted directly with providers. Still in its infancy was the idea of selecting plans based on quality and outcomes.
- Although the phenomenon may be temporary, premium increases among HMOs were leveling off.
- There are major changes occurring in healthcare organizations and structure, but they are not yet visible to consumers.[27]

■ Summary

This chapter has introduced the reader to a brief account of how American organizational structure and management have evolved and changed since the 1950s and to a picture of the current paradigms. The fate of traditional managers was recognized, as well as the changes required of them if they are to succeed on the new business scene. The meaning and importance of employee empowerment and its place in today's organizations were noted. Teamwork, its problems, and its potential in the organization were discussed. The interesting reversal in priorities of humanness and technology in management today was presented. Managed care was defined generally and specifically. Chapter 15 focuses on issues related to occupational therapy practice in the transitioning managed care environment.

REFERENCES

1. Kanter, RM: The Change Masters. Simon & Schuster, New York, 1983.
2. Bridges, W: JobShift: How to Prosper in a Workplace without Jobs. Addison-Wesley, Reading, Mass, 1995.
3. Senge, P: The Fifth Discipline. Doubleday/Currency, New York, 1994.
4. Boyett, JH, and Conn, HP: Workplace 2000. Dutton, New York, 1991, p 18.
5. Stewart, TA: The search for the organization of tomorrow. Fortune 125(10):93, May 18, 1992.
6. Stewart, TA: The king is dead. Fortune 127(1):34, Jan 11, 1993.
7. Stewart, TA: GE keeps those ideas coming. Fortune 124(4):41, Aug 12, 1991.
8. Huey, J: Where managers will go. Fortune 125(2):51, Jan 27, 1992.
9. Tetzli, R: A day in the life of Ed Deming. Fortune 127(1):74, Jan 11, 1993.
10. Kotler, P, and Clarke, RN: Creating the responsive organization. Health Care Forum, May/June 1986, p 41.
11. Stewart, TA: The search for the organization of tomorrow. Fortune 125(10):96, May 18, 1992.
12. Study shows job-redesigning, not job-cutting, works best. Advance for Occupational Therapists 11(28):14, July 17, 1995.
13. Markels, A: A power producer is intent on giving power to its people. Wall Street Journal 96:1, Southwest edition, July 3, 1995.
14. Huey, J: Sam Walton in his own words. Fortune 125(13):98, June 29, 1992.
15. Block, CM: Self-directed work teams thrive in new workplace. Advance for Occupational Therapists 11(35):96, Sept 4, 1995.
16. Labich, K: Elite teams get the job done. Fortune 133(3):90, Feb 19, 1996.
17. Sabbigh, K: Twenty-First Century Jet. Charles Scribner's Sons, New York, 1996.
18. Drucker, PF: Post-Capitalist Society. HarperCollins, New York, 1993.
19. Komp, D: Daily Guideposts. Guideposts, Carmel, NY, 1996, p 39.
20. Hodgin, DL: Critical care pros say teamwork is essential. Nursing & Allied Healthweek: Greater Dallas/Fort Worth Edition 1(10):21, May 20, 1996.
21. Kohn, A: No Contest: The Case Against Competition. Houghton Mifflin, Boston, 1986.
22. Naisbett, J: Megatrends. Warner Books, New York, 1982.
23. Cooper, PD, and Robinson, LM: Health Care Marketing Management. Aspen, Rockville, Md, 1982.
24. Todd, MK: Networking: IPA, PHO, & MSO Development Strategies. Business Network, Nashville, Tenn, 1993.

25. Fowler, FJ: Alliances in subacute rehabilitation. Rehab Economics (suppl)3:6. In Rehab Management, Oct/Nov, 1995.
26. Burcham, MP: Surviving utilization review. Rehab Management 7(5):102, Aug/Sept, 1994.
27. Ziegler, J: Snapshots of change in US health care. Advances, Robert Wood Johnson Foundation, Issue 1, 1996.

RELATED READINGS ON MANAGEMENT

AOTA: Managed Care: An Occupational Therapy Sourcebook. AOTA, Bethesda, Md, 1996.
Bair, J, and Gray, M (eds): The Occupational Therapy Manager. AOTA, Rockville, Md, 1992.
Donnelly, JH, Gibson, JL, and Ivancevich, JM: Fundamentals of Management, ed 5. Business Publications, Plano, Tex, 1984.
Drucker, PF: Management: Tasks, Responsibilities, Practices. Harper & Row, New York, 1973.
Drucker, PF: An Introductory View of Management. Harper's College Press, New York, 1977.
Drucker, PF: Managing in Turbulent Times. Harper & Row, New York, 1980.
Ducanis, AJ, and Golin, AK: The Interdisciplinary Health Care Team. Aspen, Germantown, Md, 1979.
Haimann, T: Supervisory Management for Healthcare Organizations. The Catholic Health Association of the United States, St. Louis, 1989.
Liebler, JG, Levine, RE, and Rothman, J: Management Principles for Health Professionals, ed 2. Aspen, Rockville, Md, 1992.
Longest, BB: Management Practices for the Health Professional, ed 4. Appleton & Lange, East Norwalk, Conn, 1990.
Metzger, N: The Health Care Supervisor's Handbook. Aspen, Rockville, Md, 1988.
Phillips, JJ: Improving Supervisors' Effectiveness. Jossey-Bass, San Francisco, 1985.
Schwartz, D: Introduction to Management. Harcourt Brace Jovanovich, New York, 1980.

CHAPTER 15

Occupational Therapists as Managers

CHAPTER OBJECTIVES ▪ ▪ ▪ ▪ ▪ ▪ ▪ ▪ ▪ ▪

- To understand the ways in which the occupational therapy work environment has changed.
- To recognize why a marketing attitude is essential in effective management.
- To identify the problems and opportunities in managed care.
- To view the functions of management through a marketing approach.
- To realize the importance and achievability of a positive image.
- To recognize the diverse viewpoints of organizational behavior.
- To appreciate how to use complaints to foster growth.
- To determine why employee motivation and job satisfaction are critical to effective management.
- To understand the demands on an occupational therapist in a case manager role.
- To realize the potential for self-development as an occupational therapy manager.
- To provide a gauge for self-appraisal of the emotional maturity required to become an effective manager.

Many excellent books deal with the functions of management, some by and for occupational therapists and numerous others from diverse sources, several of which are listed at the end of the previous chapter. This book is confined to an introduction to healthcare delivery today and to the often overlooked and mis-understood role of *marketing* in the daily life of the occupational therapist man-ager. This chapter demonstrates that the marketing process is at the foundation of an effective manager's performance.

A marketing approach should be among the basic management attitudes and skills of all occupational therapist managers. Problems can be solved in a sys-tematic, rewarding manner with a marketing approach, and it can become an ex-citing part of daily transactions and an assurance of finding a place in the health-care delivery system today and tomorrow. Occupational therapy practitioners who are managers can develop marketing attitudes by learning the language and techniques and by applying that information to their management problems.

What the Therapist Manages

Occupational therapy practitioners who hold management positions of *any* kind need an understanding of the marketing process to be more effective and satisfied with their personal performance. In a manner of speaking, all occupa-tional therapy practitioners who are responsible for accomplishing objectives are managers and can benefit from consideration of the marketing process as critical to their successful daily operations. Naturally, the higher the level of management, the more complex the marketing processes at work and the more critical that the strategy, tools, and mix be understood.

Rather than base professional confidence on being able to perform clini-cal and technical skills better than those being supervised, a manager's confi-dence should be based on the ability to build teams, motivate staff, and excel in other management functions. The idea is not to be better than your followers but to lead them. The definition of *management* used here as a point of depar-ture is: "Management has been defined as the process of getting things done through and with people. It is the planning and directing of effort, the organiz-ing and employing of resources (both human and material) to accomplish some predetermined objective."[1]

The Challenges of a Changing Environment

The changing environment of healthcare delivery, as characterized by Todd,[2] includes several aspects: (1) Incentives are changing, with payment for services resulting from capitation, fee for service, and packaged pricing; (2) metrics are changing, with value meaning quality in relation to cost, and quality identified by outcome; and (3) structures are changing as health care moves toward group formations, alliances, and integrated provision systems. In general, *managed care* means a system of healthcare provision that addresses the needs of a specific population by controlling the cost of, access to, and quality of health care. It consists of a spectrum of alliances from the very controlled model of the health maintenance organization to a loose network of providers[3] (see Chapter 14).

OCCUPATIONAL THERAPY AND THE PROGRAM MANAGEMENT MODEL

How occupational therapy is adapting to the collapsing pyramid can be shown in a contemporary illustration. Typical of what has happened across the United States, managers of one rehabilitation hospital dissolved their clinical management structure for occupational therapy, physical therapy, speech, psychology, and social work; a program management delivery model was adopted. With client needs declared the primary focus of care, clinicians were first aligned with program teams designed to focus on particular types of rehabilitation clients and to develop client-centered strategies. In anticipation of Medicare's potential use of functional related groups in the future, occupational therapists and physical therapists share the same gym, and social workers, psychologists, speech therapists, and program directors are located geographically close to the gym areas of the programs they serve. Department directors were replaced by program directors and clinical coordinators who focus their resources on the needs of specific patient groups.

Such reengineering of the traditional hospital organizational structure is clearly not without its challenges, regardless of where in the country the transitions have taken place. Through the literature and by means of personal visits and experiences, students are advised to become familiar with such changes taking place nationwide.

Making changes is difficult for all affected; *integrating* and *maintaining* changes are at least equally challenging. Administrators of many hospitals that have shifted to the program management model have found it helpful to increase their emphasis on total quality management (TQM) and continuous quality improvement (CQI) processes to ensure that all staff members keep in mind that patients are the first priority.

OCCUPATIONAL THERAPY AND MANAGED CARE: WHERE TO START

Occupational therapy practitioners can personalize all this information to their own situations in practice by applying lessons, principles, and practical suggestions. To negotiate within the managed care environment, the occupational therapist first needs to have correct diagnostic information when asked for it by a third-party payer. Without this information, you cannot predict what you can do or establish treatment goals or costs built on predictions. As noted in Part

Three, often occupational therapists fail to correctly diagnose limitations and disabilities because they have not sought to really know clients' preferences. Collecting outcomes data is an objective and credible way of demonstrating the value of occupational therapy services to individuals and of supporting their cost-effectiveness and impact on reducing overall healthcare costs. Managed-care payers are seeking those providers who consistently produce the best services for the best price.

According to AOTA President Mary Foto, to provide these services occupational therapists must:

- Produce outcomes that are functionally relevant and utilitarian to meeting the clients' and families' needs in their living environment.
- Produce outcomes that are sustained over time.
- Provide services that are based on comprehensive clinical pathways that are tied to specific outcomes.
- Provide a continuous quality and cost-management system.[4]

Furthermore, the two main steps for developing successful partnerships with payers are to focus more on outcomes than on services and to have internal systems of utilization and case management in each department. With each occupational therapist acting as a case manager, care is managed rather than just services delivered. Foto went on to specifically advise every occupational therapist to communicate with employers and insurers, be able to do cost-benefit analyses, determine per-case costs, determine capitation rates, and have prevention and disability management programs in place.

All occupational therapy practitioners are advised to continuously seek updated information. Articles about current activities of colleagues and announcements of continuing education opportunities (print materials, videotapes, workshops) may be found in *OT Practice, OT Week*, state association publications, *Advance for Occupational Therapists,* and *Allied Healthweek.*

CRITICAL PATHWAYS

Underwood[5] provided a commonsense approach to assist the occupational therapist who wishes to begin developing critical pathways.

1. Determine which major diagnoses are treated in your facility according to frequency.
2. Rank each diagnosis in terms of treatment differences, that is, differences in length of treatment and in treatment outcomes, perhaps by examining data from peer review.
3. Based on this list, determine for which ones third-party payers request the most information regarding progress and outcomes.
4. Identify for which diagnoses you have the most current or potential competition.

5. Post your action plan to ensure involvement and commitment of all staff.

Before developing a critical pathway, Underwood[5] cautioned therapists to consider whether they planned to include it as part of the facility's computerized data system. Because the end goal is to use the critical pathway for documentation, the information systems department should be involved early. Clinical documentation can be automatically entered into a database. With that in mind, first address the different areas about which you need to include information, explore the methods by which you plan to measure outcomes (or progress made) during the process of treatment, decide the time frames within which you will set up the critical pathway, and determine the content in each of your categories along with the time frames.

Information presented graphically is easier to grasp and allows comparisons over time, as in utilization review. Outcomes research can be both professionally and personally gratifying. It validates what you do, and, if you are asked by a third party to justify the costs of devices or procedures, you already have the data. You will have become compatible with managed care, and the leaders into the 21st century may well be those with the best outcomes documentation.

IF YOU ARE CONSIDERING PRIVATE PRACTICE

Entry-level occupational therapists considering private practice are advised to prepare themselves carefully by seeking business and legal training, advice, and experience. After conducting a needs assessment, you might inquire into the AOTA practice management courses, the Small Business Administration development centers found on college campuses, SCORE (volunteer retired executives who help inexperienced business aspirants write business plans and solve other business problems), or local Chamber of Commerce workshops. Besides developing a strong business foundation, keeping current on taxation policies, healthcare legislation, and Medicare, Medicaid, and other insurance issues is recommended. Other considerations are the amount of money needed to start, the investment of time and energy required for ongoing business, and the particular need for communication skills.

Finally, networking is an important part of developing any business. A valuable opportunity exists among peers who are part of the Private Practice Subcommittee of the Administration and Management Special Interest Section of AOTA.

▓ The Manager's Role in Transition

Accountability, competition, and survival have become everyday realities to occupational therapists as new roles and locations of practice appear daily. More responsibility must be taken for marketing one's own services, assuming more risks in program development, learning more nontreatment functions, and thinking, acting, and managing in a businesslike way. This includes developing a marketing attitude and systematically investigating the needs and wants of everyone with whom daily transactions are conducted. Command-and-control management has become less feasible, while a coach-and-cajole leadership that unleashes employees' creativity is increasingly recognized as more effective.

Occupational therapists have a responsibility to provide information to all with whom they relate. To do this effectively, first the assets of their businesses—occupational therapy services—must be understood and specified. What the service *is* does not matter to the client as much as what it *does*.

The Importance of Image

The main assets are not buildings or programs, which are, of course, important, but it is the occupational therapy image that supports its uniqueness. The way occupational therapists feel about themselves profoundly affects that picture, for attitude creates the visible foundation of impressions and perceptions made on the public. The image of occupational therapy is created by occupational therapists themselves.

The importance of the impression you make cannot be underestimated. The forms that a negative impression can take are myriad; however, being conscious of their potential can help you control this aspect of marketing. If you sent people incognito into your place of business today, what level of service would they find? When they asked for directions or information, would they encounter people who are courteous, informed, and friendly? Would employees gladly stop what they are doing to help? Would the way your visitors were dressed influence the way they were treated? All of these encounters, these "moments of truth," add up to the perceptions held by those visitors to your organization. By thinking carefully about the quality of all personal encounters, telephone calls, and business correspondence, you can control much of the image projected. External marketing makes promises; internal marketing keeps promises. It is the *spirit* of service that defines success.

Clients can all evaluate the quality of service they receive. Even though they may not know the professional skill of the practitioner performing the service, they know when they are not being treated with concern, consideration, and politeness, and they will never forget it. Because the competitive edge in today's healthcare environment can be critical, and because the new generation of customers has high expectations and is well informed about choices, it is the quality of service that they will publicize and remember when deciding whether to return.

Excellent service attracts more than clients. Physicians, donors, volunteers, and employees want to be part of an organization that serves them well. The manager of an organization is the person responsible for providing the impetus for commitment to a high quality of service. One course of action the manager might consider is taking the following steps:

1. Make clear to all that service is the business of the organization.
2. Ensure that customer satisfaction is the highest priority.
3. Convince all internal groups, such as employees and boards, that commitment to service excellence is a requirement.

When the philosophy has been established, the steps used to implement it must be repeated often:

1. Use every communications avenue possible to repeat messages about service.
2. Train employees about service expectations and how they will be measured.
3. Develop the methodologies by which service will be measured.
4. Set rewards for those who have met and exceeded expectations for service.
5. Encourage creativity.[6]

Management That Incorporates Marketing

Marketing helps one decide what services to offer, whom to serve and how, and issues of pricing, referral, and access. Marketing is a major policy-making function that belongs in all levels of management, and marketing techniques can be learned by occupational therapists in the context of today's healthcare environment, enabling them to promote their services, increase referrals, improve their image and visibility, and compete successfully.

Market-based management means flexibly filling the needs of people in an integrated environment. Such an organization is culturally integrated, sharing mutual values and ethics. Nonhierarchical, it consists of people making decisions collectively; all employees understand the economics of the organization and adapt to changes or sudden events that affect them. This is in no way germane only to occupational therapy organizations. Even the largest corporations today are moving in a similar direction. When questioned about the future of big corporations, Drucker responded that "the Fortune 500 is over." He went on to assert that big corporations will not cease to exist, but he thinks that they will "slowly and painfully transform themselves into a new kind of creature that combines the clout of a giant with the nimbleness of an entrepreneurial elf."[7]

Though mentioned elsewhere, it bears repeating in a management context that many occupational therapists, like most healthcare providers, to this point have delivered professional services they themselves decided clients needed, a nonmarketing approach to managerial planning and development. Occupational therapists will be pleasantly surprised by the many benefits derived from (1) recognition of the commonality among the concepts of marketing, public relations, and a systems approach; (2) analysis of markets as to structure and consumers; (3) understanding the rationale underlying application of marketing concepts and techniques in management; and (4) development of occupational therapy marketing programs for target populations. Going into the new century, marketing is the name of the game, and occupational therapy managers must be resourceful and cognizant of this trend to be ready to provide the most needed services in the most appropriate environments.

Mutual Exchanges within Management Functions

Regardless of the exact words used, management textbooks agree that the functions of a manager typically include planning, organizing, staffing, directing, and controlling (see Chapter 14). Each of these management functions in which occupational therapy managers engage encompasses a number of potential mutual exchanges or constituencies. For instance, the function of *planning* is carried out in any place of employment through systematic interactions with staff, colleagues, administrators, boards, and consumers. To be universally effective, managers must pay as close attention to the quality of life of their workforce as they do to that of their clients. Each constituency or public is an important spoke in the wheel of every manager's ongoing mutual exchanges.

One way in which an occupational therapist as manager might visualize those target markets with whom he or she maintains mutual exchanges is presented in Figure 15–1. By visualizing the occupational therapist performing each of the five functions of management for which she or he is responsible and by further picturing just some of the constituencies or publics with whom mutually satisfactory exchanges might be made, the idea of the marketing process can be introduced into daily management operations.

Internal Marketing in Occupational Therapy Management

McGourty[8] offered an excellent example of what could be described as a marketing approach with one spoke of a typical manager's wheel of constituencies or publics. In this case, the specific constituency or public was the entry-level staff occupational therapist, and the question was whether to include that individual in the program development projects of the organization. The decision was that it was not only possible but also a good idea. Based on the assumption that new therapists usually have many new ideas or perspectives but often are

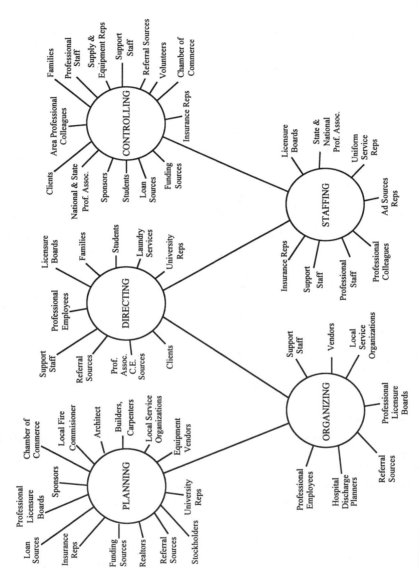

FIGURE 15–1. Marketing constituencies of the occupational therapist manager-owner of a private hand therapy clinic.

afraid to express them, involvement in program development provides a safe avenue for expression of ideas and participation that helps new therapists build trust, rapport, and team skills.

By describing what she felt were advantages to staff involvement, McGourty illustrated what could be gained by each party in this mutually beneficial activity. Each participant in the transaction shares in responsibility for the success of the organization, a goal in common. Following is a summary of what McGourty viewed as gains from involving staff in program development. Individual staff members gain:

1. Knowledge—building broader thinking, better analysis skills, role analysis.
2. Sense of power and control—an active rather than passive role, ideas that are valued, a manager willing to share power.
3. Self-esteem—self-recognition of skills and abilities, confidence building through having a valued role.
4. Teamwork skills—opportunity to work with other staff members, receiving feedback and working for idea implementation, communication and cooperation skills, learning early that teamwork is expected and not optional.

The manager gains:

1. New and better ideas—fresh perspectives of new staff accustomed to researching ideas, developing projects, and writing papers; involvement with subsequent commitment to the new program.
2. Time—staff assumption of tasks, thus releasing manager to accomplish more and other work.
3. Committed team working together with reinforced trust and positive team behaviors, loyal staff.

McGourty, co-owner of a private practice, provided specific suggestions to managers who wished to accomplish these mutually satisfying exchanges. One can readily see the amalgamation of strategic planning with the marketing process in McGourty's advice to first have a flexible, ongoing, general master plan of where the department is headed, allow for individual input and unexpected opportunities, hold meetings with staff members to listen to ideas and assign concrete responsibilities, set objectives that fit into the master plan, develop a timetable and assign responsibilities, hold follow-up meetings to monitor progress and problem-solve, and see that time is allotted to accomplish the planned program development. A final admonition was to ensure that credit is given to those who have done the work that completed the project. Neglecting to give credit where credit is due undermines the trust built during the project, for it is one more essential part of a mutually satisfying exchange between manager and employee.

▓ Complaints: Criticism or Information?

Marshall Field, the famous department store founder, is credited with having said, "Those who enter to buy, support me. Those who complain, teach me how I may please so that more will come." The natural first reaction of most people to criticism or negative complaints is usually not a positive one. It does not take research so much as common sense to know that being the recipient of complaints may contribute to excessive worry, burnout, tension, and even physical reactions. Yet contained within a simple complaint is a richness of information.

Furthermore, for every customer who complains, Field felt that there are 26 more somewhere out there who have similar dissatisfactions that you do not ever hear. Those customers simply disappear, leaving you wondering why. For that reason many corporations are taking a chance on encountering some discomfort by becoming more like the responsive organizations and using the information secured through complaints proactively as stepping-stones to success. Although a complaint is not necessarily a crisis, it can well be leading toward one that is impending. This is one more reason for using this *free advice* for self-improvement rather than perhaps paying a consultant to tell you about the same problem.

LEARN FROM THE CODFISH

Codfish are a big commercial business in the northeastern United States, and there is a national market for them. Those who ship them across the country first tried freezing them, but the freeze took away much of the flavor. So they experimented with shipping them alive in tanks of seawater, but the cod not only lost its flavor but also became soft and mushy. Finally, the shippers placed the live codfish in tanks of water along with their natural enemy, the catfish. From the time the cod left the East Coast until it arrived in the farthest western destination, the catfish chased the codfish all over the tanks. When they arrived at their destination, there was no loss of flavor or of texture.

Every organization has a few "catfish" who customarily irritate, complain, and criticize. By learning to overcome and learn from these irritations and tensions, one can emerge with the right attitude, a stronger and more effective manager who is able to grow through finding value in criticism and complaints.

PROBLEM SOLVING AND SKIP THINKING

It is possible to meet with a complainer and still maintain composure, minimize physical discomfort, and learn a great deal from the complainant. Some organizations have accomplished this by instilling in all their employees creative problem-solving skills, a change of mind, and future thinking. One company found that groups of employees who were trained in creative problem solving out-performed untrained groups about three to one on the number of high-quality ideas that resulted from encounters with complainers. Employees were given ways to distance themselves from the complaint: Set it up like a problem state-ment, remove the negative energy, and focus the mind for gathering informa-tion. Complaints were handled effectively in this way. From the psychologists' viewpoint, this is known as "skip thinking." The negative emotion is "skipped over" as the individual moves to the solution phase directly from the complaint stated as a problem. After skipping the negative energy stage, ideas are gener-ated to solve the problems identified, and then those ideas are implemented.[9]

HANDLING COMPLAINTS

A related approach to assuring consumer satisfaction, and thus continued pa-tronage, is to look at the handling of criticism and complaints as a five-step process that begins with not promising what you cannot deliver and setting re-alistic expectations for the consumer. Next is to acknowledge that there is a rea-son why the client complained and not to deny it, for *in the consumer's percep-tion* this is a unique complaint and should be treated as such. Third, after accepting that this complaint is unique, why it happened and whether it is a symptom of a bigger problem should be explored. The fourth step is to react, doing your best to suggest the right solution for what is perceived as being wrong and then evaluating whether the solution will actually accomplish what it should. (Occasionally the difficulty lies with the person who is complaining, but you must determine that.) Finally, follow up to be sure that the problem has been solved and the person who complained has been satisfied; then verify that the organization has used the information provided by the complainer to ensure that the problem does not happen again. Complaints can never be eliminated, but an organization can plan so that they are minimized and used to advantage.[10]

▓ The Employee as Number One

Kelly and Kelly, in *What They Really Teach You at the Harvard Business School,* stated that the ability to anticipate and manage organizational behavior issues is one of the major characteristics that differentiate an effective manager from a mere administrator. Among the organizational constituencies or publics of a manager are support staff. Many occupational therapy managers are unaware of how to go about developing desired mutual exchanges with this con-stituency. In *Why This Horse Won't Drink,* Ken Matejka declared that if horses don't want to drink, they won't.[11] He used this assumption as an analogy to em-ployees' behaviors, saying that "owners often spend their time looking at be-havior from their own viewpoint instead of from that of a horse. . . . Most horses drink best when allowed to drink what they want, when they want, and how much they want. . . . Further, not all horses are the same. . . . Too many managers see employees' behavior from their own viewpoint and don't know (or care) what goes on in the minds of those they try to manage. . . . Motivation and performance must be approached from the employees' point of view."[11]

THE OCCUPATIONAL THERAPIST MANAGER AND MOTIVATION

Motivation and job satisfaction have been the subject of thousands of research studies over the years. Notable early researchers dealing with the topic of motivation included Maslow[12] and Herzberg.[13] Managers will do well to become familiar with these and later works to better understand this area of such importance to effective management of employees.

The ability to motivate others is the ability to get people to feel, think, or act as you wish; however, no one person can force motivation on another. Others can be urged to work harder or to learn a new task, but ultimately the most that can be done is to help others motivate themselves. The simple act of listening to employee concerns enhances their self-esteem and their perception that you hold them in esteem. An open attitude on the part of a manager will lead to employees' increased openness to suggestions and information, as well as more willingness to examine issues realistically.

▧ A Manager's Personal Development

Not only do authors such as Stephen Covey[14] offer guidance helpful for personal self-development as managers but also the suggestions given can be used to good advantage in all interactions. Covey believed that organizational behavior is individual behavior collectivized, a good beginning step toward being a manager today. Covey asserted that highly effective people have seven habits in common:

1. Be proactive. Be responsible and take the initiative.
2. Begin with the end in mind. Any endeavor—a meeting, a workday—should start with a mental image of the outcome.
3. Put first things first. Subordinate feelings, impulses, and moods to your values.
4. Think win-win.
5. Seek first to understand, then to be understood. Listen with the intent to empathize, not reply.
6. Synergize. Create wholes that are greater than the sum of their parts.
7. Sharpen the saw. Cultivate the physical, mental, emotional, and spiritual dimensions of your character.[14]

To foster this same work spirit among individuals for whom you have responsibility in your organization, you first should establish a shared, articulated purpose. A supportive organizational culture acknowledges good performance in workers, encourages risk taking and entrepreneurial behavior, and does not punish people who do so, for mistakes can enhance motivation as well. Finally, developmental supervision, viewing employees as growing human beings with unique strengths and talents, can channel individuals' abilities toward meeting organizational goals. At the same time, as a manager it is critical to stay aware of how satisfied your staff members are with the conditions of their employment.

JOB SATISFACTION

Research studies concerning work satisfaction among occupational therapists have revealed moderately high levels of work satisfaction in both clinical and academic settings. Parham's[15] study of occupational therapy educators revealed satisfaction with such intrinsic aspects of their work as environment and opportunities for autonomy, advancement, and contributions to the profession. Rozier, Gilkeson, and Hamilton[16] focused on occupational therapists' teaching satisfaction in academe, finding faculty generally satisfied with teaching, specifically valuing lack of constraints in the higher education environment. Brollier[17] looked at hospital-based occupational therapists and concluded that their styles of management greatly influenced the work satisfaction of their staff members. Florian, Sheffer, and Sachs[18] learned that their sample of Israeli occupational therapists spent most of their time on direct client care at the expense of other duties such as supervision. This, they predicted, could lead to decreased job satisfaction and burnout.

In a study of factors affecting job satisfaction of occupational therapists,[19] Bender found that employees believed their most important job responsibilities—also the ones that produced the most personal satisfaction—were those that allowed them to make their own decisions. Because understanding what constitutes job satisfaction is a key factor in successful exchange transactions with employees, managers are advised to learn more about this topic in planned self-study of current literature and other forms of information.

MARKET ANALYSIS AND THE EMPLOYEE POINT OF VIEW

Chapter 5 noted that the first step in a market analysis or audit is to determine the status of each constituency. As a manager, you should be seeking to determine the status of satisfactory exchange with each support staff member—*from that employee's point of view.* Really knowing and caring about what is wanted and needed should become second nature as you develop each marketing exchange associated with the role of manager. It must become an attitude, a frame of mind for approaching each potential exchange, each daily interpersonal relationship. Attention to employee morale can mean big efforts such as establishing a wellness program or simply wording a criticism differently. For example, instead of saying, "You made a fine presentation today, but," try "You made a fine presentation today, and you would do even better if." Both short-term and long-term results will more than reward the effort expended, and the "habit" soon becomes a part of the daily routine.

People are not likely to change their behavior for you to operationalize your vision unless you reward them for it. A key principle of compensation is to link more of it directly to performance. This principle appears to be obvious, but the two factors that usually carry the most weight are an employee's title and length of service. Thus compensation becomes an entitlement, not an incentive, and your weakest performers get a free ride. At the same time you are encouraging your best employees to polish their resumes and look elsewhere. In short, adopt a marketing attitude in matters of management and institute the marketing process. Continually assess the status of each exchange with each of your internal constituencies or employees and adjust relationships.

Case Management

A leadership role for which an occupational therapist is well qualified is that of case manager. As managed care grows, the occupational therapist should be more frequently found in this position. In 1991 AOTA described minimum qualifications for OTRs and COTAs who aspired to be case managers in its "Statement: The Occupational Therapist as Case Manager." It declared that occupational therapists "with five years experience, of which three years are within a specific practice arena, are qualified to assume job positions as case managers" and that advanced certified occupational therapy assistants "with five years experience, of which three years are within a specific practice arena, who have attained skills in management, communications and systems may assume a case management role with persons in long-term care settings."

By successfully passing a voluntary certification examination, originally sponsored by the Certification of Insurance Rehabilitation Specialists Commission (CIRSC) and now a designation of the Commission for Case Manager Certification (CCMC), occupational therapists may use CCM (certified case manager) after their names. The CIRSC has defined *case management* as "a collaborative process which assesses, plans, implements, coordinates, monitors, and evaluates the options and services required to meet an individual's health needs, using communication and available resources to promote quality, cost-effective outcomes."

Case managers work for a variety of employers, including hospitals, home health agencies, community residential programs, insurance companies, mental health centers, and independent case management companies. The number of certified case managers by 1996 had grown to nearly 17,000 nationwide.[20]

Occupational therapists would seem to be especially well suited to work as case managers because of their education in elements of potential cases, such as task analysis, psychosocial aspects of illness, and rehabilitation techniques.

The ultimate benefits of case management can include increased productivity, decreased workers' compensation expenses, lower turnover, and decreased retraining costs.

An occupational therapist contemplating a case manager position is advised to first become familiar with the Certified Case Manager (CCM) Certification Guide from CCMC. Application must be made and an exam successfully completed. It would also be helpful to become informed about the criteria for a Certified Rehabilitation Counselor (CRC) and for Certified Insurance Rehabilitation Specialist (CIRS). (For information, write the Commission for Case Manager Certification, 1835 Rohlwing Rd., Suite D, Rolling Meadows, IL 60008.) As with any other new position you consider, learning about the conditions surrounding a prospective job makes the transition smoother.

Maturity Is Required for a Management Position

Students who are contemplating positions requiring responsibility and independent performance can assess whether they are ready to assume such posts by defining maturity in relation to themselves. Maturation is a protracted business, mixing the physiological, psychological, and social. Freud has been quoted as saying that maturity is the ability to postpone gratification.

There are some behaviors that can be expected of a mature individual:

- Cerebral response: The immature are spontaneous and unconsidered, while a mature person can "disengage viscera before speaking mind." The responses of a mature person are carefully considered and framed when reacting.

- Containment: More mature people keep their emotional reactions directly related to their objects, but the immature allow personal feelings to cross over into all interpersonal relations.

- Attenuation: The immature lack a "negative feedback loop" that keeps emotional excitement from getting out of hand.

- Perspective: A big part of maturation is recognizing that the views of others have as much legitimacy as one's own.

- Proportion: Although the immature may be moody with no reason and have no priority in their actions, those who are mature react objectively and appropriately according to the gravity of the situation.

- Goal-seeking: Mature persons are able to sustain long-term and multipurpose action, but the immature are less focused and more drawn to immediate goals.

- Insight: Mature people recognize and manage their own strengths and weaknesses.

- Intimacy: Those who are mature can create and sustain high-quality relationships.[21]

The last two characteristics are particularly significant to the success of managers. Accepting responsibility calmly, without forgetting its cost and value or suffering undue stress as a result of the actions taken, is something effective, mature managers do daily. Maturity supplies what is needed to face up to choices, make them, and live with the consequences. It also appears to be helpful if a manager has endured failure or overcome adversity, as the maturing process seems to be accelerated by emotional suffering. The Chinese philosopher Mencius said, "Life springs from calamity; from ease, only death. Men of special virtue and wisdom are wont to owe those powers to the trials they have endured."

In all things there must, of course, be balance. A person totally mature in all of these behaviors might be thought dull and predictable. Being too grown-up is inflexible, even irresponsible, in a totally mobile world. So, as in all things, understanding what is involved may help a person to make one more decision, this one evaluating one's own level of maturity and appropriateness for a particular management position. It is indeed a personal decision, and each of us has, as part of our individuality, a relative level of maturity.

As for being able to deal maturely with associates on the job, it is useful to know why people behave or misbehave as they do if it is your responsibility to have your goals carried out by others. Because few blueprints in human relations can be followed precisely, managers generally have to rely on mature judgment to gauge their actions with each situation. Considerate leadership reflects sound management.

BEGIN BY CHAIRING MEETINGS

One place where the new therapist can begin developing management and marketing skills is in meetings. Learn how to conduct effective, productive meetings by observing such rules as when chairing a meeting begin promptly, clearly state the purpose of the meeting, make sure that all members have previously received the information necessary to the discussion, retain control but don't stifle comment, and keep adequate minutes. Assistance and guidance can be found in sources such as Haimann's *Supervisory Management for Healthcare Organizations*[22] or *Management Principles for Health Professionals* by Liebler, Levine, and Rothman.[1]

How the High-Achieving Manager Evolves

There are five distinct stages in the evolution of high-achieving managers. In the first, or *initiation*, stage, a new manager learns to identify with the role of manager, especially after a nonmanagerial history as an occupational therapist. By not accomplishing this stage, the person may display anxiety around subordinates and procrastinate. At the next level, termed the *fear of success* stage, a new manager may begin to perform so well that he or she actually becomes afraid of prospering on the job and apprehensive of the consequences of all this success.

The new manager moves then to the *team-building* stage and is fully committed to the management position. The problem now is difficulty in developing new leaders among key subordinates and in forming a tightly knit team among peers and employees because of inability to relinquish control.

During the fourth stage, the *affiliation* level, the individual realizes that productivity depends on the work of others but the responsibility for management remains the manager's alone. (Familiar humorous ways of expressing this particular situation include "the buck stops here" and "if you can't stand the heat, get out of the kitchen.") At this point the task is to develop higher-level leadership capabilities to relate effectively to all levels of the organization and at the same time acknowledge the increased importance of people-oriented leadership skills, especially delegation.

The last level is the *elevation-seniority* stage in which the individual has reached a senior management post. At this juncture the manager must learn to handle increased responsibility and distancing from subordinates because of the promotion. Primary attention moves from people to organization and from projects to strategic planning and money issues.[23] However, a marketing and people-centered attitude always continues as a priority at all stages of a manager's evolution regardless of how her or his primary constituencies change.

Other management aspects of occupational therapy practice in today's healthcare delivery scene are addressed in Part Seven.

▨ Summary

This chapter has discussed aspects of effective management and the pivotal role marketing plays. The unique challenges presented by managed care were discussed. Caution and experience were suggested before venturing into the private practice arena. The importance of image and of making high-quality service a central concern were acknowledged. How to approach the functions of management from a marketing perspective were described, as well as the essential nature of motivation and job satisfaction. The stages through which an entry-level therapist might expect to move toward leadership in management were introduced. Chapter 16 explains entrepreneurship and the difference between being reactive and being proactive.

REFERENCES

1. Liebler, JG, Levine, RE, and Rothman, J: Management Principles for Health Professionals, ed 2. Aspen, Gaithersburg, Md, 1992, p 3.

2. Todd, MK: Networking: IPA, PHO, & MSO Development Strategies. Business Network, Nashville, Tenn, 1993.
3. Aaron, DH: Private practitioners and managed health care. Administration & Management Special Interest Section Newsletter 10:3, Sept, 1994.
4. Collins, LF: Excelling in a managed care environment. OT Practice 1(1):22, Jan, 1996.
5. Underwood, R: Developing critical pathways. OT Practice 1(1):23, Jan, 1996.
6. Peterson, D: Internal marketing: Outstanding service starts here. Health Texas, June 1, 1990.
7. Drucker, P: Is big still good? Fortune, Apr 30, 1992, p 50.
8. McGourty, LK: Program development with entry-level staff. Administration & Management Special Interest Newsletter 6:2, June, 1990.
9. Firestien, RL: Effects of creative problem-solving training on communication behaviors in small groups. Small Group Research 21:507, Nov, 1990.
10. Buffington, PW: Capitalizing on complaints. Sky, June, 1991, p 33.
11. Matejka, K: Why This Horse Won't Drink: How to Win—and Keep—Employee Commitment. AMACOM, New York, 1991, p xii.
12. Maslow, A: Motivation and Personality. Harper & Row, New York, 1954.
13. Herzberg, F: Work and the Nature of Man. Thomas Y Crowell, New York, 1966.
14. Covey, SR: The Seven Habits of Highly Successful People. Simon & Schuster, New York, 1989.
15. Parham, D: Faculty perceptions of rewards in occupational therapy education: Implications for improving research productivity. Occupational Therapy Journal of Research 7:195, 1987.
16. Rozier, C, Gilkeson, G, and Hamilton, B: Job satisfaction in occupational therapy. Am J Occup Ther 45:160, 1991.
17. Brollier, C: Managerial leadership and staff OTR satisfaction. Occupational Therapy Journal of Research 5:170, 1985.
18. Florian, V, Sheffer, M, and Sachs, D: Time allocation patterns of occupational therapists in Israel: Implications for job satisfaction. Am J Occup Ther 39:392, 1985.
19. Kerr, T: Most OTs well satisfied with career choice. Advance for Occupational Therapists, Mar 6, 1995.
20. Marmer, L: Making the case for a case manager job. Advance for Occupational Therapists, Apr 8, 1996, p 12.
21. Thorne, P: Just what is emotional maturity? International Management, July/Aug, 1987.
22. Haimann, T: Supervisory Management for Healthcare Organizations, ed 4. The Catholic Association of the United States, St. Louis, 1989.
23. Garfield, CA: Peak Performance. Tarcher/Houghton Mifflin, Boston, 1984.

CHAPTER 16

Reactive vs. Proactive Approaches to Change

CHAPTER OBJECTIVES

- To understand the critical need for occupational therapists to be proactive rather than reactive regardless of employment setting.
- To comprehend how management, leadership, change, and entrepreneurship can be synthesized for successful performance.
- To acknowledge and identify examples of entrepreneurship.
- To recognize current dilemmas in practice and education and to see examples of resourceful solutions.
- To recognize the importance of improving efficiency in organizations.
- To appreciate the growing potential for occupational therapists of opportunities for innovative practice.
- To be aware of the added expertise that is needed by occupational therapy practitioners if they are to become more effective manager-leaders.

Barbara Jordan is credited with having said that "the stakes are too high for government to be a spectator sport." The same can be said about occupational therapy. The stakes are too high for any occupational therapy practitioner to stand by waiting for others to announce decisions and to spend time simply reacting to those decisions. Emerging trends and issues do not announce themselves. Being unaware and unprepared when changes come about can seriously affect, even destroy, a career or an organization. It is incumbent on a professional to become as proactive as is feasible.

The primary aim of this chapter is to begin synthesizing the ideas of change, leadership, entrepreneurship, and management, all processes about which occupational therapy students should have already begun to learn. How an occupational therapy practitioner can anticipate and successfully deal with change is discussed from a variety of perspectives. By absorbing and practicing the ideas suggested, an occupational therapy practitioner can be well on the way to developing a proactive stance in his or her professional life.

▓ Entrepreneurship

Entrepreneurship can be defined as the ability to take sensible risks and implement innovations. It is, of course, understood that doing so follows a careful survey of intended buyers or users to find out if others want that product or service in the form you plan to offer it. Then plans must be altered based on the feedback you get from those potential consumers. Rather than wasting resources by using them to pursue past goals, the smart occupational therapy entrepreneur is too busy finding ways to institute new consumer links by designing the organization and the product around the intended consumer.

The entrepreneurial organization is identified by its willingness and eagerness to change with the times. Rather than observe what is happening and wondering why, the entrepreneurial organization makes things happen. Its future is under control as it negotiates successful changes. An entrepreneurial organization has high motivation and ability to recognize and exploit unforeseen opportunities and turn them into successful enterprises.[1]

IN PRODUCTS

An example can be taken from the corporate world, where it usually takes a plucky individual to exploit markets that don't yet exist or are not actually yet apparent to others.[2] Philip Knight was regarded as a nerd—as were all runners—in 1964 when he co-founded Nike and launched a new U.S. industry. The company ran no national TV ads until Nike passed $1 billion in sales; prior to that, says Knight, "We used word-of-foot advertising."

In the auto industry, history records an example of what results when a business is caught being reactive, not proactive.[2] Volkswagen sold 330 Beetles in 1950, 32,662 in 1955, and 61,507 in 1959. At that point Detroit executives became aware of a new presence on the scene, with one remarking, "We are never going to let the public catch us off base again." The title of the article from which these two anecdotes were extracted has a message for occupational therapists: "To Avoid a Trampling, Get Ahead of the Mass."

The creativity of individuals is demonstrated daily and in unexpected places. Here are just four examples of some new ideas destined to develop into successes.[3] What they have in common is that each was based on an identified need. First is a machine that can design and print labels, on-demand business cards, tags, invitations, and tickets in seven different languages and on paper, aluminum, or acetate. Second, by forcing water through a nozzle the diameter of a human hair at 2.6 times the speed of sound, a superhigh-pressure water-cutting tool can cut through most materials faster than any knife and with no broken blades to repair. Third, a special sticky tape has been designed to make breathing easier by holding nasal passages open, a boon for snorers or professional football players who want to increase their oxygen intake. Finally, a delivery company has already swallowed up 33 smaller delivery companies by accommodating corporations' outsourcing of their distribution and delivery services, picking up canceled checks from bank branches, delivering catalog orders, providing just-in-time warehousing, and making home deliveries.

Selling cosmetics without mass media advertising seems impossible, much like sewing without a needle or preaching without a pulpit. Anita Roddick, founder and managing director of the Body Shop International PLC, has proved that a successful marketing plan need not include costly ad campaigns.[4] Instead, she relies on unique products, good public relations, a highly trained staff, and a well-defined sense of values to operate her 470 stores. Furthermore, she asserts that any entrepreneur can learn similar strategies. In her case, she used nontraditional marketing methods to create a cosmetics company with a social conscience.

Beginning with rejecting animal testing, using natural and biodegradable ingredients, keeping packaging to a minimum, and using recycled materials, she creatively used both her store windows and the media for publicity about social issues campaigns. Public relations firms keep her profile high; she is quoted almost as often on her views on the environment and other issues as she is on her business. All this publicity is free, of course, and carefully orchestrated.

IN MANAGEMENT

Proof that being proactive does pay off was illustrated when representatives of four small companies were interviewed. The four companies were profiled in 1992 as among the 200 best small companies, and then followed up in 1994 to see whether they had continued to be as successful.[5] The young entrepreneurs who had launched the four new companies by using energy, luck, brains, and fierce determination were found to be doing well still. They all had one thing in common to explain this continued success: "an alertness to changes in the marketplace and an uncommon ability to move fast in response to that change." A person's economic security depends not on a job itself or on a career but on employability, adaptability, and willingness to learn and change throughout a lifetime. That includes occupational therapy practitioners who can use their marketing process skills to identify new needs within the community and design responses. Occupational therapy practitioners who remain alert to changes in their personal marketplaces and move quickly to respond to those changes will be the successful leaders and managers of the future.

IN NURSING

Jane S. Wynn, RN, established a successful business because she saw a need and responded with an entrepreneurial solution by thoroughly investigating circumstances and potential problems before launching out to establish Air Medical Alliance.[6] Noting that there were gaps in health plan coverage for patients who were injured or became ill far from their nearest approved care provider, she assembled a preferred provider organization of air medical transport programs across the United States. Wynn included strong quality assurance and central data collection programs in her company. By 1996, there were 16 programs participating in the network and offering air medical transport services to HMOs, PPOs, insurance companies, associations, and corporations.

A marketing approach can be identified throughout Wynn's experience. She receives the fruits of her success in exchange for providing throughout the United States high-quality air medical transport programs that take excellent care of the patients. (All programs that participate in her network had to be accredited.) As for her employees, in return for their good performance on the job, they not only share in the profits but also have a bonus incentive program, leading to a mutually satisfactory exchange arrangement.

Wynn recognized that many people hesitate to choose to start a business because there is no secure paycheck, and, if the idea does not work out, they see that as failure. From Wynn's viewpoint, it is not failure; it is learning and building personal experience. If it does not work out, at least she would always know she tried.

AMONG WOMEN

Because the majority of occupational therapists continue to be women, publications related to entrepreneurship among women are of great potential assistance. For professional women who wish to learn how to start, finance, and manage a successful new business, books such as *The Woman Entrepreneur,*[7] which offers specific guides and tips, a list of networks and trade associations, suggested books and periodicals, and a glossary, can be quite helpful.

Another valuable book is *The Female Entrepreneur: Overcoming Chal-*

lenges in the Business World,[8] whose author observed that "women who have tried to climb the corporate ladder see that the glass ceiling is real, but you can find alternatives." Sitterly[9] further stated that "70% of all new businesses are started by women. Therefore women are the force changing the way we do business—and business itself."

The preceding examples of entrepreneurship in products, management, nursing, and among women are widely varied. However, all are relevant to healthcare delivery: Each represents identification of a need, innovative thinking, response to the need, identification of still more new opportunities, and sensible risk taking. This is entrepreneurship as defined at the beginning of this section.

Dilemmas and Problems in Rehabilitation Facilities

Changes in organization and service delivery, as well as the urgency to increase productivity with fewer resources, are complicated by fluctuating inpatient census levels, increased demands for outpatient rehabilitation services, and shortages of rehabilitation professionals. This picture is found, to a greater or lesser extent, in most rehabilitation facilities. Managers in these locations cannot last long by using wholly reactive measures to increase productivity and control costs. Combining astute business practices with creative, entrepreneurial ideas is enabling organizations to succeed.

IMPROVE EFFICIENCY AND REDUCE COSTS

Attention to systems management is one way to reduce costs while significantly improving the provision of high-quality rehabilitation services. First of all, the most efficient ways to provide services must be identified. Healthcare professionals must concentrate on achieving changes that streamline systems, improve consumer satisfaction, use resources appropriately, and lead to lower costs. In addition to the fact that direct client care is the central concern, effective management, consumer-sensitive support services, information systems providing user-friendly, accurate, and timely data, and interdepartmental cooperation are essential for effective management. Scheduling, admitting, documentation, and communication—systems that support direct care—all influence the cost-effectiveness of services delivered and client satisfaction. Duplicated, ineffective, or unnecessary performance of tasks affects costs. Such details as scheduling clients for therapies before admission, establishing appointment times convenient to clients to ensure better attendance, and coordinating appointments are but a few methods with which to begin making changes within a facility. The best way to begin is to identify opportunities for improvement by asking those directly involved: patients, families, employees, physicians, and all other constituencies who work together to provide optimum care.

Undertaking a quality improvement process, often called continuous quality improvement (CQI) or total quality management (TQM), mandates a total organizational change from hierarchical decision making to employee problem-solving teams (see Chapter 14 for related details). Extensive planning, investment of time, and commitment are required of top managers who themselves must fully understand and accept the principles of CQI. All members of the organization need to learn new skills while contributing their individually unique and valuable information and insights. Reliable data from multiple sources, rather than intuition, generalized conclusions, or anecdotes, are increasingly used by management to drive decision making.

AVOIDING DISASTER DURING CHANGE

An occupational therapy manager comes into his or her position expected to calmly handle change and is indeed considered incompetent if unable to do so. Bennis[11] offered some practical advice to managers when he introduced 10 ways to avoid disaster during periods of change:

1. Recruit with scrupulous honesty, for when expectations are too high and promises too grand, disillusionment is inevitable.
2. Guard against the crazies, making sure that the people you recruit are change agents and not agitators.
3. Build support among like-minded people, whether or not you recruited them, as there can be no change without history and continuity, and a clean sweep is often a waste of resources.
4. Plan for change from a solid conceptual base, understanding how to change as well as what to change, for planning changes is always easier than implementing them; also, it is essential to be hypersensitive to ideas whose time has come and to know when ideas are antithetical to your organization's purposes and values.
5. Don't settle for rhetorical change; rather understand the relationships and best "fit." (Marketing and its primary attention to constituencies is evident in this leadership directive.)
6. Don't allow those who are opposed to change to appropriate basic issues, making sure that those affected are clearly aware of what is to come.
7. Know the territory, the politics.
8. Appreciate environmental factors. (Again, the process of a marketing analysis are apparent in 7 and 8.)
9. Avoid future shock by keeping an eye on the past, present, and future at the same time so as not to neglect any one of them.

10. Remember that change is most successful when those who are affected are involved in the planning.

Reading Chapter 12 in conjunction with this chapter can provide a more complete perspective.

HOW SOME HAVE ADDRESSED THEIR DILEMMAS

Rausch Rehabilitation Services in Chicago conducted a survey of managers and supervisors, primarily occupational therapists, from 86 Chicago area hospitals, outpatient centers, and skilled nursing facilities in 1994.[12] These managers and supervisors were coping with changes in reorganization, higher productivity expectations, new patient care programs, and new staff. Among the actions being taken were (1) allocating less time for staff development, (2) use of multidisciplinary managers and supervisors, (3) more part-time and flex staff, (4) larger caseloads, (5) expanding hours, especially by extending weekday and Saturday hours, and (6) work redesign. As an indicator of the marketing process at work, managers were attending to increased needs of the staff for support and education to maintain morale, prevent burnout, and aid retention as the organization moved through these industry changes.

A proactive approach was used by therapists in the Work Injury Network (WIN) program to decrease workers' compensation costs and build worker productivity.[13] The three phases of the WIN program address prevention, acute intervention, and chronic intervention, with the primary focus on the workers. Care is taken in how clients are approached and how the therapists talk to clients. Filling the needs of the client to be involved and to feel part of his or her own rehabilitation yields results that are mutually satisfying to client, therapist, and employer.

▓ Proactive Alliances

Regardless of setting or area of expertise, resourceful occupational therapy practitioners are capable of entering into successful proactive alliances. An important key is being open to opportunities and new perspectives when problems and changes occur.

IN PRIVATE PRACTICE

During the 1980s, physical and occupational therapists developed many small single and multisite outpatient therapy centers. Some have subsequently joined larger multilevel systems, and others have aligned themselves with similar smaller providers to form networks of providers. Such horizontal integration provides for multiple access sites, standardized pricing for contracts, some autonomy and control, and ultimately lower costs for the payers and public.

As with any configuration of service provision, there are, of course, problems, but these providers are realizing significant gains in market presence and profitability through such contracts. Some general suggestions for therapists considering horizontal alliances include:

1. Set reasonable expectations. Know what you want to achieve through the alliance, and then understand that it will take time, energy, and capital. No contracts should be sought until all legal aspects, financing, strategic positioning, business plan development, and pricing strategies have been completed.

2. Understand your employer market. Be aware of the size of employer organizations in your locale. Larger employers will probably move earlier into managed care and conduct their own negotiating; smaller employers tend to wait longer and to prefer directed buying. National employers may be contracted on a national or regional basis, but local networks are the best choice for a more locally driven market. Employer clinics are still another factor affecting your overall success.

3. Build your alliance around the managed care market needs in your local area.

4. Choose alliance partners carefully. Gather members with different strengths and expertise, if possible, and from different geographic locations. Develop criteria early to evaluate promising network members and their potential contribution. Fiscal and operational closeness is essential to cohesiveness.

5. Structure the alliance for long-term success by setting a high cost for entry and exit, developing a holding company organizational structure, and pooling the assets of the providers into a new organization.

6. Keep track of the larger multilevel systems in the area while using lower pricing and systems to compete against those vertical systems.

7. Use outside help when needed for legal assistance, organizational development, business plan development, audits, pricing, and marketing.

Horizontal alliances can be successful. For example, one midwestern provider group has eight rehab centers providing capitated care to more than 185,000 beneficiaries.[14]

IN EDUCATION

Varied sources have observed that the customarily slower adaptation of higher education to change has resulted in warning signs. According to The Robert Wood Johnson Foundation, some indications requiring attention are (1) a crisis in values among students, administrators, trustees, and faculty; (2) "weeding out" of students rather than educating them; and (3) production of uneducated graduates.[15] These statements refer to higher education in general.

An effective accreditation process, implemented by competent volunteer reviewers and managed by equally capable Accreditation Council for Occupational Therapy Education (ACOTE) staff, has gone far to ensure the best possible curricular content for well-prepared occupational therapy graduates. Most occupational therapy educational programs in the United States have demonstrated timely, innovative attention to students' needs, from flexible weekday class scheduling to weekend programs for assistant level, baccalaureate, master's, and doctoral level students.

Distance learning at the Medical University of South Carolina, use of retired educators as instructors at the University of South Dakota, international academic consortiums at Tufts University and at the University of Texas–San Antonio, work-study arrangements at New York University, living accommodations for single mothers with children at Texas Woman's University, interdisciplinary curricula instituted at Kirksville College Southwest Center, a weekend professional master's degree configuration aimed at adult learners offered at Mercy College, and a problem-based curriculum at Shenandoah University are but a few illustrations. Faculty such as those at the University of Kansas have found innovative ways to integrate research activity into their teaching schedules as they assume responsibility for validation of the profession. Examples abound as educators think creatively and work with college administrators to institute what is needed (see Chapter 10). A proactive approach must continue to be assumed by occupational therapy educators as well as AOTA in this critical aspect of the profession: educational preparation for practice.

IN COMMUNITY MENTAL HEALTH

A consumer-run mental health self-help program, ACT NOW (Advocacy Consumer Training for New Opportunities to Work), in Philadelphia helps clients find jobs as one key to prospering in an era of managed care and budget cuts.[16] Occupational therapists can teach consumers self-management and self-care skills in this and other consumer-run projects, as well as provide emotional support and practical advice in a nonjudgmental, nonthreatening atmosphere. After classroom training in interviews and job searches, clients are referred to established businesses for work internships with the understanding they will be offered permanent employment if they are successful. During 1995, 70 percent of the interns graduated, and nearly all were hired.

In San Francisco, Glenda Jeong, MA, OTR, exemplifies success with a similar client population.[17] After working in a day treatment program, Jeong founded a vocational program in collaboration with a colleague who now runs the business side of the enterprise: CVE/Keystone. The primary goal of the organization is to provide vocational counseling, coaching, and support to its clients, offering employment to 80 to 90 people at any given time. Clients' diagnoses include paranoid schizophrenia, major depression, bipolar disorder, dual diagnoses with substance abuse, traumatic brain injury, and stroke with psychiatric and cognitive symptoms. Rather than experiencing a hospital environment, which implies what a client cannot do, CVE/Keystone enables clients to feel that they have options and choices.

Support services are offered in Spanish, Cantonese, French, and English, and clients' experiences are tailored to their needs (once more, the marketing approach leading to success). Weekly peer work support groups, monthly workshops about the impact clients' employment might have on benefits, and job-seeking skills are among the topics addressed. In addition, quarterly workshops are held for providers such as clinicians, therapists, and counselors. Throughout the process, the role of the occupational therapist is *consultative*, performing customary duties such as writing assessments, guiding self-assessments, and completing work-site assessments.

It is Jeong's opinion[17] that many new opportunities await occupational therapy practitioners, but that much depends on how occupational therapy practitioners package themselves; they do not have to be in occupational therapy positions to do occupational therapy. She suggests that they look at employee assistance and wellness programs. Jeong herself, for instance, exemplifies an emphasis on getting involved in the wider community and publicizing occupational therapy.

For an introduction to information sources about mental health, the reader is referred to the end of the chapter.

IN RURAL SETTINGS

In Columbia, Missouri, a proactive occupational therapist is hard at work providing leadership among farmers.[18] As therapeutic services coordinator for the Missouri AgrAbility Project, Doris O'Hara, OTR/C, holds a consultative position she has developed outside the medical model. O'Hara uses both prevention and rehabilitation to assist both male and female farmers and their family members. The AgrAbility Project coordinates a variety of services to farmers with disabilities that will allow them to remain active on farms or in farm-related occupations. The project is funded through the Extension Service, the U.S. Department of Agriculture, and National Easter Seal Society. O'Hara's clinical background in technology and work evaluation and her work in rural home health and in small long-term facilities serve her well in her position. She works closely with the University of Missouri–Columbia Occupational Therapy Program, and provides opportunities for students to gain experience in a rural setting. Diana Baldwin, MA, OTR/C, program director, says it is unique in this country to have an occupational therapy program involved in an AgrAbility grant. Baldwin and O'Hara state that their involvement in this type of project will provide a model for other areas in the collaborative potential for occupational therapists. They are studying how occupational therapists are involved in AgrAbility training and ways of teaching students to work in farm settings by incorporating farm experiences into fieldwork assignments.

O'Hara coordinates therapeutic services, including occupational therapy, in the region, by acting as resource liaison and presenting educational training sessions to give clients the services they need. The occupational therapists specialize in assessing farmers' skills and abilities and recommending appropriate modifications and methods of using available assistive technology. Agricultural and agribusiness workers may have one or more of the following disabilities or conditions: amputations, multiple sclerosis, arthritis, muscular dystrophy, back pain, postpolio syndrome, cancer, respiratory problems, cardiac problems, spinal cord injury, cerebral palsy, stroke, deafness and hearing impairments, traumatic brain injury, mental retardation, blindness, or vision impairments. Twenty-one states have received grants for similar projects, to date.[19]

The Ongoing Potential for Entrepreneurship in Health Care

On September 13, 1994, a federal crime bill was signed into law. The law's aim is to develop a "tough and smart" crime policy with a stronger public safety approach and more efficient use of public health techniques through viewing crime and violence as health issues. Because rehabilitation professionals are increasingly more focused on preventive measures, it has been posited that they can therefore direct their energies toward treating crime and violence as "social disabilities." For example, on-the-job training and vocational development programs that teach the work ethic, how to prepare resumes, and other skills necessary for transition into the job world are but one possibility.

The new law has mandated programs focusing on youths who are at risk of committing future crimes and who need counseling and guidance to increase their self-esteem, make responsible choices, improve academic performance, build life skills, and develop natural outlets for their energy. Occupational therapists are already employed in prison systems, with many not only comfortable but also pleased to be in this setting. Progressing to the preventive aspect with this potential population would seem a natural move. Why not use the occupational therapist's knowledge and skills in preventive measures to help still another "well population" with goal setting, stress reduction, and time management?

This is but a single example of an opportunity, one potential direction to move. Look around you. Find others.

Occupational Therapists Must Clarify and Use Their Many Strengths

Occupational therapy practitioners themselves are responsible for bringing about changes in their careers and in their organizations. To do that, it is essential to begin with a good understanding of professional issues and of the nature of healthcare systems. Knowledge of organizational theory, research, leadership theory and techniques, strategic planning, finance, resource allocation, and information management systems is required if occupational therapists are to be recognized as effective leaders and managers. Occupational therapists need to understand new roles by seeing the big picture, looking at health care as a business, marketing their skills, and gaining new skills and experience.

By visualizing themselves in what might as first seem to be unusual roles, occupational therapists can begin immediately to practice their innate creativity and to proactively move into new professional opportunities. Many in occupational therapy are, in fact, assuming "educational" positions in the community that require guiding, facilitating, directing, and encouraging rather than traditional caregiving in hospitals and rehabilitation centers. Client-centered practice performed in communities, homes, or schools actually makes greater use of the strengths and expertise of occupational therapists, as it enables people to engage in occupations and activities that are meaningful to them. With society's growing appreciation of preventive measures as well, the "roads not yet taken" are open and should be obvious for the proactive occupational therapist.

▨ Summary

This chapter has clarified the need for occupational therapists to develop proactive attitudes and approaches to practice. Specific suggestions for managers today about how to manage change were outlined. Dilemmas and problems existing in healthcare systems were recognized, and examples of some successful solutions shared. The presence and excitement of entrepreneurism were illustrated in the origination of innovative products and services. Examples of entrepreneurism at work among some healthcare professionals were described. Evidence of proactive, innovative occupational therapy educational programs was noted. Finally, occupational therapists were reminded of the infinite number of opportunities for innovative practice of which they must take advantage. Strategic planning as an entrepreneurial and proactive skill is further discussed in Part Seven.

REFERENCES

1. Kotler, P, and Clarke, RN: Marketing for Health Care Organizations. Prentice-Hall, Englewood Cliffs, NJ, 1987, p 118.
2. Sellers, P: To avoid a trampling, get ahead of the mass. Fortune, May 15, 1995, p 201.
3. Schonfeld, E: Companies to watch. Fortune, Sept 4, 1995, p 137.
4. Wallace, C: Lessons in marketing—from a maverick. Working Woman, Oct 1990, p 81.
5. Hayes, J: Two hundred best small companies. Forbes, Nov 7, 1994, p 222.
6. Schwermer, A: Winds of change lead nurse to start air medical business. Nursing & Allied Healthweek–Dallas/Fort Worth 1:2, Jan 29, 1996.
7. Hisrich, RD, and Brush, CG: The Woman Entrepreneur: Starting, Financing, and Managing a Successful New Business. DC Heath, Lexington, Mass, 1986.

8. Sitterly, C: The Female Entrepreneur: Overcoming Challenges in the Business World. Crisp Publications, Menlo Park, Calif, 1994.
9. Business courses designed for women and entrepreneurs. TWU Update 18:(47):2, July 22, 1996.
10. Rehkamp, N: Paying the price of high-quality care. Rehab Management 4(5):103, June/July 1991.
11. Bennis, W: Why Leaders Can't Lead. Jossey-Bass, San Francisco, 1989, p 147.
12. Grace, IA: Charting changes in rehab. OT Week 9(7):16, Feb 16, 1995.
13. Reichley, ML: Employers and employees "WIN" with pro-active approach. Advance for Occupational Therapists 11(26), July 3, 1995.
14. Fowler, FJ: Making horizontal alliances work. Rehab Economics(suppl) 3(5):98. In Rehab Management, Aug/Sept 1995.
15. Wingspread Group: An American Imperative: Higher Expectations for Higher Education? The Robert Wood Johnson Foundation, Princeton, NJ, 1993.
16. Hettinger, J: Helping clients become wage earners. OT Week 10(9), Feb 29, 1996.
17. Tapper, BE: New opportunities for mental health OTs. OT Week 10(9), Feb 29, 1996.
18. Keely, M: The Missouri AgrAbility Project: Getting farmers back on the job. Connections. University of Missouri–Columbia, Spring, 1995, p 3.
19. The Missouri AgrAbility Project: The Missouri AgrAbility Project Training Manual. Author, Columbia, Mo, 1995.

Additional Sources for Information about Mental Services

Although new information continually becomes available, someone seeking facts must start somewhere. Students just beginning their search for more information are advised to start by choosing among the following.

Advocacy

Bazelton Center for Mental Health, 1101 15th St., NW, Suite 1212, Washington, DC 20005-5002. At this writing, assistance may be found through its publications *Managing Managed Care for Publicly Financed Mental Health Services*, 1995; *At Home–Strategies for Serving Older People with Mental Disorders in the Community*, 1995; *Opening Public Agency Doors*, 1995.

Communication

Wellness Reproductions Inc., 1-800-669-9208 (distributors for Nurseminars Inc. videotapes). *Understanding and Communicating with a Person Who Is Hallucinating*, 1989; *Understanding and Communicating with a Person Who Is Experiencing Mania*, 1989; *Understanding Relapse: Managing the Symptoms of Schizophrenia*, 1989.

Alzheimer's Disease

Gibbs Associates, Boulder, Colo. Publication: *He Used to Be Somebody: A Journey into Alzheimer's Disease through the Eyes of a Caregiver*, 1995.

From AOTA

Wellness and Lifestyle Renewal: A Manual for Personal Change, by Rosenfeld, 1993. *Psychosocial Occupational Therapy: Proactive Approaches*, by Cottrell, 1993. *Occupational Therapy Treatment Goals for the Physically and Cognitively Disabled*, by Allen et al, 1992.

Additional telephone numbers:

National Depressive and Manic Depressive Association (312) 993-0066.
National Alliance for the Mentally Ill (703) 524-7600.
National Alliance for Research on Schizophrenia and Depression (312) 641-1666.
Alzheimer's Association 1-800-272-3900.

PART SEVEN

STRATEGIC PLANNING

*We are not passive TV viewers watching
the human story unfold. We are living the
story and we have a fair chance to bring the
story to a successful resolution.*

Yankelovich, *New Rules*

CHAPTER 17

■▓▓▓▓▓▓▓▓▓▓▓▓▓▓▓▓▓

Systematic Decision Making

CHAPTER OBJECTIVES ▓ ▓ ▓ ▓ ▓ ▓ ▓ ▓ ▓ ▓

- To know what strategic planning means.
- To identify the link between marketing and strategic planning.
- To realize the importance of simultaneously looking backward and forward in the strategic planning process.
- To appreciate the vital lessons that can be learned from others' business failures.
- To recognize how organization development is related to strategic planning.
- To follow the process of making sound decisions.
- To recognize how to use the nominal group technique and Delphi process to make good decisions.
- To note the steps in beginning a strategic plan.

Grandmothers are so wise! Like most teenagers growing up, I seemed to be constantly wrestling with ponderous (to me) problems that needed decisions. My grandmother's advice was to simply ask, "Will it matter 10 years from now?" Can you honestly think of a better way to prioritize the time you spend in daily deliberations? Doesn't that simple question put your perspective where it belongs? Common sense dictates that all growing and developing individuals, organizations, and professions alike must adapt and change to survive, let alone achieve success, however that is measured. The decisions affecting and determining the extent and direction of that growth are what constitute futuristic, strategic planning. The ability to discern the simple from the critical and to expend the appropriate amount of time and energy in information gathering and deliberation before making the decision is at the heart of the matter. This chapter deals with that fundamental topic, describes the decision-making process, and offers specific ways to make effective decisions.

Ask the Right Questions

Before strategic planning was accepted as a useful methodology, administrators approached planning by beginning with "what if": What if the neighboring hospital adds more beds? What if our competitor decides to manufacture more splints? Through use of strategic planning, a comprehensive analysis of your strengths, of what you do best, is made. Resources are allocated to greatest advantage to fulfill the objectives you have made for your future activities.

Strategic planning goes beyond traditional healthcare planning, and it requires good marketing data and analysis. One way to begin *your* strategic planning is to ask:

1. In what am I a leader?
2. What are my strengths?
3. What are my unique strengths?
4. What are my weaknesses?
5. What are my potential threats?
6. How can I build strength on strength?

Drucker,[1] from a slightly different view but with a similar purpose, suggested beginning by asking yourself three other questions:

1. What is my business?
2. What will it be?
3. What should it be?

As you contemplate decisions abut the future, either of these heuristic beginnings is a right way to start. Wise decision making eventually separates effective and ineffective managers. Futurity built into decision making is the vital ingredient, and keeping the raison d'être of the business in mind at all times is how to reach that future. Begin with the vision, with what you want to have happen. Develop your forecast, what you think is going to happen. Then develop your strategic plan, what must happen if you are to achieve the goal you have set.

Strategic Planning vs. a Strategic Plan

Strategic planning is a constant ongoing process, whereas a strategic plan is the result of stopping and taking a still picture of the present and future environments. Strategic planning is the "continuous process of making present risk-taking decisions systematically and with the greatest knowledge of their futurity; organizing systematically the efforts needed to carry out these decisions; and measuring the results of these decisions against the expectations through organized, systematic feedback."[2]

A strategic plan, by contrast, is a black-and-white document (or a scheme outlined in your computer) describing your intentions. No two strategic plans are alike; however, there are characteristic components in all strategic plans:

1. A mission statement
2. Major objectives
3. An action plan
4. A description of resources needed to fulfill the objectives
5. A procedure for monitoring performance
6. An evaluation system[3]
7. A plan using the results of the evaluations to modify the original objectives and make revisions as indicated.

Strategic Planning Means Strategic Decision Making

Strategic planning is an entrepreneurial skill, according to Drucker, and for a manager it is the essential first step toward making decisions that have a long futurity and are made on a systematic basis. It is the only way to prevent committing today's energy and resources to continue supporting past decisions. For that reason, Drucker used *strategic decision making* as a synonym for *strategic planning* to put an unmistakable emphasis on its importance in any enterprise. The implication in Drucker's question 3 (on the previous list of questions) is that there *will* be change involved and that risks *will* be taken. The trick is to know which changes to make, which risks are the right ones to take, and what new and different ways there are to reach your new objectives. Entrepreneurial decision making is always more responsible and more likely to be effective if it is rational, organized, and based on knowledge rather than on intuition or prophecy.

▨ Looking Back While Looking Ahead

Drucker's contention was that ridding ourselves of what is no longer needed from the past is the first thing to do to attain the objectives of tomorrow. Strategic planning is looking for new and different ways to attain objectives rather than believing that simply doing more of the same will suffice. In his words, "Systematic sloughing off of yesterday is a plan by itself,"[2] yet getting rid of yesterday is the decision many long-range plans seldom attack. As a result, new plans never become reality, and nothing changes. Drucker's quote is quite familiar to all management students. One of its implications is not as evident as it might be, though; in order to systematically slough off yesterday, one must first *look at yesterday* and weigh which parts of yesterday are too vital to lose. Those parts are the legacy of yesterday that are to be appreciated, valued, and built into the decision being made today, the decision that will directly affect tomorrow. For instance, the great and enduring concept of occupational therapy has an underpinning of core values and a sense of timeless purpose that should never change. If these bedrock principles are given up, a great idea will be overlooked. The answer is, over time, to successfully adapt daily practice to a changing world without losing those core values.

Bennis[4] concurred with Drucker on the importance of building on successful past experience while looking to the future. In addition, he stated that at least part of the problem with American business resides in its elevation of obedience over imagination; he noted that the very businesses suffering the most, such as the auto industry, were founded by people who were more imaginative than obedient. America itself grew out of both disobedience and vision. Bennis suggested being hypersensitive to ideas whose hour has come while prudently keeping in mind the old, but always true, adage that those who ignore history are destined to repeat it.[4] Earlier, two American philosophers said it another way: "The present is the past rolled up for action. The past is the present unrolled for understanding."[5]

WHAT CAN BE LEARNED FROM BUSINESS FAILURES

A study was conducted based on the premise that lessons can be learned by paying attention to why some successful organizations get into trouble.[6] Questions concerning business failures were asked in 1994 of corporate executives, management consultants, venture capitalists, turnaround specialists, equity analysts, and portfolio managers. A summary of their responses identified six key situations, related to business failures, that they recommended be avoided:

1. Identity crisis. Aside from simply inept management, the most frequent cause of failure was determined to be the inability to understand the

very fundamentals of the business itself. What is the business's core expertise? What are the key services or products that earn the profits? Without a thorough understanding of what the enterprise is all about, decision making becomes capricious, and the company drifts. Trying to make quick fixes and demanding too many successive changes exacerbate worker resistance. Moving too far from essential core skills and expertise also creates problems because the very "reason for being" has been forgotten.

2. Failures of vision. For a company to survive, imagination and creativity must be part of strategic planning and sensing future trends. Getting stuck with yesterday's technology has been one of the most common disasters of shortsightedness. The price of not paying attention can be steep when managers go to sleep.

3. The big squeeze. Watch out for overwhelming debt from which it is impossible to recover.

4. The glue sticks and sticks. Comfortably maintaining outmoded models and past glories breeds complacency and bloat with no one working very hard. Pure human nature has come into play, as workers see no need to move beyond a technique or strategy that worked well in the past. It could be that success today has in it the seed of future failure, a notion expressed by one of the survey's participants. When those responsible for the organization cannot abandon strategies that no longer work, that same attitude will undoubtedly spread throughout the organization. In short, arrogance and relying on past success can blind people. Trouble starts when you have good people whose ideas do not reach the top.

5. Stay close to the customer. Regardless of constant reminders of how essential this fact has become, many companies continue to fail because they have lost touch with their most important customers. Following up on key customers to determine why they discontinued using products or services gives valuable information affecting the future because one can learn more from mistakes than from successes. It is pretty hard to solve problems and satisfy customers' needs if you do not know what you are doing wrong.

6. Enemies within. What has been declared tantamount to managerial malpractice are such problems as managerial hypocrisy, that is, encouraging risk taking and then punishing good-faith failures, preaching one doctrine and practicing another, or announcing the importance of teamwork and rewarding individuals who work at standing out from the crowd.[6]

This summary of observations based on lessons learned from failures contains wise advice for occupational therapists. Armed with a clear retrospective view and decisions already made about what should be "sloughed off," the manager then approaches the organization development phase of strategic planning.

Strategic Planning and Organization Development

Hand in hand with strategic planning goes organization development. The strategic planning process provides a framework for risk-taking decisions. The subsequent actions that must be taken to implement a decision require changes in an organization. Organization development is a process set in motion in response to change, an educational strategy intended to change the beliefs, attitudes, values, and structure of organizations to enable them to adapt to new technologies, markets, challenges, and change itself.[7]

Two most important aspects of organization development are (1) as a way of managing change and (2) as a way of focusing human energy toward specified desired outcomes. Fundamental to organization development is the fact that the individual members of the organization must be given opportunities to grow, which continues this book's ongoing emphasis on an employee-centered environment. Continuing support for this assertion comes daily from multiple sources, as successful companies acknowledge that success or failure depends on the attitude of the employees.[8] Furthermore, organization development is a practical approach. Much has been written about organization development, and detailed information is available in the business section of the library.

Strategic Planning Links with Marketing

Kotler and Clarke[9] defined *strategic planning* as "the managerial process of developing and maintaining a strategic fit between the organization's goals and resources and its changing market opportunities." Here is the important link between strategic planning, or strategic decision making, and marketing. The admonition to be constantly alert for opportunities is implied in each of the definitions of *strategic planning* discussed here. Being watchful for opportunities can also be detected in the advice that strategic planning is an entrepreneurial skill.

MacStravic[10] concurred with Kotler about the integral nature of the strategic planning process in the development of marketing plans and built on the work of Drucker and others to illustrate the point. MacStravic considered such planning to be the first essential step in managing all marketing efforts. He likened it to the manner in which reporters reach their objective: the story. Before ever beginning, the reporter asks what, who, where, how, when, and why.

Similarly, in marketing an environmental assessment is done first (the marketing audit), followed by decisions about marketing objectives and strategies (see Chapter 4). Regardless of definitions and terms, marketing plans that will continually meet new and changing challenges rely heavily on strategic thinking and logical decision making.

How to Make Sound Decisions

Because this chapter is about decision making, it is logical to include an introduction to the basic process of making good decisions. Whether the decision is selecting a brand of toothpaste or entering into an alliance with another private practice group, making decisions is a fact of everyday life. Common sense tells you that one decision can be made almost automatically, while the other decision will have far-reaching effects for years to come. In general, the potential consequences determine the amount of effort you put into making a decision. Yet in every case you are receiving information, thinking of alternatives, comparing options, selecting one, and putting your choice into action.

Volumes have been written about the decision-making process, and all agree that there are basically six elements involved: (1) identifying the problem, (2) gathering information, (3) analyzing information, (4) choosing an alternative, (5) implementing the chosen alternative, and (6) following up on implementation.[10] The more complex and far-reaching the problem, the more important each element becomes. Following are brief explanations of what each step in the decision-making process means:

1. Identifying the problem. Elementary as this may seem, it often is the most overlooked, misunderstood, and difficult. Is there in fact a problem? Is it truly the problem, or is it a symptom of a problem? Your first task before you can proceed any further is to specify in words exactly what the problem is.

2. Gathering information. With a specific purpose in mind, get as much information as you think you need to help you make an intelligent decision. Remember that no one can tell you how much information is "enough," and it is up to you to decide whether the amount of effort is commensurate with the potential impact of the decision you have to make. Finally, work only with facts, not opinions or rumors.

3. Analyzing information and forming it into alternatives. Guard against endlessly gathering information. Knowing you have answered as many questions as possible and found as much reliable data as are available, realize that you may never feel wholly comfortable. At some point it is incumbent on you to take a stand and assume some risk. In the case of decisions with significant potential consequences, the needs of the organization, the department, the clients, and you yourself all enter into your deliberations, but most often it is impossible to satisfy all. The next step is then to arrange all your decision factors into alternatives among

which you must choose. Using some criteria can narrow your list to three or four.

4. Choosing an alternative. Make your decision based on which best fills your needs and suits your preferences. Test your selection by questioning whether it deals with the problem directly, creates a policy, or has adverse effects on any other aspects of your operations.

5. Implementing that alternative. This is action, and from here the decision maker can proceed to use the basic management functions of planning, organizing, directing, coordinating, and controlling.

6. Follow-up. This is usually the weakest part of the process, even though it is the most critical if the effects of your decision are to be measured before you continue. Monitoring is essential, and so are clarifying instructions, assessing timing, making adjustments, and supervising the effort.

Associated with forming alternatives and making choices are constraints to take into consideration, most commonly time, money, quality, personalities, and politics.[11]

▨ The Role of Brainstorming in the Decision-Making Process

In the decision-making process, it is often helpful for a small group to brainstorm what strategic action can take advantage of available opportunities and what risks are involved. The alternatives for each risk or opportunity may be considered and the related advantages or disadvantages acknowledged. As a result of this process preferred options may be selected.

FORMAL AND INFORMAL GROUPS

Formal groups may be classified into two types: command groups or task groups. The *command group* fits into an organization chart and consists of subordinates who report to a given supervisor, for example, a chief of the rehabilitation unit and those for whom that person is responsible. A *task group* is made up of employees who work together to complete a particular task or project, for example, a group including a nurse, occupational therapist, and physical therapist assigned to resolve a transportation scheduling problem.

Informal groups are natural groupings of people that evolve in response to social needs. One specific kind of group is the *interest group*. The objectives of such groups are not related to those of the organization. An example is employees grouping together to present a unified front to management for more benefits. A *friendship group* is formed because the members have something in common such as age, political beliefs, or ethnic background.

In general, formal groups are designated by the formal organization and are a means to an end. Informal groups are important for their own sake, satisfying a basic need for association.[12]

DELPHI TECHNIQUE

Two techniques that increase the creative capability of a group in generating ideas and understanding problems in order to arrive at better group decisions are the Delphi and nominal group methods.[13] If generation of ideas and consequent consensus are done by mail, the Delphi process has been effective. Conducted by mail, this technique involves the solicitation and comparison of anonymous observations on the topic of interest through sequential questionnaires mailed out to participants and interspersed with summarized information and feedback of opinions from earlier responses. Participants independently generate their ideas to answer the first questionnaire and return it. Staff members summarize these as group consensus and then return this summary along with a second questionnaire with new, more focused questions. After several rounds of anonymous group judgment, the belief is that the consensus estimate will result in a better decision.

THE NOMINAL GROUP PROCESS

The nominal group process is a structured group meeting in which a group of 7 to 10 members sit around a table but do not speak to each other. Instead, each person writes ideas and, after 5 minutes, a structured sharing of ideas takes place. Each person, in turn, presents one idea while one individual who was designated as recorder writes the ideas on a flip chart in full view of the entire group. This process continues until all participants have no more ideas to share. The resulting list of ideas is used for structured discussion in which each idea receives attention before voting. To accomplish this, members clarify or state their degree of support for each idea. Independent voting next takes place as each member, in private, selects priorities by ranking or voting. The group decision is the mathematically pooled outcome of the individual votes.[13] Conflict is often encountered during group interactions toward decision making, and a helpful reference to address this situation is contained in *Management Principles for Health Professionals.*[3]

▪ Summary

This chapter discussed the definitions and elements of strategic planning, including its association with marketing. A generalized description of the decision-making process was outlined. The role of brainstorming, specifically the nominal group technique and the Delphi process, was introduced. The importance of heeding history while looking ahead was emphasized and illustrated by using some lessons learned from recent business failures. Chapter 18 continues the discussion of strategic planning as related to healthcare delivery services in general and to occupational therapy specifically.

REFERENCES

1. Drucker, PF: An Introductory View of Management. Harper & Row, New York, 1977, p 118.
2. Drucker, PF: An Introductory View of Management. Harper & Row, New York, 1977, p 119.
3. Liebler, JG, Levine, RE, and Rothman, J: Management Principles for Health Professionals. Aspen, Gaithersburg, Md, 1992.
4. Bennis, W: Why Leaders Can't Lead. Jossey-Bass, San Francisco, 1989.
5. Durant, W, and Durant, A: Lessons from History. Simon & Schuster, New York, 1968.
6. Labich, K: Why companies fail. Fortune, Nov 14, 1994, p 52.
7. Bennis, WG: Organization Development: Its Nature, Origins, and Prospects. Addision-Wesley, Reading, Mass, 1969.
8. Sellers, P: Can Home Depot fix its sagging stock? Fortune 133(4):139, Mar 4, 1996.
9. Kotler, P, and Clarke, RN: Marketing for Health Care Organizations. Prentice-Hall, Englewood Cliffs, NJ, 1987, p 90.
10. MacStravic, RE: Marketing Health Care. Aspen, Germantown, Md, 1977.
11. McConnell, CR: The Effective Health Care Supervisor. Aspen, Rockville, Md, 1982.
12. Gibson, JL, Ivancevich, JM, and Donnelly, JH: Organizations: Behavior, Structure, Processes. Business Publications, Dallas, 1976.
13. Delbecq, AL, Van de Ven, AH, and Gustafson, DH: Group Techniques for Program Planning: A Guide to Nominal Group and Delphi Processes. Scott Foresman, Glenview, Ill, 1975.

Suggested Sources for Additional Information about Strategic Planning

Camillus, JC: Strategic Planning and Management Control. Lexington Books, Lexington, Mass, 1986.

Capon, N, Farley, JU, and Hulbert, J: Complete Strategic Planning. Columbia University Press, New York, 1987.

DeGreen, KB: The Adaptive Organization: Anticipation and Management of Crisis. John Wiley, New York, 1981.

Drucker, PF: Managing in Turbulent Times. Harper & Row, New York, 1980.

Drucker, PF: Management, Tasks, Responsibilities, Practices. Harper & Row, New York, 1985.

Jaffe, EG, and Epstein, CF: Occupational Therapy Consultation: Theory, Principles and Practice. Mosby–Year Book, St. Louis, 1992, pp 76–80.

Schwartz, D: Introduction to Management: Principles, Practices, and Processes. Harcourt Brace Jovanovich, New York, 1980.

The Futurist. The World Future Society, Bethesda, Md.

CHAPTER 18

■▬▬▬▬▬▬▬▬▬▬▬

Strategic Planning and Occupational Therapy

Strategic planning is a constant, ongoing process, a habit that should be formed, and an approach and way of thinking that should become part of all occupational therapy practitioners' everyday routines. Rather than dealing with future decisions, strategic planning deals with the futurity of those important decisions being made at present and with which the decision makers will have to live. This chapter is targeted toward *all* occupational therapy practitioners, whether in institutions or the community, in education or private practice, whether shaping their own careers or shaping an occupational therapy program. It includes examples of the strategic planning in process in national corporations, in AOTA, in educational institutions, among nurses, and in occupational therapy practice; emphasis on the critical role played by effective, committed leaders with vision; an explanation of stretch targets; and a way to assess the stage of penetration of managed care in your own region.

Begin with a Vision

Occupational therapists need vision to reach their full potential. The same holds true for the organization and for the country of which they are part. Missions, whether personal or organizational, need to be big enough to make everyone stretch and grow. Visionary bosses can see the threat over the horizon and act before it is too late. It then takes adroit management to enlist those who are responsible for carrying out the action to join in the mission and the work needed to bring it about. What managers get paid for is to make tough decisions and then to carry them out. No decision is fraught with more anxiety than shedding old lines or businesses and plunging into new ones. The same is true of radically altering the way an organization goes about doing what it already is prepared to do.

To illustrate, examples of managers who handled anxiety-producing decisions and the futurity of those decisions can be drawn from the corporate world.[1] In every case, careful attention to detail, risk taking based on solid factual information, and astute study of trends went into each strategic plan.

1. In 1985 General Motors decided to add new and different product components, the acquisition of which caused ripples throughout the company for the next 5 years.

2. Gould, Inc., clung against odds to a plan to transform the company, maintaining that you must either believe in your idea or not.

3. Gannett Company, founder of *USA Today*, planned for the new publication with great care. By 1980 it had surveyed 400,000 households to determine whether there was a need or desire for such a publication before devising its strategic plan and marketing plan.

4. Warner-Lambert, in 1980, believed in strategic planning, but CEO Ward Hagan admitted having difficulty afterwards in making all the little decisions that went into making the big decision happen.

5. Rolm Corporation CEO Kenneth Oshman firmly believed that any manager's job is "to peer intently three to five years into the future looking for problems."[1]

The same can be said about occupational therapy practice and many of the directions in which it is being propelled while deliberately moving. Wise strategic planning and perceptive decision making are critical to the future of occupational therapy.

▨ Activating the Vision

As CEO Hagan of Warner-Lambert discovered, the first question is "How do you create a vision that inspires personal responsibility among your staff?" You can tell whether you have inspired that personal responsibility when everyone in your organization has accepted the same mission and is working to achieve it, as vision is the link between dream and action only if it is carried through to fruition.

People *want* to make a commitment. In the long run, commitment and not authority truly produces results. The manager who provides the freedom and environment in which committed people can work toward a shared mission succeeds and is truly a leader. A leader is the source of the vision, a person who holds a unique combination of skills: the intelligence to create a vision and the practical capability to make it happen. Successful managers actually see themselves as leaders and have the discernment to start ventures[2] (see Part One for the relationship of management and leadership).

Any enterprise must begin with a strategic plan that includes listening to potential consumers, selecting the right target markets and constituencies, and allocating adequate resources. Marketing provides long-range direction and purpose but must be coordinated with other functional activities. As already noted, the marketing concept requires a consumer-buyer orientation; therefore, managers' decisions and activities focus on customer needs and on adapting the organizations' products, prices, promotional efforts, and other activities to meet these needs.

The well-documented experience of the Chrysler Corporation, beginning over two decades ago, illustrates these points.[3] The company appealed to the federal government in 1979 for $1.5 billion in loan guarantees in order to survive. Several reasons were given for this state of affairs, but most analysts were of the opinion that two strategic planning mistakes were made earlier in the 1970s. By 1983 Chrysler had paid off its federally guaranteed loans 7 years early and was once again profitable. The absence of a strong customer-centered marketing orientation was considered to be a prime contributor to the company's problems in the 1970s, and an improved market sensitivity reflected in a revised strategic plan was a key to the company's success in the 1980s, another example of the inseparable nature of strategic planning and marketing.

STRETCH TARGETS AND BENCHMARKS

It is sometimes beneficial as well as instructive to practice and use the vernacular of the field you are studying. One of the words being used recently in businesses is *stretch targets*. Some managers recognized that small, incremental goals seemed to invite everyone to continue doing the same comfortable processes year after year, and mediocrity was the result. Those managers with foresight further perceived that performance had to become far better to prosper or even, in the long term, to survive. For that reason, among others, the terms *stretch targets* and *stretch management* have appeared frequently in popular business literature.

Stretch targets are, quite simply, targets or goals designed to require extraordinary effort to achieve them. The first reaction of those made responsible for their accomplishment is that the goals are impossible; however, wise managers have already carefully gauged the parameters and realities of these targets.

Dubbed by some as masters of the art of stretch management, Boeing, Mead, 3M, and CSX agree that they have some basic techniques in common, although they use them to varying degrees depending upon the circumstances. First, a clear, convincing, long-term goal must be set, with honesty as the best management practice. The goal must ring true, be unambiguous, and its importance and necessity made understandable; then the goal must be translated into one or two specific stretch targets so that the aim is clearer. Second, benchmarking is used to prove that the goal, although difficult, is not impossible and that others have accomplished it. (The definition of *benchmark* is a standard, criterion, gauge, or measure with which to compare or judge.) The idea is to show that if others can do it, so can we—a powerful persuader. The third and final step is for the manager to get out of the way and let those who were designated find ways to meet the targets.[4]

▓ Nurses Who Practiced Futuristic Decision Making

Laura Vonfrolio, a critical-care nurse, was frustrated by a perceived lack of respect and appreciation and left hospital employment to set up a business to train financial corporation employees in cardiopulmonary resuscitation.[5] She is one of many nurses who have "packaged" their expertise and skills in new ways, made strategic plans, and moved successfully into new practice areas.

Many nurses today have recognized that the United States cannot afford to have a care system based totally on illness any longer; instead, a healthcare system is in order, which provides many more opportunities for nurses to have their own businesses. Some have learned advanced marketing and business skills and have started businesses that provide on-site services and wellness programs to corporations, consulting and placement firms, and many other diverse types of business, including one who established a book publishing company that also publishes *Revolution: A Journal of Nurse Empowerment.*

Reminiscent of the warning that it is a mistake to watch too long the doors that are closing and thus miss those doors that are opening, nurses who had found themselves being replaced by unlicensed personnel took matters into their own hands. They realized that they have a plethora of skills waiting to be used elsewhere, and so today nurse entrepreneurs have expanded into home health care, law, publishing, education, writing, consultation, invention, and company president positions, to name a few.

Sharing with occupational therapists the fact that formal business training is seldom found in healthcare professions educational programs, many nurses are overcoming that lack in creative and practical ways. Successful nurse entrepreneurs advise others to use careful marketing approaches, attend business workshops, and continue to work full-time or part-time while getting their ventures off the ground. One nurse set up a company that markets an intravenous site protector that prevents needles from being accidentally pulled out. Another nurse established a business that offers in-home child safety evaluations and modifications. Several nurses have established innovative and timely home health companies. They have noted with interest that the increase in home health care is a sign that nursing has come full circle, for in the early part of the 20th century nurses cared for patients in their homes.

Among the tips offered by these entrepreneurial nurses for those who are contemplating similar moves are the following:

- Thoroughly investigate all aspects of the intended business field.
- Be prepared to invest much time, money, and energy.
- Attend the best marketing workshop you can afford.
- Develop a strategic plan.
- Find an accountant, a lawyer, and a banker you can trust.
- Make and continually update long-range plans.
- If possible, continue working at a job until the business is established.
- Keep start-up expenses to a minimum.
- Do what you love, and enjoy it.[5]

Strategic Planning and Managed Care in Your Own Town

If occupational therapists are to be among the successful healthcare providers of the future, they must adapt to the changing market conditions surrounding them. The managed care, or managed cost, environment must be approached by looking for new and different ways to attain objectives rather than by believing that doing more of the same will suffice. Managed care requires efficiency and effectiveness in meeting the demands of consumers. As emphasized throughout this book, *consumers* means *all* occupational therapy consumers or constituencies, including managed care organizations.

Frances Fowler's[6] strategy emphasized the need for therapists to adopt a proactive stance in reshaping services and systems. She stressed the critical need to continuously assess the stage to which managed care has developed in your own community and to develop a timetable that lays out the sequential steps and changes you will need. Conducting all planning from a cost-reduction perspective, therapists should base adjustments on an assessment of where the market is now and where it is headed. To evaluate the stage of development of the managed care market in your own area, the author suggested envisioning five stages through which managed care in a region moves, ranging from "nonexistent" (the level of managed care is less than 10%) to the "mature market condition stage" (managed care penetration exceeds 60%). After ascertaining the stage in your area, your next moves are development of a strategic plan that leads into the changes you must make and the steps to be taken to put the plan into action

OCCUPATIONAL THERAPY POSITIONING IN AN INSTITUTION

The importance and practicality of strategic planning was highlighted by Teri Shackleton, MSc, OT(C), and Marie Gage, MSc, OT(C), when they developed and successfully implemented a strategic planning process at Victoria Hospital to be positioned in the emerging Canadian health paradigm in 1992. Using a definition of *strategic planning* that indicated "a rational method for building consensus for participation, commitment, urgency, and action,"[7] Shackleton and Gage proceeded on the assumption that strategic planning is an essential process for the healthcare industry in an age when accountability is either directly or indirectly a challenge. They understood that the benefits of strategic planning included anticipating and adapting to environmental changes; providing a means to problem-solve, make decisions, integrate actions, and coordinate resources; and positioning to take advantage of opportunities.

The outcome of the strategic planning process was a *living* document that could be updated as environmental demands changed. (Recall from Chapter 17 that the strategic *plan* is a still picture, a snapshot taken during the ongoing process.) To arrive at the stage of having a plan in hand required first examining historical data, a current departmental profile, and environmental trends. These data were used to analyze the department's strengths, weaknesses, opportunities, and threats (a SWOT analysis). The final document reflected the department's commitment to patient care, education, and research at Victoria Hospital and was titled "Building on Our Strengths." Because the strategic plan is a living document, annual reviews are conducted during which progress toward the vision is evaluated, current environmental trends are considered, objectives for the next year are decided, and actions are discussed.[7]

FUTURISTIC PLANNING IN A RURAL SETTING

Evidence of a proactive approach appears in growing numbers of reports, regardless of the type of organization. A 60-bed rural hospital in Colorado used a contract-managed medical rehabilitation unit within the hospital to provide a stroke team as well as a continuum of care for patients recovering from orthopedic surgeries, debilitating diseases, trauma, and burns. Administrators of the hospital, looking ahead, feel prepared to meet the demands of managed care as it eventuates. At the same time, a major national healthcare agency decided to provide rehabilitation services with its own employees in all its 300 facilities, but with the same eye to the future as the rural hospital: to be positioned favorably as health care continues to move into the managed care mode.

FUTURISTIC DECISION MAKING WITH A SENIOR POPULATION

A gratifyingly large number of occupational therapy entrepreneurs are emerging in creative new roles. Brenda Fraser, MSC, a Canadian occupational therapist, using funds furnished to the Canadian Association of Occupational Therapists by the Seniors Independence Program, Health and Welfare Canada, put a pilot project in place in Manitoba and Newfoundland.[9] The idea was to move away from the medical model and adopt instead a biologic, psychosocial, socioenvironmental conceptualization of health, concentrating on the senior population.

Fraser noted that a key component of the effort was collaboration, as therapists interviewed seniors about issues affecting their quality of life and then identified interventions to meet the needs that they had expressed. Promotion of the strategies they had planned took many forms, including the CAOT-created manual, *For the Health of It: Occupational Therapy within a Health Promotion Framework*. Networks were established, an outreach program to seniors' apartments was established, educational resources were provided, seniors wrote a newsletter, and information was disseminated in local newspapers, on television shows, and at health fairs. Handouts on memory, arthritis, and back care were devised, occupational therapy volunteers gave presentations at seniors' meetings, and a "Healthy Aging Game" was generated for the use of home care workers.

Of special interest here and related to entrepreneurship, strategic planning, leadership, marketing, and the occupational therapist's role, Fraser concluded with several admonitions. The first was that occupational therapists "need to break through barriers that force us to practice in a certain way."[9] By barriers she meant traditional occupational therapy practice and approaches that inhibit exploration of community practice. Further, she asserted that the initiative must come from therapists, for they must create the jobs themselves.

For many occupational therapists, working in the community presents new perspectives and challenges not experienced or learned in school. Among these perspectives is the fact that "working *in* the community is not the same as working *with* the community. You must let the community drive the process and identify *their* resources." Fraser obviously had a grasp on the marketing process when she admitted that "relinquishing control to the client is a leap for most professionals" because it is necessary to work *with* consumer groups in the community to create your own occupational therapy opportunity and demand.

▨ Strategic Planning in Educational Programs

Across the country, occupational therapy educators are a vital and moving force within the profession, and as such they, too, engage regularly and actively in strategic planning processes where they work. One example would be the cyclical strategic planning at Texas Woman's University, a state-supported institution with an enrollment of approximately 10,000 students. The University Strategic Planning Committee includes representation from the School of Occupational Therapy. All university employees were invited to submit concerns, suggestions, and observations, which were integrated into the strategic plan, along with recognition of state and national trends and mandates in higher education. As the project evolves, regular reports are shared with all employees, not only for information but also with a continuing request for reactions and concerns.

The role, scope, and mission statements are the first outcomes to be approved, followed by decisions as to which degree programs do not meet established productivity criteria in respect to past performance, needs, and trends. During 1990 deliberations, a doctoral program in occupational therapy was one of the first new programs for which support was given. This was in response to the urgency of filling a national need of the profession for doctorally prepared occupational therapists that was expressed by occupational therapy faculty.

It is logical for an occupational therapy educational program to echo and support the mission and strategic plan of the parent institution, and at the same time it is an example of the total commitment required throughout an organization to a common goal and plan, the results of which bring success and strength. With foresight, *Essentials and Guidelines for an Accredited Educational Program for the Occupational Therapist* and *Essentials and Guidelines for an Accredited Educational Program for the Occupational Therapy Assistant* require that the occupational therapy educational program must "be consistent with that of the sponsoring institution."[10] All educational program directors must adhere to that admonition and ensure that the institution's strategic plan is used as a guide for their own ongoing planning.

Strategic planning involvement and activity similar to this example can be found across the country as occupational therapists who are responsible for leading their respective educational programs through intermittent crises continuously evaluate their strengths and remain alert for potential threats. Opportunities and demands, whether internal or external, must be anticipated and recognized, if students are to be provided with the preparation to go into the current healthcare scene as entry-level occupational therapists.

AOTA, State Associations, and Strategic Planning

Strategic planning by AOTA was begun formally in the early 1980s and has been continuing ever since. For example, in 1990 the ongoing strategic planning process mapped out a plan for the upcoming 5 years to address the specific issues of personnel shortages, reimbursement, public recognition of the profession, research, education, practice, minority issues, leadership development, technology and information management, international activities, and consumer collaboration. Each intervening year since then, the plan was evaluated and revised in response to changing needs and trends, and in 1995 those responsible for each of the 11 specific categories prepared analyses of progress and the current status of their parts of the plan.[11] Following is one example of the type of data used by AOTA to make decisions.

WORKFORCE PROJECTIONS AND REALITIES

The U.S. Department of Labor, Bureau of Labor Statistics (BLS), made its biennial projection for occupational therapy in fall 1995.[12] Its prediction was for a 72 percent rate of growth for therapists and an 82 percent rate of growth for assistants and aides between 1995 and 2005. Similar rates of growth were forecast for physical therapy, speech-language pathology, and audiology. These predictions were based on the size of the workforce, how the U.S. economy overall is estimated to perform, demand for services including demographic information, services generated in the past, and the level of employment within the profession. Keep in mind that BLS does not try to factor in possible changes in reimbursement for occupational therapy services; rather, the predictions are made based on the current situation. Demographics are taken seriously by BLS, especially the ever-increasing number of Americans who are 65 or older and who have a greater need for healthcare services, including occupational therapy. Therefore, based solely on the BLS data, the number of available positions for occupational therapists will continue to grow, regardless of how healthcare services are financed and delivered. AOTA continues to monitor whether the future demand for occupational therapy will indeed follow the BLS prediction and whether the profession will continue to see the kind of growth that it has experienced in the past.[12]

Meanwhile, individual occupational therapists, who should always be cognizant of what communications such as the BLS report are telling them, are advised to follow local, state, national, and international trends themselves to keep revising their own "personal strategic plans." Employment projections such as those of BLS are, of course, heartening, but occupational therapists at the same time need to keep an eye on other sources of updated information, such as predictions made in AOTA's 1996 "Workforce Study" about the possibility of an oversupply of personnel.

Most state occupational therapy associations also develop and update strategic plans. The Texas Occupational Therapy Association, for example, operates within the framework of a strategic action plan with six major goals that are based on the needs and expressed wishes of TOTA members and prioritized with that in mind. Within each goal are specific objectives designed to achieve that goal. This systematic, ongoing methodology enables board members to measure progress while remaining attuned to developing trends and changes.

AN EXERCISE: THE MULTISKILLING DECISION

One way to better understand the gravity and complexity of some futuristic decision making is to experience the process. Rather than a hypothetical problem about which a decision can be made, an actual occupational therapy dilemma existing in 1996 is used. The format is the six steps of the decision-making process as outlined in Chapter 17: identifying the problem, gathering information, analyzing the information, choosing an alternative, implementing the chosen alternative, and following up. In the following scenario, imagine yourself in the role of a primary decision maker: you are the president of AOTA and must announce your decision as soon as possible.

THE BACKGROUND. Closely associated with healthcare reorganization at this time is the idea of the healthcare generalist or the multiskilled provider, a recommendation most notably put forth by the Pew Health Professions Commission's report.[13] A decision must be made, on behalf of all AOTA members, about its official stance on occupational therapy and multiskilled providers. Practicing AOTA members need to know the official position of their professional association on this issue to help them make their own decisions in the workplace.

THE PROBLEM. A dilemma exists in that the definition of a multiskilled practitioner is unclear, and therefore no analysis is possible until the ambiguity has been removed. One question is whether *multiskilled* actually means one person who is trained to deliver multiple services previously provided by several different specialized persons. Another question is whether it is possible to differentiate, among all allied health personnel, the nonskilled and skilled services of each specialty in order to regroup and redistribute responsibilities among generalists and specialists.

GATHERING INFORMATION. One viewpoint was expressed by AOTA President Mary Foto:

The distinction between skilled and nonskilled services lies more in the medical necessity of intervention than in the intervention per se. That is, is treatment reasonable and necessary to the client's condition? Will treatment result in significant, practical improvement, and is it in fact resulting in significant, practical improvement? When the answer to these questions is yes, then the services are skilled. When the answer is no, the services are caregiving. The issue before us, then, is to develop objective criteria for the determination of the yes and no responses to these medical necessity questions.[14]

Another view concerns educational programs whose directors ask what content and curriculum changes would be required to support whatever decision is made. Does *multiskilled* mean a cross-trained therapist or a universal core curriculum?[15]

Still another opinion is expressed by the TriAlliance representatives: "It is the position of the TriAlliance [as of February 1996] that clinical multiskilled personnel at the professional or assistant level is likely to result in unacceptable levels of risk or potential negligence that could result in harm to, or poor outcomes for, the recipient of services. The use of multiskilled personnel at the aide level is an acceptable practice.[16]

In summer 1996, following an open forum held at the AOTA annual conference and publication of two articles in *OT Week,* the AOTA Cross-Training Task Force surveyed leaders within the profession for further input. The vehicle used to collect this information and to meet the needs of members was a concept paper. The purpose of the concept paper was to define the issue more clearly and present multiple perspectives of it. The paper described many of the concerns surrounding cross-training, gave definitions of key terms, and described the premises that were used in writing the paper. Advantages and disadvantages of cross-training that had already been put forth by members and in the literature were discussed, and optional strategies for dealing with requests to implement cross training were given.

Cross-training was defined as "the preparation of an individual in one profession to perform skills and tasks typically associated with another profession."[17] *Multiskilling* was considered to be preparation of an individual from one profession to be credentialed at the entry level in another profession. An example of this would be a COTA who earns an associate's degree as a physical therapy assistant.

Although there are many more opinions and more information yet to be considered, in the interest of space only one more viewpoint is included here. A number of practicing occupational therapists have expressed opinions that the uniqueness and value of occupational therapy must not be diluted or diminished by reducing it to a handful of techniques lost among those of a general helper. They feel that occupational therapy is the most timely and appropriate answer to what is being "discovered" daily in the United States: The care most needed now, and with exponential growth tomorrow, is a variety of community-based alternatives to hospitalization and nursing home care. Occupational therapy practitioners are eminently well prepared to provide exactly that. Holding back their services would be a threat to those needing occupational therapy, those who will benefit from assistance that would enable them to live satisfying lives within their own environments. Persons influence their own development, health, and environment through purposeful activity, a truth that is synonymous with occupational therapy.

Other questions asked are: Exactly what is a multipurpose professional? How can specific professional competence continue to be built? How will clients recognize these new professionals? How can qualified staff be recruited to this kind of multipurpose profession? How will this multipurpose individual actually lead to lower resource costs?

ANALYZING THE INFORMATION. This is the stage of the decision-making process in which AOTA is now engaged and from which alternatives will be formed. Subsequently a choice will be made, implemented, and followed up. How would you make the decision, and what would it be? By the time this book is published, this decision will most probably have been made, and you have the advantage of being a Monday morning quarterback. Stop a moment now and consider what decision you would make based on the preceding facts and observations. This is an opportunity for you to imagine having to make the decision based only on available information and input. What would *you* do at this point? It should now be apparent that listening and then heeding and sifting what you learn are the way the decision-making process commences. However the dilemma is resolved, it will be an example of strategic decision making on the part of those responsible. Next is some practical guidance for developing your personal strategic decision-making skills.

▨ Ground Rules for Initiating Strategic Planning

One of the first steps toward controlling your own professional future is to listen to your consumers. What services do they want? Are they satisfied with what they are now receiving, or do they wish to supplement or supplant their present services? Regardless of whether you contemplate introduction of a new service or a product, you must begin by finding out whether others really want it and in the form you have in mind to offer.

Equally important is that after you do get this feedback you keep an open mind and revise your plan if necessary. Recall the earlier explanation of the difference between market pull and market push. At this juncture, market pull is obviously being advised as the desirable approach.

Maintain your vision and goals. Look at problems as challenges and respond to them positively, and don't hesitate to ask anyone for information that may help you. Don't fear making mistakes, but do learn from them, and don't repeat the same ones. Persistence and determination are essential. Be an outgoing listener, yet keep your internal control and your belief in yourself. Take calculated risks, and don't gamble. Keep high standards of integrity and reliability if you seek long-term success. Be a team builder rather than a loner, and inspire by example those you choose as colleagues.

When making decisions, remember the pitfalls to avoid: Don't agonize over *every* decision; don't be a wishful thinker blinded to reality; don't make decisions based on intuition and without conscious attention or reasoning; don't spend a lot of energy on designing elaborate contingency plans for every possible problem; and don't get caught up in listing endless pros and cons that carry you in circles. (Review Chapter 17 for positive and practical decision-making steps.)

Choosing Potential Business Partners for Strategic Alliances

Among the strategic decisions professionals often must make is selection of business partners. Entering into a strategic alliance as an option was mentioned earlier in relation to partnerships or networks contemplated by private practitioners. At this point it seems appropriate to provide some general rules for students to remember.

DON'TS

- Don't form an alliance to correct a weakness because the party bringing a weakness to the alliance will thereafter be subservient to the other party in the alliance.
- Don't form an alliance with a partner who is in the process of trying to correct a weakness because your company will inherit that weakness.

DOS

- Form an alliance to profit from a unique strength, one that is possessed by no other competitor, because only unique strengths can be sustained and defended over time. Relative strengths can be acquired or duplicated.
- Form an alliance with someone who possesses a unique strength of his or her own, thus combining two unique strengths and giving the highest probability of success.
- Be certain that neither partner has the ability or desire to take away the other's unique strength.[18]

Finding and working with a partner requires great patience and determination. Seek compatible strengths, strategies, and cultures, which are most likely to lead to similar values and a similar appetite for risk. Both parties must make comparable contributions, something obvious and worthwhile besides money. Be certain that there are no conflicts of interest and no overlapping interests if you wish to prevent possible attempts at control. Once the right partners have found each other, be assured that two prime qualities are present: confidence in themselves and trust in each other. Innovation, entrepreneurship, and successful joint ventures are more dependent on the key people than they are on money, technology, or target markets.[19]

▓ Marketing and Strategic Planning: Inseparable

Clearly, a *marketing approach* and *strategic planning* are concepts with two different names, yet actually they are mutually supportive and inseparable. That inseparability adds continued support to the hypothesis that parallels and complements exist among the processes of occupational therapy, leadership, management, marketing, and strategic planning. Strategic planning entails futuristic decision making; so do occupational therapy, leadership, management, and marketing. Each is made up of many exchanges and transactions brought about as a result of decisions made with short-range and long-range objectives in mind. It is impossible to declare that one or the other begins here or there.

A final example of this statement is Craig McCaw, the cellular pioneer credited with pulling the cellular business out of its low-tech backwater and turning it into the growth engine of the telecommunications industry.[20] A current vision is to create a celestial counterpart to the Internet by creating a constellation of 840 satellites to transmit signals from any point on the planet to any other with the speed and capacity of fiber-optic cable. Calling the venture Teledesic, McCaw has been backed in his "crazy scheme" by Bill Gates, who stated, "I wouldn't have invested in Teledesic unless Craig was involved. He thinks ahead of the pack." Now the hard work has begun to operationalize the vision.

Chapters 17 and 18 have averred that there first must be a vision, followed by decision making, followed by a strategic plan. This, however, is only the beginning. You can come up with the best strategy in the world, but without marketing, management, and ongoing monitoring (that is, hard work and attention to all constituencies and details) for implementation, it will not move ahead. Have a vision that is based on sound data and judgment, built with innovative thinking, and processed through the logical steps of decision making. Then keep in mind that megadecisions are mined with surprises, so be prepared!

▨ Summary

Strategic planning and futuristic decision making have been further discussed in this chapter, with examples of the process in action in national corporations, in AOTA, within educational institutions, among nurses, and from occupational therapy practice in the field. Starting with a mission or vision, the amount of commitment needed to reach the goal was made clear. The critical role played by an effective leader was described, for without a fully involved organization the vision will never happen. The notion of stretch targets was explained, as well as how to assess the stage of penetration of managed care in your region. Finally, the complementary and parallel processes at work in occupational therapy, strategic planning, leadership, management, and marketing are recognized. Chapter 19 moves on to another view that must be integrated into your perceptions: globalization of occupational therapy issues, illustrating a thread of commonality among occupational therapy concerns worldwide.

REFERENCES

1. Magnet, M: How top managers make a company's toughest decision. Fortune 111(6):52, Mar 18, 1985.
2. Naisbett, J, and Aburdene, P: Re-inventing the Corporation. Warner Books, New York, 1985.
3. Guiltinan, JP, and Paul, GW: Marketing Management: Strategies and Programs, ed 3. McGraw-Hill, New York, 1988, p 9.
4. Tully, S: Why to go for stretch targets. Fortune, Nov 14, 1994, p 145.
5. Rohland, P: Nurse entrepreneurs. Income Opportunities, Oct 1995, p 12.
6. Fowler, FJ: Positioning for managed care. Rehab Economics (suppl)3(4). In Rehab Management 9(4):108.
7. Burkhart, PJ, and Reuss, S: Successful Strategic Planning: A Guide for Nonprofit Agencies and Organizations. Sage, Newbury Park, Calif, 1993.
8. Shackleton, TL, and Gage, M: Strategic planning: Positioning occupational therapy to be proactive in the new health care paradigm. Can J Occup Ther 62(4), Oct, 1995.
9. Stahl, C: OTs have to create their own jobs in the community. Advance for Occupational Therapists 11(19):9, May 15, 1995.
10. American Occupational Therapy Association: Essentials and Guidelines for an Accredited Educational Program for the Occupational Therapist. Author, Bethesda, Md, 1991.
11. Marmer, L: The five-year education plan: Is AOTA on target? Advance for Occupational Therapists 11(34), Apr 28, 1995.
12. Holland, HE: Bureau of labor statistics issues updated workforce projections. OT Week, Feb 1, 1996, p 12.
13. Pew Health Professions Commission: Health Professions Education for the Future: Schools in Service to the Nation. Author, San Francisco, 1993.
14. Foto, M: Delineating skilled versus nonskilled services: A defining point in our professional evolution. Am J Occup Ther 50(3):170, Mar, 1996.
15. Foto, M: Multiskilling: Who, how, when, and why? Am J Occup Ther 50(1):7, Jan, 1996.
16. TriAlliance of Health and Rehabilitation Professionals: Use of multiskilled personnel. OT Week 10(8), 1996.
17. American Occupational Therapy Association: White paper: Occupational Therapy and Cross-Training Initiatives. Author, Bethesda, Md, Dec, 1994.
18. Robert, M: Strategy Pure and Simple. McGraw-Hill, New York, 1993.
19. Houghton, JR: Why Corning's joint ventures endure. Planning Review, 1994, p 9.
20. Kupfer, A: Craig McCaw sees an Internet in the sky. Fortune 133(10), May 27, 1996.

PART EIGHT

FUTURISM, GLOBALIZATION, AND OCCUPATIONAL THERAPY

To put the world in order, we must first put the nation in order; to put the nation in order, we must first put the family in order; to put the family in order, we must first cultivate our personal life; we must first set our hearts right.

Confucius

CHAPTER 19

Assuming Responsibility for Your Professional Future

CHAPTER OBJECTIVES

- To comprehend the meaning of futurism and globalization.
- To acknowledge the value of monitoring trends to anticipate the future.
- To identify sources of information from which to learn about trends and changes.
- To understand how occupational therapists can have an impact on their own personal futures as well as on the future of their profession.
- To see how corporations go about expanding overseas.
- To recognize patterns of economic development worldwide.
- To realize the critical importance of understanding and listening for cultural cues.
- To realize what is happening among occupational therapists worldwide.
- To recognize some rules to follow for going to work overseas.
- To know how to have a mutually successful experience when employing an internationally educated occupational therapist.

By the time a book that reviews trends or issues is published, new occurrences have at least slightly altered the picture. For the trends that are newest and most meaningful to you, just stop and look around *you* today for, in Naisbett's[1] view, what is going on *locally* is what is going on in America. So it is your own pulse in which the surveyors of trends have an interest; however, concurrently watching the larger picture is also essential if an occupational therapist is to be proactive.

Futurism and globalization are not concepts related only to corporations; they are occupational therapy concerns, as well. They are realities of which many occupational therapists in other countries seem more cognizant than most in America. Wise therapists read international professional journals and, when possible, travel worldwide to share and learn about progress in other countries. There is a richness and diversity among occupational therapists internationally that can enhance and strengthen the profession as mutual learning takes place.

Part Eight expands the reader's views to wider horizons than those solely within the United States of America. Awareness of what is happening across America as well as around the world is essential to the worldwide future of occupational therapy. This chapter discusses futurism and globalization as two factors with which occupational therapy practitioners should be familiar. Reasons for developing a global mindset and ways to go about it are suggested. Chapter 20 then continues development of this viewpoint with more concrete and detailed examples and suggestions.

To Develop a Futuristic Viewpoint, Watch the Trends

The Environmental Scan Committee of United Way of America identified nine leading forces, which they termed *change drivers* (elements or concepts that lead future societal modifications), that can be considered key developments in American society. The Futures Task Force of AOTA looked at these same trends as they studied influences on the profession.

The first element identified by the United Way committee was (1) the maturation or graying of America, a now-familiar realization, with the second trend (2) the developing mosaic society (e.g., growing population of elderly, increasing ethnic diversity, more single-person households, increasing number of persons with disabilities, increasing immigration). By *mosaic society* the committee was referring to transformation of the society from a "mass" toward a mosaic—a society made up of many distinctive identities. The remainder of the nine change drivers were (3) the redefinition of individual and societal roles, (4) exploding information-based economy, (5) globalization (worldwide activities), (6) economic restructuring, (7) attention to personal and environmental health, (8) redefinition of family and home, and (9) the rebirth of social issues.

One status report of today's evolving business world was published in the December 13, 1994, issue of *Fortune* magazine. It observed four business revolutions taking place: globalization of markets, spread of information technology and computers, dismantling of the structure that has organized work since the mid-1800s, and a new information-age economy whose sources of wealth are knowledge and communication rather than natural resources and physical labor. The authors were far from alone in these conclusions.

During 1995 citizens were aware of the collapse of the Mexican peso, economic aftershocks of the Japan earthquake, and a looming United States–China trade war. Almost unnoticed was another major occurrence: beginnings of a global expansion of economies in developing countries, as they began assuming leadership roles as drivers of global growth.[2] In 1996, this growth continued at an average rate of 7.2 percent annually.

Futurism and Trends

In their 1990 book, *Future Work,* Coates, Jarratt, and Mahaffie[3] recognized that North America's ability to compete in world markets in the next century will rise or fall depending on the quality of its workforce. Thinking as futurists, the authors began in the late 1980s to implement an ongoing scan of the corporate environment that would identify significant emerging trends that were shaping the workforce. The focus of their book was an analysis of these trends organized into seven themes, the 37 component trends within these themes, implications of the forces contained therein, and suggested possible subsequent actions to be taken. Readers may use the book to build anticipatory perspectives into their own organizations. The seven themes, or currents, described were:

1. Increasing diversity in the workforce: making heterogeneity and flexibility work.
2. Reintegrating home life and work life: reversing a 100-year trend.
3. Globalization: facing the realities of competing in a world economy.
4. Expanding human resources planning: restructuring roles and practices to improve business-unit planning.
5. The changing nature of work: training and reeducating for a knowledge-based workforce.
6. Rising employee expectations: striking a balance between demands and costs.
7. A renewed social agenda: expanding corporate social responsibility.

In a manner similar to Naisbett's caution a decade earlier, Coates, Jarratt, and Mahaffie[3] urged a continuing awareness of bellwethers by every interested party, for it is what is happening all around you that supplies indicators of trends and their effects. The source of each piece of information should be scrutinized, as it may be shaped by a particular ideology or political interest and thus biased. Scanning means not only to read but also to sort, save, and sometimes to pitch out.

LOOK FOR THE SIGNS

Each occupational therapy practitioner should look for signs of what is happening in other cities, states, nations, and organizations and the potential effect on his or her own organization. In addition to already-familiar sources of information, look into statistical agencies' publications, abstracts publication series for shortcuts to literature sources (e.g., *Psychology Abstracts*), polls and surveys, legislative and governmental agencies' reports, futurist literature, computer databases, indexing services, abstracting services, and bibliographies. Detailed lists of specific information sources are provided at the end of the Coates et al. book.[3]

The Organization Man caused a stir in 1956 with its incisive comments and predictions about world affairs. One of the futurists noted for analyses of trends in 1970 was Alvin Toffler with his landmark book, *Future Shock*,[4] followed in 1980 by *The Third Wave*.[5] Toffler pointed out that *future shock,* or the disorientation brought on by the premature arrival of the future, can be fatal to those who do not prepare for it. In 1982 Naisbett brought out another popular work, *Megatrends*.[1] These and other publications were explosive because they sought to dramatically alter the way people viewed the world and what was happening, usually heuristically and with uncomfortable accuracy. All presented a picture of their own current America and what they foresaw in the future.

This is in no way an exhaustive list of futurist literature about America; other publications appear frequently. However, these examples merely introduce occupational therapy practitioners to the types of resources that are helpful in developing an awareness of the shifting environmental scene surrounding them. Globalization can be noted fairly universally as a critical factor in futuristic thinking and for that reason is discussed in this chapter.

Evolving to the Future: Occupational Therapy in the United States

No one arrives at tomorrow without having passed through yesterdays. Everything changes, just as the sun rises each morning without your help or influence. The future of occupational therapy is the business of individual occupational therapy practitioners, and there is much to be learned from each other globally.

THE PAST

It may seem like only yesterday that occupational therapy educational program directors in the United States were working hard to inform potential students about the profession and to attract them to enter programs of study. The main reason given then by those who enrolled in occupational therapy programs was usually related to helping others and being of service to humankind. It was tacitly understood that earning a big salary was not probable but that the rewards were many and valued in other ways. Jobs were relatively scarce. After completion of academic coursework, each student progressed to the clinical education phase of occupational therapy education, usually into hospital-based psychiatric and physical disability units. Faculty members often earned comfortable salaries compared with hospital-employed therapists.

THE PRESENT

Today, just a relatively few years later, a radically different picture has emerged in the United States. Occupational therapy has become recognized as a vital, effective healthcare profession. Students must demonstrate outstanding abilities to be considered for admission into most occupational therapy educational programs. The main reasons given by beginning students for having chosen this profession are related to high entry-level salaries and plentiful job offers. Fewer acknowledge being drawn primarily because of desire to be of service to others. Faculty members' salaries now have usually fallen below those customarily offered by employers other than public universities. Insufficient numbers of qualified graduate-level faculty are available for employment in academic programs, thus containing the supply of graduating students. This, in turn, limits the number of entry-level therapists available, increases shortages in occupational therapy personnel, raises competitive practice salaries, and makes faculty positions seem even less attractive.

Educational program faculty have continued without pause to conscientiously prepare future occupational therapists, stay in touch with rapidly changing practice trends, eliminate outdated information, and integrate current facts and concepts to prepare students to enter today's healthcare system. As practice roles change, the educational preparation for both OTR and COTA must be realigned. The healthcare revolution of the 1990s represents the largest reorganization of health care in America since the 19th century. Because it is anticipated that 80 percent of services will be provided in clinics and homes and 20 percent in acute-care hospitals, basing a curriculum on a traditional hospital model is no longer viable.

Traditional fieldwork settings as sites for the final phase of educational preparation of occupational therapy students are disappearing daily. Previously confirmed student fieldwork placements that are canceled with alarming frequency are forcing professional association policy makers to seek alternative ways to conduct this aspect of occupational therapy students' education.

HOW IT SHOULD BE AND WHERE TO BEGIN

No one can predict the future with certainty, but occupational therapy practitioners can sometimes find valuable advice in unexpected places. Charles Handy,[6] a respected philosopher for the world of business who tries to describe the future, provides an example with his recent observations. One of his predictions in the early 1980s was that by 2000 half the working population would be making their livings outside traditional organizations, an idea termed "crazy" at the time. Today more than 35 percent of Americans in the labor force are either unemployed or temporary, part-time, or contractual workers. In Europe the figure is already close to 50 percent. Handy's two best-sellers, *The Age of Unreason* in 1989 and *The Age of Paradox* in 1994, are both noted for their clarity and prescriptive nature. When asked for current tips for today's workers, he said that loyalty should go first to your team or project, second to your profession or discipline, and only third to the place where you work.[6] Another suggestion was to look for customers, not bosses.

Occupational therapy practitioners must develop futuristic and global mindsets. Observation of trends, close at hand and worldwide, and an anticipatory viewpoint that is perceptive and open are essential. Habitually reading *OT Week*, the *American Journal of Occupational Therapy*, the *Occupational Therapy Journal of Research*, the Special Interest Section Newsletters, *OT Practice, Rehab Management*, and *Advance for Occupational Therapists* as sources of information about trends within the profession in the United States is one starting place. In addition, expanding your reading habits to include occupational therapy international journals, as well as U.S. and worldwide business and marketing publications, is strongly advised. Development of political acumen and involvement should be a concurrent activity, as well.

POLITICS IS YOU

The importance of political involvement to the future of your profession cannot be underestimated. It is not only critical but also the responsibility of every occupational therapy practitioner to participate, and it can be done on every level from within your organization up to the national scene. Input is possible and needed legislatively if you wish to affect your own future. At the very least, you must vote. Then you can participate actively to make a difference in a number of other ways.

Increase your involvement and communication with government officials on both the state and federal levels. Begin with studying the issues and helping candidates locally and at the state level with their campaign needs. Seize every opportunity to be involved. One way to take an active role to shape your future is through providing testimony at public hearings. A definition of *testimony* is "a declaration or affirmation of fact or truth, as that given before a court; evidence in support of a fact or assertion; proof."[7]

Written or oral testimony is your opportunity to express your opinion on an issue. The information you give can make a real difference in the outcome of proposed or enacted policy. To learn where and when these chances are available, watch for notices (which appear in the *Federal Register* or in your state's register) on proposed, withdrawn, and adopted rules, as well as open meetings and hearings. You have the right in this country to speak out and voice your opinion and thus shape your own tomorrow.

There are some basic guidelines to assist you in delivering the most effective testimony:

- Remain informed through the federal and state registers.
- Notify your legislator that you wish to testify before a committee.
- As you enter the hearing, complete testimony cards and register in order to be scheduled and to declare support or nonsupport of issues.
- Come prepared with two accurately written texts: one detailed and one abbreviated. Leave copies for each committee member and for the press, and send copies to your legislators and to the governor, if it is a state issue.
- In giving the oral testimony, begin by introducing yourself with name, title, affiliation, credentials, bill number and title, and the position you have taken on the legislation or issue.
- When appropriate, begin by saying that you are sorry that (names) members are absent and cannot hear your testimony, thus ensuring that this fact is noted in the official minutes of the session.
- Limit your presentation to 5 minutes by keeping the message simple and brief.
- Be prepared to reference what you say.
- Enhance your credibility with outcomes and efficacy studies to support your opinions.
- Be concise and dramatic in speech, but express yourself as if in a conversation.
- Never use abbreviations, acronyms, jargon, or technical terms; assume the listeners know nothing about your profession.
- Use success stories about real people as an effective note.
- If possible, add testimony made by influential persons.
- Do your homework and know the names and hometowns of committee members because you make a positive impression if, when questioned, you can tie your testimony to their districts.
- Do not pretend. If you do not know the answer to a question, assure the committee members that you will provide the answer as soon as possible, and then follow up.
- Do not be surprised if committee members are unable to remain present throughout the entire testimony. Their schedules are heavy.
- When you have finished your presentation, thank the members and tell them that you look forward to working with them.[8]

There are a heartening number of successful occupational therapy role models throughout the United States who have worked effectively through AOTPAC and through their state affiliates to bring about legislative changes. Watch newsletters for ongoing examples of how occupational therapy colleagues, such as Teri Black in Wisconsin, habitually use all these steps to advance the profession through legislative interventions.

■ Going Overseas: When Corporations Consider Expanding

Companies that choose to enter international markets do so with varying degrees of commitment. Usually one of four basic approaches is selected to determine the degree to which a marketing program will be modified to the different environmental conditions and characteristics of foreign markets: the home country strategy, host country strategy, regional strategy, and global strategy.

The home country strategy has an export orientation that exports domestically made products to countries where buyers have similar needs and characteristics. There is no systematic research of overseas markets or major modifications of the products themselves, and relatively low risk is involved. In the host country approach, there are extensive commitments made by adapting marketing plans to the conditions existing in the different countries. Prices and promotion messages vary according to what is appropriate. A disadvantage is that the costs involved may cause prices to be uncompetitive if too many modifications are necessary.

In the regional approach, the company views the whole region or the entire world as one potential market and organizes policies and activities on a worldwide basis. The product itself is standardized, with slight variations reflecting small differences and with promotional programs developed regionally. Overall, there is a uniform image of the organization and its product. Finally, those companies using a global strategy view the world as one market rather than as a collection of many national or regional markets. Theirs is a uniform marketing approach of standardized products, meaning lower costs and more efficiency but inappropriateness in countries with strong local preferences.[9]

USING INVESTMENTS AS AN INDICATOR FOR EXPANSION

Western Europe is still the preferred location for U.S. companies that plan to expand overseas, but other sites are emerging as markets with potential. A recent study, *Manufacturing Investment Abroad,* of globally minded businesses was done by Ernst and Young.[10] It showed that China, Brazil, and Mexico were becoming challengers for foreign investment dollars. In 1994 the European Union drew 54 percent of the overseas investment by U.S. companies, down from the

61 percent of the previous year. The United Kingdom continued as the first choice worldwide, but China doubled its total of projects over the previous year to come in second, followed by France, Germany, Mexico, Japan, Canada, Italy, India, and Brazil. The most promising emerging markets for the future were Vietnam, Thailand, Taiwan, Indonesia, the Philippines, and the Czech Republic.

EUROPEAN MANAGERS AND GLOBALIZATION

Many consider Europeans to be better equipped for globalization because they are as aggressive as Americans but with a special European style.[11] Nestlé, based in Switzerland, has doubled sales in 12 years by using friendliness as an effective management technique, CEO Helmut Maucher says, doing things quietly, step by step, and avoiding friction. Looking back over 5 years, though, he then sees the radical change he has accomplished. He does not, however, rest on his laurels and is now moving into Third World markets because only 25 percent of his products are sold in the developing world, where 80 percent of the world population lives. The cultural diversity of its corporate board, said by some to resemble closely the UN Security Council, is considered a huge asset at Nestlé.

Some basic leadership and management components presented in Part One of this book can be detected in comments some European managers made about the reasons for their success. One French manager of an auto parts manufacturing company, Noel Goutard of Valeo, reported that he had put workers into teams responsible for organizing their own activities and expected every worker to make 10 suggestions a year for improvements. Further, all suggestions must be considered within 10 days. As a result, workers have accepted the changes enthusiastically and joined him in the goal of having a company that is prepared to confront environmental market conditions. Valeo gave the reasons for increasing profits by 26 percent: service, quality, and price, with even the farthest-flung outer-office secretary sounding like Peter Drucker. Finally, when asked where he had learned so much about management, Goutard replied, "Listening to customers; they can teach you everything you need to know."[11]

MARKETING, PUBLIC RELATIONS, AND
OVERSEAS EXPANSION: AN EXAMPLE

Failure to use a marketing approach can be discerned in the 1995 cancellation of a $2.8 billion project intended for construction near Bombay, India.[12] When protests began in 1992 against the proposed gas-fired power plant of a multinational consortium, the citizens' concerns were dismissed as irrelevant. The project was killed through public hostility. Environmentalists complained that the impact analysis was not complete; economists called the project too expensive; villagers saw it as a threat to their farms. Many observers believed the deal's rupture was hastened by faulty public relations, publicity, and promotion—not listening to and explaining to all affected parties what was happening. Local analysts in Bombay reiterated that the people could easily have been won over if consulted and given explanations from the start.

LISTENING FOR CULTURAL CLUES

Companies considering comparative advertising (comparing by name or inference other products or services) outside the United States must take care not to run afoul of local laws, customs, and tastes.[13] In some countries (e.g., Germany and Luxembourg) comparative ads are simply illegal. Even if comparative advertising is legal *in principle,* there are minefields of relevant legislation you may need help in negotiating. Also, in some countries comparative ads are thought to be "low class" or perceived to be like American political advertising. For example, in Great Britain the practice is treated as a rather unseemly way to do advertising. Therefore, persons coming into the country are strongly urged to familiarize themselves with the myriad regulations in place in England.

The yearly calendar of the American President Lines (APL) is prepared carefully before it is distributed to customers worldwide.[14] Saudi Arabian customers, for example, could be offended with a drawing of New Year's Eve revelers kissing or with the use of a certain color or angle of a pictured ship. It is so vital an issue that a special researcher is brought in each year to compile a list of holidays celebrated around the world. Artwork is reviewed by APL employees with diverse cultural backgrounds. To illustrate the point, the February page of the 1995 calendar honored Chinese New Year and pictured a boar for the Year of the Boar. As this picture would offend Muslims who abstain from pork, a picture of a dragon was used in some locations instead. Another example was the removal of a black border from a drawing because Chinese customers would not consider it "a gift color." One drawing of a clock was removed because it is a symbol of death in some Asian cultures. When such decisions are made, APL does not even ask for, let alone demand, explanations. Instead, they trust the cultural advisers as the experts who understand their individual cultural connections and the issues of greatest importance to them. Nothing would be worse than to offend a potential or present customer.[14]

Euro Disney was cited as an example of what might happen in the case of failure to fully investigate and accept cultural habits and nuances. In its first 18 months of operation, Euro Disney, a new theme park outside Paris, lost almost $1 billion. One report attempted to identify Disney's miscalculations in translating its theme park experiences from one culture to another. Euro Disney's ability to generate revenue is determined by the number of visitors to the park and their average length of stay. Both fell short of expectations. The causes were said to be (1) failure to note that Paris winters are particularly uninviting with nasty cold and rain between November and March, (2) Europeans will not take their children out of school to visit Euro Disney, and (3) European families favor 3- or 4-week-long vacations in summer with vacation budgets that are more modest than those in the United States. They are far less likely to spend it all on an expensive 2- or 3-day visit to Euro Disney and then return home. Many would limit their Euro Disney visit to just 1 day, on the way to their final vacation destinations.[15]

Disney management was said to rely too heavily on the Disney appeal or mystique rather than adapting their products to the needs and customs of their overseas clients. This report stated that Disney alienated many French citizens by imposing intact its American standards of dress, behavior, and morality on the operation of its French-based park. Up to its 1992 opening, an overbearing attitude was alienating the French. When considering any new market, preliminary research should be conducted to determine risks and threats to success, and the results of this research should be interpreted carefully and objectively.

More examples of the need to be constantly aware of cultural clues can be found in the American practice of publicly voicing commendation for achievements of individuals. Some employees from cultures such as Japan consider public commendation of an individual an affront to the harmony of the group. In Sweden, "the Jante Law" discourages an individual from rising noticeably above others.[16] Finally, some cultures do not approve of the idea of incentive pay, considering it to be akin to bribery. In some countries, the objections to bonuses are more fiscal than philosophical. Instead of cash, employees prefer more leisure time, access to vacation villages, or anything that cannot be taxed. Do retain your principles and beliefs, but modify them to account for cultural differences.

▨ The Need and the Feeling: The KLM Celebration

The interest of people around the world in widening their understanding and horizons was illustrated when KLM Royal Dutch Airlines launched its "Bridging the World" program as part of its 75th anniversary celebrations.[17] People from all over the world were invited to propose how KLM could help them achieve long-cherished dreams that would reflect that "the ocean of air unites all peoples." KLM would make 2000 air tickets available and pay all other expenses involved for the 10 prize-winning proposals.

An astonishing 12,000 proposals in 25 languages from 120 nations were received. Imaginations had been captured by a sense of deeper meaning in a world where too many factors separate people. American Joni Tada's prize-winning mission resulted in 150 wheelchairs being brought to Ghana, along with a 25-person training team. Three top international musicians were led to the Ukraine to teach a master class for six young talents from the Kiev Conservatory. Fifteen young soccer enthusiasts from the streets of Rio de Janeiro had their first plane ride, this time to the Netherlands to study with the Dutch professionals, thanks to a winning Dutch entry. Paula Jeane, an American who works in Morocco with blind people, led a group of her students and some Moroccan educators through the streets of San Francisco and Los Angeles to visit institutes for the blind, organizations that make Braille books, and a guide-dog center. Three Zimbabwean artists from Mutare visited the Dutch town of Haarlem where now an astonishing African mural becomes visible when the Langebrug bridge is raised. American James Watson wanted to build a clinic in Guinea, outside Conakry, and 25 construction workers and 15 tons of building materials were transported to Guinea by KLM to help local people build the clinic, which now serves 200,000. Two American missionaries in Thailand planted 75 citrus trees in Lilongwe, the capital of Malawi, as a source of fresh fruit for the students and to generate income by selling the surplus fruit at the local market. Twenty-five children from all over the world were flown to Denmark, home of Hans Christian Andersen, for a special conference on children's literature and discussion of what was important in stories from a child's point of view.[17] Recognition of the importance of a global mindset permeates the recounting of these stories, each one different, yet alike, in the feeling they represent.

▓ Globalization of Occupational Therapy

The concept of a global mindset means appreciation of the beliefs, values, behaviors, and practices of those from other regions and cultures. The occupational therapy practitioner is advised to develop this capacity for use in practice in the United States as well as overseas, along with skills in assertiveness, negotiation, networking, proposal writing, program development, and communication.

Globalization is no longer a word that can be disassociated from occupational therapy because Western society and Western history have given way today to world history and a world civilization that has been "Westernized." The primary resource in this emerging world is knowledge.[18] Failure to recognize this can, at the least, slow down and impede clear thinking; ultimately, it can inhibit professional growth.

Rita Goble, PhD, Dip OT, a professor at the Institute of General Practice, Exeter University, Devon, England, while meeting with AOTA representatives, observed that geographic and communication problems are slowly being alleviated through modern technology, and the efforts of international organizations such as the World Federation of Occupational Therapists (WFOT) and the World Health Organization (WHO) are bringing occupational therapists together on a worldwide basis. As the population around the world ages and as new advances in medical technology save lives as never before, countries everywhere will have great numbers of citizens with chronic impairments. Whether in India, the United States, Australia, or Sweden, occupational therapists are eminently prepared and qualified to work with these individuals who need to manage within their own environments, to facilitate their independent community living, and to assist them to live outside institutions.

Regardless of how it is approached, the idea of a global mindset is increasingly a part of growing and developing. Occupational therapy educational programs continue to be established worldwide, and growing numbers of occupational therapists move about on an international basis. More questions will arise about the product in common—occupational therapy services—and its nature. Issues of uniformity in frames of reference, quality of services, and models of practice are but a few of the potential concerns that will appear on the horizon. Consideration of international reciprocity or equivalency in accreditation is a future possibility. Borrowing from the international marketing terms introduced earlier, the choice and proportion of home country versus host country strategies will become considerations.

An illustration of expanding international interests can be seen in the work being done by the International Centre for the Advancement of Community-Based Rehabilitation (ICACBR) in partnership with Disabled Peoples' International (DPI), both organizations based in Canada.[19] The DPI is working in Russia to introduce occupational therapy as a new health discipline. In Russia, where health and social systems are undergoing extensive reform, institutions receive most of the resources for people with mild and moderate disabilities, and persons with severe disabilities are typically cared for at home and have no access to health, education, or social services. The ICACBR and DPI have collaborated with Volgograd Medical College 6 to establish a series of exchanges and training programs to increase the capability of Russian disability non-government organizations to advocate on behalf of the disabled community. It was projected that by the end of the project 50 students would have completed training programs in occupational therapy.[19]

New Zealand occupational therapists learn program development skills from a Japanese occupational therapist at an international conference in Dunedin. Swedish occupational therapy educational program planners join forces with those from the United States, and a Swedish occupational therapist conducts an ongoing research project to develop rehabilitation in a village in Botswana. An American occupational therapist spends 10 years working in Peru among leprosy patients; another travels to Zimbabwe to teach occupational therapists there how to make orthopedic furniture from paper products because of the scarcity of wood. A Canadian occupational therapist joins forces with a team to ease the ravages of an HIV/AIDS epidemic in Zomba, Malawi. The world grows smaller and more challenging daily, as occupational therapists worldwide share problems and solutions.

Mary Shaheen, OTR, volunteered her time on two trips to Guatemala with an organization called Heart of the Matter (HOTM) to help in the education of teachers in developing countries by training them in more effective teaching techniques.[20] A second goal was to meet students' needs for clothing, food, and medical care. Shaheen welcomed the opportunity to broaden her world view and to use her professional knowledge to help children there to ultimately think more critically and be able to problem-solve and take the initiative in making changes.

Like managers of American corporations who are expanding operations overseas, occupational therapists are discovering the critical need to adapt well to new cultures if they are to succeed. American occupational therapists will do well to learn from their worldwide colleagues how to interact and adapt internationally and understand the cultural preferences of others, if not their languages. There are potentially devastating losses in translation in spoken language and in gestures and body language. For instance, a "sharp" businessman in United States translates into a "devious or unprincipled" businessman in England. The familiar OK sign—making a circle of thumb and forefinger—used in United States introduces a totally different connotation in Latin America. On such seemingly trivial details, an overseas project may founder. In that the process of occupational therapy, to be truly effective, requires the full collaboration of clients and their caregivers, it seems logical that a host country strategy (see preceding explanation) would most often be the appropriate choice. Such decisions must be carefully made.

Occupational Therapy Practitioners, Futurism, and Globalization

In addition to the earlier advice about expanding your reading habits into a wider variety of U.S. publications and becoming involved with legislators, today's U.S. occupational therapy students are advised not to limit their reading to American publications. As stated before, globalization is found on every list of trends discussed, and the wise student develops familiarity with the excellent writing and creative suggestions in occupational therapy journals worldwide. Some have been continuously published for many years, such as the Canadian, British, and Australian occupational therapy journals. More recent publications include the *Scandinavian Journal of Occupational Therapy,* originated by Birgitta Lundgren-Lindquist in Sweden, and the *New Zealand Journal of Occupational Therapy. The WFOT* (World Federation of Occupational Therapists) *Bulletin* has been an excellent resource for many years, and the *International Journal of Occupational Therapy* was recently launched by Franklin Stein, OTR, of the United States.

Information technology, including the Internet and the World Wide Web, are still other developing resources for information (see Chapter 20).

WHEN YOU WANT TO WORK OVERSEAS

If you are an occupational therapist considering employment overseas, the World Federation of Occupational Therapists (WFOT) suggests that you ask yourself these questions:

- Do you have a speaking knowledge of the language of the host country? Whether you are dealing with clients, doctors, a landlady, or a salesclerk, you cannot understand their questions or ask your own if you do not know the words.

■ Are you able to adapt to all types of conditions? Instead of trying to change the conditions to fit your own usual pattern, can you adjust to those of the host country?

■ How good is your health, both physically and emotionally? Your system must be able to withstand changes in climate, nutrition, work hours, and other people's attitudes.

■ How good is your professional knowledge? Do not attempt to work abroad without 1 year, and preferably more, of work experience in occupational therapy. You must be strong enough to benefit from giving as well as taking, for you must be ready to accept the responsibility of representing your entire professional population.

■ Do you really know your own country? In addition to being an occupational therapist abroad, you are your own country's ambassador and should be prepared to answer every type of question, including those related to government, education, cultural patterns, and politics.[21]

WHEN YOU PLAN TO EMPLOY AN INTERNATIONALLY EDUCATED OCCUPATIONAL THERAPIST

The obverse side of the coin is being aware of what goes into the successful integration of an internationally trained occupational therapist into your U.S. organization's rehabilitation team. As the United States becomes more culturally diverse and more active worldwide, including internationally trained occupational therapists on treatment teams provides an opportunity for enhanced service delivery. Your own awareness of cultural issues and perspectives is broadened as a result.

Special needs and requirements are associated with the employment of internationally trained occupational therapists. The following suggestions are based on the experience of Cynthia F. Epstein, MA, OTR.[22]

1. Know the legal responsibilities associated with the H-1B visa process.

2. Engage an attorney specializing in immigration law.

3. Be prepared for interviews requiring extensive telephone calls in varying time zones.

4. Remember that cultural differences may limit the communication process.

5. Put overseas courier costs into your budget.

6. Hire internationally trained occupational therapists with NBCOT (National Board on Certification in Occupational Therapy) certification whenever possible.

7. Before confirming employment, make sure the therapist is approved to sit for the exam if not NBCOT-certified.

8. Plan to wait at least 2 or 3 months between hiring and arrival.

9. Expect to invest extra time to help the internationally trained therapist.

10. On the therapist's arrival, have American money ready in case it is needed.

11. Be prepared with temporary housing.

12. Have someone ready to take the therapist to obtain a social security card, driver's license, bank account, and the like.

13. Make arrangements for any required testing or credentials.

14. Realize that more personal involvement may be required with an internationally trained therapist than with an American therapist.

15. Make clear to the therapist that driving a car to and from work may be necessary.

16. Know that a longer training period than usual may be needed to familiarize the therapist with site requirements and legalities.

Epstein provided additional helpful advice for those who have assumed responsibility for managing internationally trained occupational therapists:

1. Be sure guidelines and expectations are clear and consistent.

2. Show respect for the occupational therapist.

3. Acknowledge the special skills and interests of the occupational therapist.

4. When appropriate, act on behalf of the occupational therapist.

5. Instill support and awareness of cultural diversity throughout the organization.

6. Encourage direct and honest communication.

7. Furnish avenues for creative team building.[22]

Advice such as this echoes one of the objectives of current U.S. delegates to WFOT: to ease the transition of foreign-trained therapists into U.S. occupational therapy practice and customs. In the United States the WFOT delegates are trying to help states form international committees to reach out to internationally trained therapists in every state who are going through the acculturation process. International state liaisons are being asked to assume more active roles as guides and mentors to their states' foreign-trained therapists.[23]

▒ Summary

The future is imminent. Occupational therapy is at a crossroads in the United States and worldwide: Either therapists recognize and adapt their expertise to contemporary healthcare roles, or occupational therapy may be threatened as a recognized profession. The AOTA statistics officially record patterns of employment shifts in the United States, but one need only look around to see a startling comparison to the picture of occupational therapists at work just 5 years ago.

This chapter has introduced futurism and globalization as two more topics with which students should be familiar. Occupational therapists need to know what is happening in America and around the world, as well as what to do about it. Specific suggestions for reading more broadly, developing a global mindset, and assuming responsibility for presenting testimony on behalf of the profession were outlined. Finally, examples of international activity among occupational therapists were shared. Recommendations were made to those considering going to work overseas or planning to employ internationally educated occupational therapists. Chapter 20 introduces commonalities among occupational therapists worldwide and what can be shared and learned by all.

REFERENCES

1. Naisbett, J: Megatrends. Warner Books, New York, 1982.
2. Richman, LS: Global growth is on a tear. Fortune, Mar 20, 1995, p 43.
3. Coates, JF, Jarratt, J, and Mahaffie, JB: Future Work. Jossey-Bass, San Francisco, 1990.
4. Toffler, A: Future Shock. William Morrow, New York, 1970.
5. Toffler, A: The Third Wave. William Morrow, New York, 1980.
6. Rapoport, C: Charles Handy sees the future. Fortune, Oct 31, 1994, p 155.
7. The American Heritage Dictionary. Houghton Mifflin, Boston, 1982.
8. Rose, BW: Testifying: Essential advocacy for occupational therapy. OT Week 7(24):14, June 17, 1993.
9. Wind, Y, Douglas, SP, and Perlmutter, HV: Guidelines for developing international marketing strategies. Journal of Marketing, Apr, 1973, p 141.
10. White, M: Ear to the ground. World Trade, Jan, 1996, p 69.
11. Hofheinz, P: Europe's tough new managers. Fortune, Sept, 1993, p 113.
12. Jayaraman, N: The end of a deal. World Business, Sept–Oct, 1995, p 111.
13. Fitzgerald, N: Compared to what? World Trade 9(1):58, Jan, 1996.
14. Levine, DS: When the dragon slew the pig. World Trade 9(1):27, Jan, 1996.
15. Spencer, EP: Educator insights: Euro Disney—What happened? What next? Journal of International Marketing 3(3):103, 1995.
16. Wennblom, M: Personal communication, Gothenburg, Sweden, June 9, 1996.
17. MacDonald, G: Bridge across the nations. Holland Herald, Sept, 1995, p 54.
18. Drucker, PF: Post-Capitalist Society. HarperCollins, New York, 1993.
19. Marmer, L: Changing the sobering statistics on disability. Advance for Occupational Therapists, 11(38):13, Sept 25, 1995.
20. Stancliff, BL: OT travels to the "heart of the matter." OT Practice 1(3):57, Mar, 1996.
21. Stancliff, BL: Professional support at home and abroad. OT Practice 1(3):15, Mar, 1996.
22. Epstein, CF: Hiring an internationally trained occupational therapist. OT Practice 1(3):21, Mar, 1996.
23. Stahl, C: One world of OT. Advance for Occupational Therapists, Apr 29, 1996, p 22.

CHAPTER 20

Occupational Therapy Global Problems in Common: Learning from Each Other

CHAPTER OBJECTIVES

- To understand how a country's economic status affects healthcare delivery.
- To realize the importance to occupational therapists of learning about global economic trends.
- To know that governments everywhere are seeking ethical, effective solutions to complex healthcare delivery problems.
- To become familiar with community rehabilitation practice in other countries.
- To acknowledge unique occupational therapy problems in developing countries.
- To realize how creative and adaptive occupational therapists are solving problems globally.
- To recognize how American occupational therapists are helping to meet needs

abroad while internationally educated therapists are helping to meet needs in the United States.
- To seek opportunities for better understanding and respect for the cultural values of all ethnic groups.
- To understand how occupational therapy educational programs develop abroad.
- To recognize unique characteristics of international occupational therapy education and practice.
- To appreciate international occupational therapy professional journals as well as the potential of information technology.

"Misery loves company" is a wise saying from past years. So it is with problems and issues among occupational therapists worldwide. Regardless of the form that healthcare delivery takes or the national economic system in place, and despite varied geographic and environmental circumstances, commonalities among problems and their solutions do exist. It seems that every country is experiencing some kind of healthcare crisis. None seems able to keep pace with medical innovations and public demand while balancing the fiscal problems created by both.

It is heartening, yet daunting, to acknowledge and appraise worldwide approaches to problem solving and progress. There are different variations of solutions everywhere, regardless of the kinds of government and healthcare systems in place. It is impossible to discuss here in detail all the factors affecting occupational therapy practice around the world. Instead, a few representative examples are included here to demonstrate that occupational therapists around the world share much with those in the United States, and all of us have much to learn from each other's experiences. In every case described, there are elements of marketing, management, and leadership in common with U.S. occupational therapists. Worldwide, occupational therapists use innovation, marketing, and decision-making skills to deal with problems germane to their cultures and situations. Through communication and mutual understanding, much can be shared, learned, and applied to problem solving at home.

▩ Valuing Cultural Diversity

First, there must be acknowledgment and respect for all cultures, beliefs, and healthcare methods found around the world. For years there have been advocates for the recognition and integration into occupational therapy of techniques of healing used in other cultures. For example, in 1976 an article in the (then) AOTA *Occupational Therapy Newspaper* pointed out the need to recognize and value other forms of therapeutic approaches such as those used by *curanderos*.[1] Occupational therapy literature before and since has offered similar suggestions, that is, to explore more relevant interaction methods among non-

English-speaking occupational therapy clients, to provide more meaningful services, and to perceive and respect the unique cultural values and interpretations of different ethnic groups.[2–5]

During a recent alternative healthcare conference, "Enhancing Practice through the Millennium," organized by Michael Pizzi, MS, OTR, CHES, FAOTA, many forms of alternative techniques of healing were explored.[6] The ideas and methods presented were not new but instead were rediscoveries of ancient techniques. The general purpose and tenor of the conference were encapsulated in Pizzi's opening remarks, that "healing and health are a constant interplay of person, environment, and culture." *Reiki* from Japan, acupuncture from China, and *chakras* from India were among the alternative techniques of healing that were explained to attendees.

Chi-Kwan Shea, MS, OTR, a native of Hong Kong, received her occupational therapy education in the United States and has been at St. Francis Medical Center in Los Angeles since 1984. Most of her clients today are African-American or Hispanic. Shea agrees that occupational therapy practitioners need to be able to establish mutually comfortable relationships with all types of patients.[7]

Another example can be found in association with Navajo values. Advance care planning poses a serious conflict, as it is felt to be a dangerous violation of traditional Navajo values and ways of thinking.[8] Ethnographers who have studied the Navajo identify it as breaching one of the culture's central concepts. Therefore, the requirements of the federal Patient Self-Determination Act present a serious dilemma for healthcare personnel caring for Navajo clients.

■ Creativity and Adaptation Around the World

Argentine occupational therapists have unique problems but approach their solutions in the same way as therapists in Botswana, Sweden, Peru, Malaysia, New Zealand, and elsewhere: with creativity, enthusiasm, and adaptability. Comparing stories is energizing and encouraging, such as the ways in which Argentine occupational therapists are proudly promoting their profession and effectively treating their patients despite financial instability and equipment shortages.

In Venezuela, occupational therapists are persevering against great odds to meet the increasing demands for practitioners, specialization, and technical competence in a society where the profession is in transition.[9] The Federacion Venezolana de Terapeutas Ocupacionales now legally represents all 23 state associations of Venezuela. Registration and licensure were introduced in 1992, and occupational therapists are working hard to upgrade education there. The first college offering training for occupational therapists opened in Caracas in 1959, and there are now three programs graduating between 50 and 65 practitioners annually. Occupational therapy services are presently concentrated in the capital, Caracas, despite a great need in rural areas.

Because Latvia needed help in developing rehabilitation services for its individuals with handicaps, the Swedish Professional Organization for Occupational Therapy sponsored a project in Latvia. The purpose of the first step was to reeducate nine Latvian physicians to become occupational therapists. The next step is to start a 4-year educational program there.

Occupational therapy treatment of patients with cognitive disorders in Denmark focuses on the individual and is based on thorough assessment of dysfunction in relation to ADL. Treatment is directed toward the daily life of the person and his or her current activities in personal ADL, work and leisure, social environment, and quality of life.[10]

The team approach of a psychiatrist and an occupational therapist was found to be an effective way of providing a maintenance program in the community for schizophrenic patients in Johannesburg, South Africa.[11] Relatives are educated to accept that the illness will be chronic with no chance of return to the previous state. The occupational therapist uses activity groups, art therapy groups, outings, and individual counseling. Occupational therapy intervention in the community consists of three different categories: rehabilitation, maintenance, and education.

AMERICAN OCCUPATIONAL THERAPISTS HELPING ABROAD

An American occupational therapist, Miranda Janeschild, OTR, traveled to El Salvador to instruct therapists there in the techniques needed to provide therapy for children with neurological, orthopedic, and developmental disabilities.[12] Therapists who attended the course came from the city of San Salvador, from shelters for abandoned children, and from the countryside. Problems among the pediatric physical and occupational therapists, noted Janeschild, were (1) lack of communication among them, (2) range of motion as the primary modality of therapy, (3) few therapists with skills in analyzing abnormal movement, (4) functional goals not established with clients, and (5) parents not included in the decision making or treatment sessions of their children. Instruction was modeled after a basic course in neurodevelopmental treatment and incorporated contemporary theories and approaches for working with children with cerebral palsy.

Christine Trexel, OTR, a Level III occupational therapist at St. Luke's Rehabilitation Institute in Spokane, spent 6 weeks in Vietnam presenting occupational therapy workshops to Vietnamese physical therapists.[13] Occupational therapy does not exist yet in Vietnam, but Vietnamese physical therapists and nurses recognized the importance of incorporating activities of daily living, fine motor coordination, and traditional occupational therapy domains into treating the whole patient. Cultural mores, such as the unquestioned role of the adult children to care for elderly or infirm parents, bring unique challenges to introducing the value of independence in activities of daily living. Traditionally the hospital patient's personal needs are all met by family members while the individual is in the hospital and subsequently at home. Therapy services are seldom available in rural areas.

Gale Haradon, PhD, OTR, now a program director at University of Texas–San Antonio, gave valuable service in Romania by helping orphans in dangerous conditions there. Maude Malick, OTR, CHT, a pioneer of psychiatric and hand rehabilitation in the United States during World War II, is presently in Bosnia to assess rehabilitation needs among the war victims there and direct supplies where they are needed most. Linda Lehman, OTR, another U.S. occupational therapist, has served nearly a decade in Brazil to assist those diagnosed with leprosy. You are advised to read occupational therapy professional publications to learn about similar opportunities overseas and for information about other occupational therapists who continue to assist their colleagues and disabled populations abroad.

Occupational Therapy Community Practice in Other Countries

An effective way to increase your personal knowledge about how occupational therapists resolve problems worldwide is to become familiar with situations from those therapists' viewpoints. With the advent of growing community practice in the United States, sharing of such experiences is invaluable. Community-based rehabilitation involves measures taken at the community level to use and build on the resources of the community. This includes the disabled persons themselves, their families, and their communities as a whole. Whether the setting is urban, rural, in a small town, a western or eastern country, or an established or developing country, the definition of community-based rehabilitation is the same, even though there are issues and problems unique to each setting.

CANADA

In 1992 about one-fourth of Canadian occupational therapists worked in community-based settings; by 1995 the number had risen to one-third. Results of a survey of community occupational therapy practitioners there indicated that they felt inadequately prepared for the relatively new and growing role of community consultant and its concomitant skills.[14]

The Canadian International Development Agency (CIDA), believing that community development is a major issue internationally, supported development of community rehabilitation programs in Canada as well as international linkages for a consortium of community-based rehabilitation partners.[15] The concept of community-based rehabilitation formally appeared when the World Health Organization (WHO) introduced a model whereby member states collaborated with members of WHO to address the needs of people with disabilities and their families. It is their contention that as the home emerges as the setting for management of chronic illness, disability, and problems related to aging, families and community networks must assume greater responsibility for preventive care and rehabilitation.

One of the six centers funded through CIDA is the International Centre for the Advancement of Community-Based Rehabilitation (ICACBR) based in Kingston, Ontario. In addition to Canada, ICACBR's charter members include India, Indonesia, Bangladesh, and more recent members from Asia and Russia. Even though fully committed to technology advancement, ICACBR introduces only devices that are socially, culturally, and economically acceptable to the people in the communities in which they will be used. Most health problems in most areas of the world are not just biologic, but have, in addition, strong psychological, social, and cultural causes. ICACBR makes it clear that they have no intention of trying to replace the healthcare systems in other parts of the world but intend only to work with existing resources and to augment the services already in place. The ICACBR representative asserted that the aim is to support different approaches to community-based rehabilitation. If one approach can be applied to Sweden or Bosnia or Latin America, that model is documented and analyzed to determine the core elements of successful community-based rehabilitation and styles of healthcare systems.[15]

NEW ZEALAND

In 1990 healthcare services in New Zealand were increasingly provided in the community as opposed to the previously customary hospital settings.[16] It was decided that action has to be taken in four key directions in order to adequately prepare occupational therapists and to effect change:

1. Theory development to show what it is that makes occupational therapy unique.
2. Education to prepare students to be responsive to healthcare needs while remaining true to the important values and qualities inherent in occupational therapy.
3. Management skills in communication, motivation, teamwork, program planning, forecasting, budgeting, marketing, networking, and data analysis.
4. Risk taking and innovation to develop new roles as service delivery managers, consultants, and educators.

Looking toward the future, New Zealand occupational therapists concluded they needed a philosophy that relates to the values and cultures of their clients and that they must be creative, innovative, and prepared to move away from the sheltered environments of established services.[16]

Client-centered care and the marketing process are readily detected in an account of community occupational therapy in Otago Province on the south island of New Zealand.[17] Therapists responded to individual differences in communities and used members of the communities to assist in providing support, prevention, and information. This approach is taught in the occupational therapy educational program. One of the four community program facets is Project Enable, a disability resource center for laypersons and professionals that is staffed by an occupational therapist and a mechanical engineer. Working as a team they go out to solve problems, such as a seating difficulty, and create adaptations. A librarian is also on staff to locate answers to problems with a modem that is connected to international sources.

Another aspect of the program is Community Integration Service (CIS), funded by the New Zealand Intellectually Handicapped Group, whose goal is to provide people of all ages with support in home and community. This support, using community resources, is individualized in a lifestyle plan based on a person's interests and life goals and includes assistance for parents and caregivers. The objective is to help clients become part of the community while developing their strengths and helping them with their weaknesses.

The Friendship Network provides an opportunity for friendship for people with limited social networks who are at risk for social isolation, while the Parent to Parent part of the program is a telephone support and information system staffed by volunteers trained in listening skills and appropriate responses. This community program, after recognizing the variety of needs requiring individual responses, respects these differences. By doing so, the power is given back to the people.[17]

Other New Zealand occupational therapists closely examined the close relationship of occupational therapy and health as a global concept.[18] They urged peers to adapt community occupational therapy to the demands of clients by providing efficient service while being accountable and cost-effective. They noted that New Zealand was unable to continue to afford all the health care that was expected. It was further explained that carrying out cost containment with an emphasis on health promotion should be encouraged, as it is in line with international trends.

The preceding information has demonstrated that occupational therapists around the world are, like those in the United States, practicing in increasing numbers in the community. There is therefore an obvious need for occupational therapy students to be prepared for new practice alternatives and to gain more experience in community-based sites.

COMMUNITY-BASED REHABILITATION IN DEVELOPING COUNTRIES

By the year 2000 four-fifths of persons with disabilities will live in developing countries, an increasing rather than decreasing figure.[19] Malnutrition and bronchopulmonary infections are the main causes of death among children with disabilities in developing countries. Adults with disabilities have generally lower incomes than able-bodied adults and consequently are more likely to suffer from poverty. Children with disabilities have less opportunity to attend school. Adults are often excluded from leadership positions and thus from planning and decision making in their societies. They receive less education and vocational training and are often unemployed. Fewer of them marry or form families.[20]

A recent study in Botswana by two occupational therapists had the goal of developing Community Based Rehabilitation (CBR), a concept developed by WHO. During 1990 these therapists carried out a door-to-door survey in Moshupa village.[21] Many of the facts uncovered helped them better understand the nature of the problems in this particular population. Of the disabled, 22 percent were younger than 15 years of age; moving difficulties were identified as the most prevalent diagnosis, similar to findings in Zimbabwe. Of people with disabilities, 30 percent had parents who were related. Most caregivers were single mothers, and the mother was the center of the family in this society because most fathers were away working in the mines in South Africa for long periods. Many women do not marry so as to keep the rights to their own property and wages.[21]

By understanding these and other relevant data, a community-based program of rehabilitation that best fit the needs and resources of this population was successfully established, one more example of occupational therapists' extending their knowledge and support abroad. In this case the occupational therapists were from Sweden.

▓ Comparative Development of Occupational Therapy Educational Programs Worldwide

Steadily and gradually, the number of occupational therapy educational programs is growing globally. Numbers of students in past years have come to the United States to enter occupational therapy educational programs and then return to their native countries to initiate educational programs and clinical practices. Others, graduated from programs outside the United States, have come to the United States to practice. Exact data are available from AOTA and the National Board for Certification in Occupational Therapy (NBCOT, formerly AOTCB). The spectrum of occupational therapy educational programs is as broad as there are countries in this world. Each country has much of which to be proud, and students should look forward to learning about other nations and their unique origins and histories.

The World Federation of Occupational Therapists (WFOT) plays a key role in enforcing standards for occupational therapy education worldwide.[22] If occupational therapy programs in any country want their graduates to be recognized universally as well-prepared professionals, they must be approved by the educational committee of WFOT according to the minimum standards developed by WFOT. Most occupational therapy programs worldwide are WFOT-approved, but WFOT does withhold approval from some programs that appear to have deficiencies. To be a member of WFOT, a country must have at least one WFOT-approved school. For updated information about WFOT, request from AOTA the names of the current AOTA representatives to the WFOT organization.

For educational programs, finding fieldwork sites and alternatives to traditional fieldwork is but one related problem that faculties have in common internationally. With growing awareness resulting from globalization, occupational therapists worldwide can learn from each other, share information and experiences, and spread the influence and richness of occupational therapy among all who can benefit from it. There is a wide variance in the stages of development and growth of occupational therapy educational programs around the world. Following are some representative facts about occupational therapy education worldwide.

The first school in Japan was started in Tokyo in 1963 and is called National Chest Hospital, School of Rehabilitation. At the time of this writing, there are 58 occupational therapy programs in Japan and more being developed. Most are 3-year diploma programs, and eight award bachelor's degrees. A number of students from Taiwan have enrolled over the years in U.S. occupational therapy programs and then returned to their native land to establish successful practices as well as educational programs. One Thai student, who was sponsored by the Thai government to secure occupational therapy education in the United States, now teaches the occupational therapy program at Chieng Mai University in Thailand. These two instances are representative of many such students who come from other countries and graduate from occupational therapy programs in the United States and then return to their respective countries to initiate educational programs and practices.

Mutual exchanges of information and support among U.S. occupational therapy educators and those in Canada and the United Kingdom have been occurring for decades. Canadian educational guidelines highlight the fundamental concepts of occupation, meaningful activities, and a client-centered approach to practice, similar to those of the United States. Curricular content about home, or domiciliary, care has been modeled for years by professional colleagues in the United Kingdom, and instances of collaboration between U.S. and Canadian educators are many.

Another illustration of mutual exchange is that of Swedish and Australian occupational therapy educators, who have done much to further international exchange of research and practice by traveling broadly to seek new opportunities for their students and colleagues. In a manner similar to some U.S. programs, the University of Newcastle in Australia established its occupational therapy program with a problem-based learning model.

Occupational therapy education in Puerto Rico began in 1952 as a combined OT/PT certificate course, which continued until 1970 when the two separated. The bachelor of science in occupational therapy program is fully accredited by AOTA and is the only program of its kind on the island, graduating

30 students each year. There are two occupational therapy assistant programs as well.[23]

Costa Rica is the only Central American country that has a university degree program in occupational therapy. However, Nicaragua is presently developing an occupational therapy program with some assistance from U.S. therapists.

A self-financed team of six healthcare professionals, including an occupational therapist and four physical therapists, traveled to Kenya in 1994 to teach a weeklong series of workshops to occupational and physical therapists. Arriving to find the whole healthcare system in disarray, they joined Kenyan physical and occupational therapists in curriculum development, scholarship awards, technology dissemination, and provision of access to current rehabilitation techniques.[24]

Australia and Universal Health Insurance

Since the 1980s, Australia has provided its residents with a universal health insurance plan funded through a payroll tax of 1.4 percent on gross incomes over $7,400 (U.S.), which is known as the Medicare levy. Free room and board and treatment in public hospitals by staff physicians is provided by Medicare to all Australian residents. Most outpatient care and physician visits are free, and pharmaceuticals are subsidized. Medicare users can choose their own physicians; the government sets costs but does not limit the charges that physicians make. Private insurance companies supplement the public system, and there are encouraging examples of cooperation between the public and private sectors.[25]

Caring for Australia's elderly and disabled is increasingly becoming the domain of the private sector. Provision of long-term health care is handled by the government by basing it on the rationing of institutional as well as residential care while simultaneously increasing home and community healthcare services. Approximately 12 percent of Australia's population is at least 65 years old, a number that is expected to double by 2025. Yet few territories (equivalent to U.S. states) plan to add significant numbers of public nursing homes or beds. To be admitted to a skilled nursing home, a potential resident must first be evaluated by a geriatric assessment team that looks at medical stability, ability to perform ADL activities, and availability of an alternative caretaker. The government plans to contain healthcare costs by reducing reliance on nursing home care and inpatient rehabilitation, the most expensive components of geriatric care. To achieve this goal, Australia is planning to expand its provision of retirement homes and geriatric hostels.

In summary, the Australian system of health care is an example of government-provided basic care, with ancillary care available on a limited basis from public sources. To control costs, the Australian government is leaving the growth of rehabilitation and long-term care to the private sector.[25]

▨ Economics and Its Effect on Health Care in Nordic Countries

Just as in the United States, national economic factors affect all aspects of healthcare delivery in countries around the world. *Nordicum,* the Scandinavian business review, in late 1995 announced that Nordic countries must make structural reductions in spending.[26] It was noted that growth of private consumption had slowed in Denmark, the unemployment rate in Finland was very high, and new budget cuts were expected in Sweden. To help the student understand that the United States is not alone in its search for an effective model of healthcare delivery, the healthcare-related circumstances in Sweden are described here as an example of worldwide shared dilemmas. The critical role played by economic factors is evident, even though the history of health care in Sweden is dissimilar from that of the United States. Nevertheless, current similarities and complexities become evident as responsible citizens in both countries continue to seek satisfactory conclusions.

SWEDEN'S QUANDARY WITH HEALTHCARE CHANGES

In Sweden greater reliance on noninstitutional care and use of "local" facilities instead of more sophisticated, expensive hospitals was advocated as early as 1986.[27] Sweden is a relatively sparsely populated northern European country. The population of 8.7 million, 18 percent of which is at least 65 years old, is mainly concentrated in the coastal and southern regions. Responsibility for Swedish inpatient and ambulatory health care lies with 23 county councils and 3 large municipalities that are not part of the county council areas. The counties also operate the public dental service and services for the mentally retarded, with 80 percent of the county council activities devoted to healthcare and medical services. Swedish health care has been hospital oriented for the past 40 years, with 70 percent of the cost of health care covered by taxes levied and administered by the county councils. The tax assigned to health care is comparable to a universal public health insurance covering the individual's costs for medical care (Fig. 20–1).

THE FEELING OF CHANGE

Long considered a model of comprehensive health care that is available to all citizens of all ages, Sweden would appear to be quite different from the United States in the nature of its healthcare problems. This may, indeed, be the case as far as the current structure and financing of health care are concerned; however, discussion of the problems and issues among occupational and physical therapists in Sweden produced a surprising number of commonalities. The first

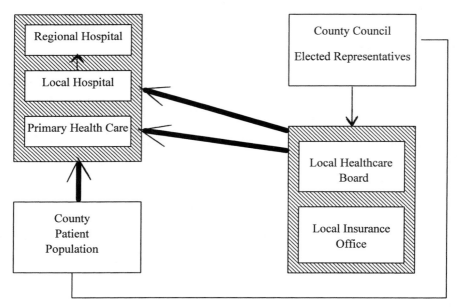

FIGURE 20–1. Method of tax distribution in a county in Sweden.

apparent shared perception was the feeling of change, of transition that appeared imminent. As in the United States, economic realities in Sweden are a major factor affecting healthcare services.

THE SITUATION

The Swedish healthcare system is engaged in an organizational reappraisal. Morbidity and mortality data, as well as health status, continue to indicate that Sweden is one of the world's healthiest populations. An infant mortality rate of 5.8 per 1000 live births and an average life span of 74.2 years for men and 80 years for women place Sweden near the top of lists of comparative health statistics.[28] In spite of this superior performance on collective indices, a growing crisis has appeared in Sweden at the healthcare service delivery level. One example is the increasing demand for care from the rapidly growing number of older citizens, requests that cannot be met because of pay schedules that are too low to attract new personnel in a tight labor market. This problem was created by the successful cost-containment policy enacted a decade earlier.

At the same time there are pressures to increase hospital resources, to keep up with new technology, and to shorten lengthy waits for elective procedures, as well as demands for more services in the primary care and home care sectors.[29] Before improving continuity of care, especially for elderly persons, an obstinate dilemma must be overcome: whether primary care services should be integrated with county-administered hospital services (the present situation) or with municipally administered social services, as in Finland.[30]

There are still more facets of this complex situation. In order to remain industrially competitive in a period of rapid economic integration, Sweden must reduce tax levels that are among the highest in Europe. Also, widespread economic success has created an affluent population that is increasingly less willing to accept a stratified healthcare system perceived to be beyond the influence of individuals.[31]

PROPOSALS FOR ALTERNATIVE SOLUTIONS

These and other quandaries have been creating demands for major change in the Swedish healthcare system and resulted in a broad range of proposals, from neoconservative suggestions to replace the present public system with a set of privately operated financial and provider markets[32] to an adamant defense of the present structure by those who believe the solutions lie in providing increased resources to a strapped delivery system.[33] One of the most important proposals was advanced by the Social Democratic party in its preliminary national program for the 1990s,[34] which suggested that certain market-oriented mechanisms be introduced inside the existing publicly operated system. Patients would be given free choice of sites and providers both within and across county lines (said by some to be giving patients permission to "vote with their feet"), and providers would find budget allocations as well as salaries tied to their ability to attract patients and to serve them efficiently. This proposal was said to reflect that part of the Social Democratic tradition that asserted pragmatism in the face of a changing political environment.[35] During the ongoing Swedish debate, two key issues surfaced: (1) the proper role of competitive behavior in a restructured health system and (2) whether private-sector providers, insurers, or both ought to be incorporated within an accepted new model.

Two specific examples of proposals tried in the early 1990s were those in Stockholm County and Kopparberg County. Cautious incrementalism is exemplified in the Stockholm County model, which resembles more closely a public competition model and calls for patient choice of both primary care and hospital providers, combined with a primary health center–based budgeting structure.[36] Personnel salaries were linked to productivity, including population and patient-based measures of effectiveness, with poorly performing providers evaluated by social as well as economic criteria. The Stockholm experiment thus fell short of introducing strictly market-based financial competition.[31] The Stockholm County Council embarked in January 1992 on this new way of financing and organizing health care, and the new model was fully implemented in 1995.

By contrast the Dalamodel, adopted in principle in Kopparberg County in 1990, was more radical, combining a patient-driven primary care system with a manager-driven, contract-based system for hospital services. The Dalamodel called for the creation of 15 primary health boards controlling both primary care and hospital budgets for district inhabitants, under the presupposition that this financing arrangement would generate pressure for greater efficiency inside primary health centers and in the publicly operated hospital clinics. Private as well as publicly operated providers were entitled to compete for contracts from primary health boards.

These two models indicate the wide range of reorganization alternatives under consideration in Sweden. Perhaps the most important difference is the character of the new market to be established and the relative decision-making balance between patients, on the one hand, and administrators and politicians on the other. In the Stockholm model, the driving force was the patients who would serve to prioritize quality and continuity of care by bringing institutional budgets and personnel salaries with them. In contrast, the Dalamodel, emphasizing cost containment, created a roughly similar type of public market in primary care, but the hospital sector had a mixed public-private market based on short-term contracts, with the driving force the administrators and politicians who negotiate these contracts. In both instances, market elements would be incorporated into the public system as a means through which to reinforce the achievement of public sector goals and objectives.[31]

Efforts to introduce public competition in Sweden are being watched with much interest by other countries. Although demographic and fiscal pressures in these countries may not be quite so intense, policy makers in the United Kingdom,[37] Italy,[38] and Spain[39] share with Sweden similar problems concerning efficiency levels within publicly operated institutions, waiting times for elective procedures, low salaries for professional personnel, and inadequate responsiveness to patient preferences. The Stockholm and Kopparberg experiments are of international interest also in that they retain public accountability over service outcomes while introducing market-style mechanisms to encourage more efficient provider performance. If the present reform process is successful and the dramatic changes do eventuate, Sweden may well reassert its traditional role as an international model for publicly operated health systems in Europe.[31]

Why This Must Concern U.S. Occupational Therapists

What is important to those who read this description is that the outcome of the Swedish debate may contain lessons about the capacity of publicly operated health systems to effectively integrate normative objectives with performance-oriented goals. Governments around the world are wrestling with the infinite complexities of healthcare delivery problems. Watching and listening to the experiences of others who are searching for ethical, effective solutions to mutual problems is a wise, commonsense assist for your own deliberations.

In response to a question about how she meant to approach the changing roles and needs appearing within the healthcare delivery system, one Swedish therapist replied that "the thing is to get used to change as a constant factor. Trends about organizations and economic incentives will come and go. The question is to take the best out of it, challenge the future by taking independent steps and not just wait for somebody else to tell you what to do."[40]

▓ Where to Seek Information

The WFOT is the best source for all current information about occupational therapy education and practice worldwide, and occupational therapy practitioners are strongly encouraged not only to contact them for current information but also to become active members. When possible, attend the exciting WFOT conferences, held worldwide, to meet enthusiastic, energized professional colleagues who represent practice internationally.

INTERNATIONAL PROFESSIONAL JOURNALS

One has only to read occupational therapy journals other than *The American Journal of Occupational Therapy,* such as those from Canada, New Zealand, Scandinavia, the United Kingdom, or Australia, or to peruse WFOT publications to realize that change and adaptation, threat and innovation, flexibility and creativity are found worldwide. Actions are being taken around the world to ensure that the full promise of occupational therapy is realized.

The editor of the *Scandinavian Journal of Occupational Therapy,* Birgitta Lundgren-Lindquist, launched the first issue of this new journal in 1995 with a commentary about the purpose of the publication. Among the topics anticipated were health, adaptation and well-being, conceptualization of activity and occupation, relationships between health and occupation, critical analysis, how occupational therapy can meet the challenges imposed by social problems, high unemployment rates, escalating healthcare costs, work in a changing and more diverse culture, and need for cost-effective models of training. In addition, articles were invited that would encourage scientific inquiry and provide a forum for research, which includes qualitative methods, case studies, and conceptual and theoretical articles that synthesize state-of-the-art ideas from colleagues throughout the world. A person might have thought this journal was a copy of *The American Journal of Occupational Therapy* because so many commonalities with U.S. occupational therapists' interests and dilemmas were evident.

INFORMATION TECHNOLOGY

The information age has built the need for rapid dissemination and control of information. One visit to e-mail quickly establishes this fact: Online, a director of occupational therapy in London urges every occupational therapist to develop leadership skills. Also online, a Canadian professional suggests that a strategic planning approach and the capacity for being proactive are essential for today's occupational therapists, while a Swedish occupational therapist sends out a plea worldwide for a therapist needed in Latvia. Interchange of ideas among occupational therapy practitioners worldwide is a valuable and informative activity and an international sharing of occupational therapy talent and creativity. One example would be the service created for members of the Technology Special Interest Section of AOTA; another is Canadian-based Occup Ther.

Because this is a book and the information in a book cannot be updated weekly or monthly, as is the case with a journal or news magazine, only general introductory information is presented here to launch the reader into the realm of electronic services. The World Wide Web and Internet have quickly become useful means for occupational therapy practitioners to keep in touch with new services and to enhance the diversity of resources available to them. A definition of *World Wide Web* (WWW) is a universal database of information linked together by computers. It provides users with the means to access a variety of media by way of software interfaces. *Internet* is a worldwide network of computers, literally a "network of networks" scattered throughout the globe. While the WWW is a body of information, the Internet is the physical side, a mass of cables and computers. Access to the Internet means having access to electronic mail, interactive conferences, information resources, network news, and the ability to transfer computer files.

Because no one owns either the Internet or the WWW, there is no single governing body. Internet networks are funded and managed locally according to local policies. From one organization to another, availability and sophistication of electronic equipment may vary widely and at times fluctuate for many reasons. Among the causes of this variability are financial resources of organizations, the level of computer literacy of those in decision-making positions, and the relative importance assigned to updated technology purchases. By seeking alternatives and using creativity, occupational therapy practitioners can successfully adapt to such changing situations.

▨ Summary

This chapter has asserted that occupational therapists around the world have much to share and learn from each other. A global mindset should be deliberately developed by American occupational therapy practitioners if they are to continue to grow as informed professionals. Examples of the variety of stages of growth among occupational therapy educational programs worldwide were described, as well as sources from which more specific information can be secured. Occupational therapy practitioners were advised to read international professional journals as well as those published in the United States and thus to learn from the experiences of therapists in other countries who are adapting to changing healthcare situations. It was further suggested that all occupational therapy practitioners develop familiarity with and use information technology as it becomes available. Given the movement in the United States toward more community health care, two countries' responses to this same issue were described. Finally, heartening and generous indications of the ways in which occupational therapists in the United States have already addressed issues of cultural diversity both here and abroad were described.

REFERENCES

1. Gilkeson, GE: Commentary: Renewed medical liaison. Occupational Therapy Newspaper, July, 1976, p 3.
2. Christiansen, C: Multicultural competencies in early intervention: Training professionals for a pluralistic society. Infants and Young Children 4:3, 1992.
3. Dillard, M, Andonian, L, Flores, O, Lai, L, MacRae, A, and Shakir, M: Culturally competent occupational therapy in a diversely populated mental health setting. Am J Occup Ther 46:721, 1992.
4. Litterst, TAE: The foundation: A reappraisal of anthropological fieldwork methods and the concept of culture in occupational therapy research. Am J Occup Ther 39:602, 1985.
5. Mauras-Neslen, E: An Hispanic perspective. OT Week 4(49), Dec 13, 1990.
6. Joe, BE: Striking an alternative chord. OT Week 10(1), Jan 4, 1996.
7. Joe, BE: Celebrating Asian-American month. OT Week 7(12):7, May 13, 1993.
8. Carrese, JA, and Rhodes, LA: Western bioethics on the Navajo reservation: Benefit or harm? JAMA 274(10): 826, Sept 18, 1995.
9. Sinclair, K: Meeting the challenge in Venezuela. OT Week 9(46), Nov 16, 1995.
10. Sorenson, LV: The O.T. treatment of patients with cognitive disorders in Denmark. WFOT Bulletin 32, Nov, 1995.
11. Rodseth, D, and Crouch, RB: A program for the maintenance of the schizophrenic patient in the community. WFOT Bulletin 32, Nov, 1995.
12. Janeschild, M: Pediatric OT in El Salvador. OT Week 9(35), Aug 31, 1995
13. Trexel, C: Vietnam sees value in rehab. OT Week 9(8), Feb 23, 1995.
14. Marmer, L: Community-based OTs short on needed skills. Advance for Occupational Therapists 10(21), May 8, 1995.
15. Marmer, L: Changing the sobering statistics on disability. Advance for Occupational Therapists 11(38):13, Sept 25, 1995.
16. Hanschu, B, and McFadden, S: Out on a limb: A novel approach for occupational therapy practice. Australian Journal of Occupational Therapy 28(2):39, 1981.
17. Sher, B: What's new in New Zealand: Respecting individual differences in the community. WFOT Bulletin 31, May, 1995.
18. Fechner, CI: Community occupational therapy and the changing concepts of health. New Zealand Journal of Occupational Therapy 42(2):4, Summer, 1991.
19. Safilios-Rothschild, C: Disability and rehabilitation: Research and social policy and developing nations. In Albrecht, GL (ed): Cross National Rehabilitation Policies: A Sociological Perspective. Sage, Beverly Hills, Calif, 1981.
20. Helander, E: Rehabilitering for alla WHO's program for rehabilitering i u-lan derna. NU nytt om u-landshalsovard 2:3, 1987.
21. Lundgren-Lindquist, B, and Nordholm, L: Community based rehabilitation: A survey of disabled in a village in Botswana. Disability and Rehabilitation, August, 1992.
22. Thiers, N: WFOT approval is crucial for foreign schools. OT Week 8(15), Apr 15, 1994.
23. Irizarry, D: Puerto Rico's unique aspects of practice. OT Week 8(38), Sept 22, 1994.

24. Jeter, E, and Kilmarx, M: Bringing Kenya and America together. OT Week 9(5), Feb 2, 1995.
25. Murer, CG: Australia's health care model. Rehab Management 8(3):102, Apr/May, 1995.
26. Korhonen, I: Nordic economic trends. Nordicum 2, 1995, p 2.
27. Forni, PR: Health care delivery in Sweden and Finland: A challenge to the American system. Journal of Professional Nursing, July–Aug, 1986, p 234.
28. Nordic Statistical Secretariat (ed): Yearbook of Nordic Statistics, 1989/90. Nordic Council of Ministers, Copenhagen, 1990.
29. Calltorp, J: Privatization and decision making in health care questions. Uppsala University, Uppsala, Sweden, 1989.
30. Saltman, RB: National planning for locally controlled health systems: The Finnish experience. Journal of Health Politics, Policy and Law 13:27, 1988.
31. Saltman, RB: Competition and reform in the Swedish health system. The Milbank Quarterly 68:4, 1990.
32. Johnson, A: Turn Services Loose: A Service Society's Myths and Possibilities. Svenska Arbetsgivareforeningen, Stockholm, 1986.
33. Anderson, OW: How can Swedish health care meet demands on costs, technology, and equality? Lakartidningen 86(33):38, 1989.
34. Social Democratic Party (SDP): Program for the 1990s. Tidens Forlag, Stockholm, 1989.
35. Tilton, TA: Why don't Swedish Social Democrats nationalize industry? Scandinavian Studies 59:142,
36. Brogren, PO, Hessselback, B, and Karlsson, A: Community Population Responsibility in Health Care. County Council, Stockholm, 1989.
37. Ham, C, Robinson, R, and Benzeval, M: Health Check: Health Policy in an International Perspective. King's Fund Institute, London, 1990.
38. Fattore, G, and Garattini, L: Allocation of financial resources in the national health care system: A theoretical introduction and a practical solution. Economica Publica 11, Nov, 1989.
39. Garcia Vargas: We should introduce competition in the public sector. Expansion, Madrid, Mar 9, 1990.
40. Wennblom, M: Personal communication. Gothenburg, Sweden, July, 1996.

PART NINE

THE LOGICAL PROGRESSION

Example is not the main thing in influencing others. It is the only thing.

Albert Schweitzer

CHAPTER 21

Occupational Therapy Leaders

- To realize that leaders are found in every occupational therapy role category.
- To recognize just a few persons who are examples of contemporary occupational therapy leaders.
- To identify within the lives of these individuals their attitudes of adaptation to change, their recognition of the opportunities hidden within problems, their open minds that found ways to fill the needs they detected, and their ability to hold on to their visions and values as they move toward their goals.
- To see the value of selecting, consciously or unconsciously, appropriate marketing tools, whether personal selling or publicity or promotion, to achieve the variety of goals represented by these leaders' examples.

Ingrained habit and custom can supply confidence and reassurance. The "habit and custom" of occupational therapy, with its client-centered caring and its core of therapeutic occupation, should be so woven into the fabric of therapists' lives and thinking that in a constantly changing world of healthcare service delivery it indomitably continues, adaptive and discernible in all its forms of application. On the transitional scene of health care, occupational therapy is a growing force because members of the profession have continuously worked to make it so. Throughout this book those occupational therapy practitioners who have been used as examples, as well as those whose publications have been referenced, have been included because the author gratefully recognizes and acknowledges them as leaders in the profession.

The intent of this chapter is to illustrate what the preceding chapters have collectively asserted: The qualities and attributes of leaders are present among hundreds of occupational therapy practitioners who serve as role models and as mentors for today's entry-level occupational therapy practitioners. To demonstrate that assertion, in this chapter several persons have been selected as examples. Age is not a criterion, for the ages of leaders in occupational therapy are as varied as the persons themselves, whether age 20 or 80. Nor is level of education a sole determining factor, as the educational credentials of occupational therapy leaders range from associate's to doctoral degrees.

Some names are immediately recognizable, and others are not yet as well known. Leaders in occupational therapy are found everywhere—as researchers, educators, clinicians, managers, businesspersons, and in newly created categories of practice. What singles out these individuals as leaders and what they have in common are their attitudes of open-mindedness, flexibility, vision, creativity, independence, intelligence, and all the other characteristics enumerated in previous chapters on leadership. By developing these attributes, you, too, can become a leader and build your own and your profession's future.

▨ Role Models Then and Now

One leader after another has recognized needs and proactively blazed the trail of occupational therapy through the years. Whether it was Clare Spackman and evaluation and treatment of physical dysfunction, Eleanor Clarke Slagle and an early model of treatment for the mentally ill, Susan Tracy and the importance of interpersonal relationships, A. Jean Ayres with a neurobehavioral orientation, Mary Reilly offering occupational behavior education, Adolf Meyer and a vision of an occupational therapy philosophy, Wilma West with early proposals for the role of occupational therapy in prevention and for movement of practice into the community, or Gail Fidler with continuing guidance for psychiatric occupational therapy practice, the list is long and illustrious. In every case, needs were identified and solutions put forth, a traditional response among occupational therapy leaders.

It is, of course, impossible to name all the members of the occupational therapy profession who have used marketing approaches, consciously or unconsciously, and who have become successful leaders. For that, a separate book would be needed, as occupational therapy is fortunate to have a history that includes so many distinguished leaders in America and around the world. Here are a few examples of occupational therapy practitioners who have demonstrated leadership and marketing as they turned obstacles into opportunities and always accepted personal responsibility for the future—their own and that of the profession of occupational therapy.

▨ Where Leaders Are Found

Leaders are present throughout the occupational therapy profession. One way to typify leaders is through the occupational therapy roles categories furnished by the Occupational Therapy Roles Task Force of the American Occupational Therapy Association (AOTA) in *Occupational Therapy Roles.* (This document, when approved by the Representative Assembly in 1993, replaced two rescinded documents from 1985 and 1990.) Using this categorization, the potential roles include OTR practitioners, COTA practitioners, educators (consumer, peer), fieldwork educators (practice setting), supervisors, administrators, consultants, fieldwork coordinators (academic setting), faculty, program directors, researchers, and entrepreneurs (see Chapter 3). The author recognizes that categories of occupational therapy personnel were published in 1996 in the AOTA policy manual as Association Policy 1.44; however, the categorization of roles just listed has been deliberately selected for use here.

In the vernacular and categorization of *Occupational Therapy Roles,* the leaders selected as examples for this book cumulatively fall within all the classifications. It would be overly simplistic and stereotypical to consider any occupational therapy leader as occupying only one category because those with vision and dedication tend to occupy multiple roles over a lifetime, even simultaneously. Whether "officially" classified as practitioners, researchers, fieldwork educators, program directors, or entrepreneurs, the influence of leadership can be felt throughout the profession in these persons' secondary roles as well.

Because leadership is a function of both personality structure and situational interaction, additional characteristics that leaders have in common include intelligence, risk taking, a positive regard for self and others, enjoyment of lifelong learning, empathy, clear values, a need to achieve, active listening and communication skills, skills in marketing, politics, motivation, trust building, empowerment, and the ability to evaluate current trends and foresee long-term significant developments that could potentially affect their organizations and themselves. Could leadership also be an *e* word? A leader, after all, is enthusiastic, energetic, earnest, effective, ethical, enterprising, empowering, encouraging, essential, enabling, empathetic, elastic, enlightened, enquiring, and enduring. So, isn't leadership an *e* word? As you share highlights of the following occupational therapy practitioners' lives, keep in mind the characteristics of leadership, and note the leadership attributes that can be identified in the accomplishments of these admirable exemplars.

Six Contemporary Leaders

Leadership has been portrayed in this book as being found throughout the profession and at all levels of practice, whether local, state, national, or international. The following occupational therapy leaders exemplify this statement. Without them and their many counterparts, the profession would not be the viable, robust entity it is today. Included here, in alphabetical order, as contemporary leaders are Sue Byers-Connon, Helen Hopkins, Joan Rogers, Sally Ryan, Fred Sammons, and Shirley Wells. All are known and respected for a primary role, but each has also served in one or more additional capacities. One person is known *primarily* as founder and head of a corporation, one as a researcher, one as an educator, one as a representative of Certified Occupational Therapy Assistant (COTA) affairs, one as a representative of cultural diversity issues, and one as an author.

SUE BYERS-CONNON, BA, COTA, ROH

Sue Byers-Connon is presently an instructor in the Occupational Therapy Assistant Program at Mt. Hood Community College in Oregon, an AOTA accreditation council evaluation specialist, cochair of the AOTA ad hoc committee on COTA issues, and immediate past COTA representative on the AOTA Executive Board. She has held many other posts over the years, beginning in 1980 as an AOTA alternate student representative, has given numerous presentations, and written several publications. Among her honors are the AOTA/COTA Award of Excellence, AOTA Roster of Honor, and Employee of the Year recognitions.

Her responses, when asked what she considered to be the most important decisions affecting her career, indicate devotion to the profession as her main concern. In 1983 Byers-Connon worked on the public relations committee for the AOTA conference and attended the COTA Forum, where she was exposed to the COTA leaders who then served as role models for this beginning practitioner. The following year she presented a paper at the AOTA conference. Shortly afterwards she agreed to complete a 1-year term on the Commission on Practice, and next was asked to be a COTA representative on the Accreditation Committee. To this she also agreed, seeing both as opportunities to learn better how to serve her chosen profession. Believing strongly in OTR-COTA partnerships, she has cochaired several committees on the state level with OTRs. She now encourages students to become involved early in state and national associations, and many have indeed done so. In her clinical practice she also works closely with all levels of practitioners. Byers-Connon says:

Being involved in my state and national professional organizations is a way to grow and to give back to a profession that has provided me with a rewarding career. I am continuing to pursue a degree in adult education to expand myself as an instructor. As a member of a professional organization I feel a responsibility to be involved and to effect change. To do this I am willing to continue to learn from others, to accept feedback as a way of learning, and to form multiple professional partnerships. I am not afraid of taking risks, for I have been inspired by COTA leaders who have paved the way and encouraged and mentored me. I want to make a difference.[1]

HELEN L. HOPKINS, EdD, OTR, FAOTA

The name Helen L. Hopkins is perhaps most familiar to occupational therapy practitioners from the cover of *Willard and Spackman's Occupational Therapy.* She was coeditor with Helen D. Smith from 1975 to 1993 for four editions of this publication. Helen Willard and Clare Spackman had edited the first textbook on occupational therapy written by occupational therapists in 1947, with a second edition in 1954. Hopkins's involvement with the book began in 1967 and 1970, when she was asked by Spackman to write two chapters for the third and fourth editions. She states that "this opportunity was the beginning of my research and writing for the profession." In addition to editing the occupational therapy textbook, Hopkins has served in many capacities in her state and national professional associations, including being treasurer of the AOTA, president of the Western Pennsylvania OT Association, and delegate to the AOTA Representative Assembly.

Hopkins had always wanted to be a teacher and began her work life as an elementary schoolteacher. Not satisfied that she was fulfilling her interests and potential in that area of teaching, she was attracted to occupational therapy because it did include teaching. However, it was teaching people how to function after illness or trauma by using arts and crafts that she loved. She graduated from an intense certificate program under Helen Willard at the Philadelphia School of Occupational Therapy in 1947, accepted a job sight unseen at Indiana University Medical Center during the time that the polio epidemic was at its height, and had the good fortune to work with Winifred Kahmann, the first occupational therapist to be elected president of AOTA. She credits Kahmann with providing the opportunity to meet and to observe as role models many of the profession's leaders. This, in turn, kindled her interest and future activity in state and national associations.

On the job, ingenuity in finding ways to respond to needs of the patients was not only encouraged but required; no devices were available commercially and had to be made with whatever a therapist could find at hand. Problems were many, and as a result she assumed the responsibility to develop equipment that solved many patient problems. When working in New York City at the Institute of Rehabilitation Medicine with Muriel Zimmerman, they published a series of books that were circulated around the world and showed some of the ideas. This eventually led to the commercial manufacture of rehabilitation devices and equipment.

At this time AOTA was beginning to recognize a need for advanced education in occupational therapy. Realizing this was another way to serve her profession and that her commitment was necessary, Hopkins took advantage of living in New York City to work on a master's degree at night after work for 2½ years. Meanwhile, she was on several national AOTA committees. After receiving the degree, she taught at the University of Pennsylvania with Willard and Spackman. She was then asked to start an occupational therapy department at St. Francis Hospital in Pittsburgh and accepted this new challenge. While there, she began her writing career with the *American Journal of Occupational Therapy* and in *Orthotics, Etc.* by Licht.

In 1967 she responded to a request to help establish the occupational therapy educational program at Temple University, where she was a faculty member until 1986, serving the last 7 years as chair of the department. While there, she accepted opportunities to be involved in the administrative governance of the university and to represent the unique contribution of occupational therapy to the health and well-being of people of all ages.

At the same time, being aware of ongoing change and needs within occupational therapy for graduate education if the profession was to be regarded as a viable health profession, she embarked on coursework toward a doctoral degree in curriculum theory and development. After 8 years of full- and part-time study, she earned the degree and then used it to develop occupational therapy master's degree programs at Temple University.

Hopkins retired from Temple University, which means that her leadership has continued in new directions. She has since coedited two editions of *Willard and Spackman's Occupational Therapy;* been a board member and volunteer at a community mental health, mental retardation, and aging program in Philadelphia; been a book reviewer; been a consultant to educational occupational therapy programs; and is the assistant state coordinator for long-term care in the Health Advocacy Division of AARP in Pennsylvania. When asked her opinion of how she achieved her multiple goals, Hopkins replied:

> I tried to take advantage of the opportunities that were given to me and do my very best to accomplish results needed to further the profession of occupational therapy. I have tried to think ahead regarding what would be needed so that the profession would be understood and known by the institutions and public with whom we work. It is my belief that human beings must be active and involved in their world to grow and obtain satisfaction from their existence. I have tried to do the best possible job that I could. I met each new challenge and tried to foresee what would be needed in the future by keeping in touch with the trends of the times through listening and reading. Whenever I approached a new task I remembered what my grandfather told me as a child, "All that you do, do with your might; things done by halves are never done right."[2]

JOAN C. ROGERS, PhD, OTR, FAOTA

The main vision and goal in Joan C. Rogers's professional career was to become an accomplished researcher. Mainly for her achievement of that goal, she has earned visibility and respect as a leader in the occupational therapy profession. Among the honors she has received are the Eleanor Clarke Slagle Lectureship (the highest academic award of the AOTA), charter member of the Academy of Research and chair in 1995, and the Award of Merit (the highest award of the AOTA). Her list of publications fills nine pages, grants awarded occupy three more pages, and six more sheets record presentations only since 1985.

Rogers recognized her strengths and interests in undergraduate school, as her views of scholarship were heavily influenced there and later confirmed during her graduate studies. She began her professional career in clinical practice with acute care clients. Although she liked her job and did it well, she looked forward to intellectual stimulation and a research environment. In retrospect, Rogers feels that her academic appointments as a faculty member at three successive universities represent her search for a research-supportive environment. Although each of those universities placed a high value on research, the social and financial resources were not in place for allied health faculty. Her goal, however, was ultimately achieved in her current position in the Department of Psychiatry at the University of Pittsburgh. She regards as the greatest mistake of her research career that she did not take advantage of a postdoctoral fellowship and says it is unfortunate that "young" OT faculty continue to not appreciate the value of this experience.

Since 1984, Rogers has been director of Geropsychiatric Occupational Therapy at Western Psychiatric Institute and Clinic (WPIC) of the University of Pittsburgh Medical Center as well as a faculty associate of the Geriatric Education Center of Pennsylvania, Temple University, and University of Pittsburgh. Having set her goal, to become a funded researcher, she joined one of the premier U.S. research institutions in mental health. She reports that "my learning at WPIC took place in the school of hard knocks," as she had no mentor but did have access to—and took advantage of —senior scientists there. "Prior to submission, all grants at WPIC undergo (1) a scientific critique—2–3 researchers critique the proposal, the investigator has the opportunity to revise the proposal or respond to the criticism, and all reviewers must approve the project before it is sent out for external funding; (2) a human subjects review; and (3) a financial review. There is opportunity to learn how to meet these various standards, including how to write a well-justified budget." She knows and appreciates WPIC as "a tough environment," as she must meet the performance standards set for faculty in the Department of Psychiatry.

Rogers's final comments seem to be further evidence of a leader who listens, learns, and values criticism and who always keeps in mind the ultimate goal of her work. She noted, "I regard my 12-year survival here as among my greatest achievements. My greatest surprise was one day waking up and discovering that

I was among the most heavily funded faculty in the geriatric module. Further, that researchers from other disciplines on campus recognized and valued my work sufficiently to ask me to collaborate on their projects."[3]

SALLY E. RYAN, COTA, ROH

Sally E. Ryan is currently the coordinator of Level I fieldwork in the Department of Occupational Therapy at the College of St. Catherine in St. Paul. Among the accomplishments for which she is primarily known is as editor of the books *Practice Issues in Occupational Therapy* and *The Certified Occupational Therapy Assistant.* Ryan graduated from the first occupational therapy assistant program at Duluth in 1964 and has worked continuously on behalf of the profession and of certified occupational therapy assistants (COTAs) since then, as she has given keynote addresses and presentations nationally and internationally. She has served in clinical practice, supervision and management in long-term care, consultation, and as a faculty member. Leadership positions she has assumed include treasurer and vice president of the NBCOT, Minnesota representative to the AOTA Representative Assembly, a member-at-large on the AOTA Executive Board, and a member of numerous state and national committees. Among the honors given to Ryan were her selection as the first COTA to receive the AOTA Award of Excellence and as one of the first recipients of the AOTA Roster of Honor.

Although she has continued to further her education in areas she deems helpful to her future, Ryan says that she made the decision to remain in the profession as a COTA and not pursue higher occupational therapy degrees because she felt that "COTAs need a voice, and I can be of the most help and influence in behalf of them if I am one of them."[4] She feels that she was never parochial in her affiliations and met everyone she could, both locally and nationally.

An overarching view, in retrospect, she said, is that whenever an opportunity appeared, she took it, remembering that one of her teachers had told her class, "*You* are your professional association." Ryan said that she has tried to put that advice into practice whenever possible.

> If you want to be a leader you must have and keep a vision. You must put yourself and your personal interests aside, for the true leader must always be looking for or to the greater good of all stakeholders. . . . I didn't plan to be a leader, just wanted to make a difference. So I learned how to deal in and with politics, operated in more than one circle, and learned everything possible from those who were expert in those areas in which I had an interest. I worked as a team player, as well as independently, controlled my own future, and took responsibility for my own affairs and for implementing my vision.[4]

FRED SAMMONS, OTR, PhD, FAOTA

Fred Sammons is best known among occupational therapists for having founded and built a business primarily for development and manufacture of orthopedic and daily living assistive products. Sammons is known formally today as chairman of Sammons Preston Division of Bissell Healthcare Corporation. Among the honors that have been accorded him are an honorary doctorate, the AOTA Award of Merit, presidential commendation from both AOTA and AOTF, and lifetime board member of AOTF. He has held several offices in the Illinois Occupational Therapy Association, served on the AOTA conference committee for 1959, and has attended every AOTA conference since that year. The Fred Sammons Conference Center at AOTA national headquarters building in Bethesda, Maryland, is an ongoing reminder of his generosity.

Over the years Sammons set a priority on building his business by finding and filling the niches and needs of clinical occupational therapists and their clients while simultaneously applying his productivity and management skills to raising money for occupational therapy research through the AOTF. He has also contributed thousands of dollars personally for scholarships and in support of an endless number of projects benefiting students and the profession in general. A pervasive attitude of viewing problems and change as opportunities is clear. Endless enthusiasm for his work and in behalf of his chosen profession is self-evident, and client-centered interests can be seen as instrumental in both occupational therapy practice and in business.

Sammons grew up on a farm in Pennsylvania and says that his inclination toward worldwide traveling began when he worked as a boy on iron ore freighters on the Great Lakes during World War II. He received an industrial arts education with courses in printing, photography, electricity, and drafting and accepted his first job as a high school shop teacher. Later he read an article by Wilma West, OTR, in an industrial arts journal that told of shop teachers who became occupational therapists, thus planting a first seed for the future. With GI Bill support for service in the Korean War, he graduated from an occupational therapy program and began his first position at the Rehabilitation Institute of Chicago (RIC), where he developed skills in working with amputees.

Seeing a growing need among occupational therapists for devices and products, he invented his first device: a button hook for use by amputees and stroke clients to fasten and unfasten the sleeve buttons on their unaffected arms. To manufacture this product, he made a wooden rack that held 12 suction cups and wire loops in position while liquid epoxy resin became hard. He now had a product and production line, so next he made an ink rendition of the hook, had the first brochure printed, and continued developing other new products.

At the 1959 AOTA conference, he purchased a booth and handed out "purple ditto" fliers to attendees. The post office box he rented that year he used for 35 years. Next he devised the company logo "Be OK" and the company name "Fred Sammons Inc." In 1960 he sent a six-page mimeographed catalog to all OT departments listed by AOTA with new products such as built-up spoons, forks, knives, and stainless steel food guards. Later catalogs were printed on newsprint and used photographs that he took and developed in his home darkroom. Catalogs were sent to all students studying in occupational therapy programs, and faculty often used the catalog as a textbook.

Product selection increased rapidly as ideas for new devices came from therapists and clients. Manufacturing was kept separate from the distribution throughout, with production contracted out to specialized job-shops. When the completed item was received, instructions were added, and the product packaged and added to the inventory. Over the years, the steady increase in numbers of occupational therapists meant new departments and clients, emerging disability groups, and new products needed to accommodate these new demands.

Sammons cited two product innovations that were important to his company and the profession. The first was Velcro, a hook and loop fastener that replaced snaps and buckles. The second was low-temperature splinting material that therapists could mold against the skin to make temporary, low-cost splints. Splint fabrication became a major part of the orthopedic side of occupational therapy. This led many therapists to specialize in hand rehabilitation.

The main 380-page Sammons Preston catalog for 1996 offered thousands of orthopedic supplies and products for performing activities of daily living, 350 of which were new since the previous year's catalog. It was of highest quality production, offered three ways to order, gave a special number for ordering that would accommodate hearing-impaired customers, and promised same-day shipping. Sammons said:

> From the beginning I determined that the individual occupational therapist was my customer and that the catalog was to serve as my sales agent. . . . I attended a lot of state therapy conferences because I always felt that I got an opportunity to meet local therapists and to stay in touch with their needs and preferences. I regularly sat in on the conference lectures to keep up with changing trends in the profession. My little niche market was growing. I was offering whatever the occupational therapists wanted, so sensed a need to expand the business. . . . I needed additional manpower, so offered short term employment to working therapists to represent Sammons Company at state and national conferences. In that way we had clinicians who used the products in their clinics as our sales persons. . . . As for advertising and promotion, I used the space on the back cover of *AJOT* for building the image of the company and for introducing product ideas. . . . My most popular promotional idea has been the "Free Foto With Fred." At conferences I use a Polaroid to produce the souvenir photographs. When I visit colleges and universities, using a 35mm camera, I photograph as many as four students at a time, copy and return prints to the students. . . . We also publish a catalog called *Enrichments,* which therapists give to their clients and which we send to the general public. . . . For more than twenty years, special education students have come to our warehouse to learn and practice working skills. Most of them are now gainfully employed in our community. . . .
>
> I made the first products in the basement of my house in my spare time, typed the invoices and took the packages to the post office. . . . Later, an insurance man advised me to concentrate on marketing while contracting the manufacturing to

outside vendors. After the purchase of my first business computer we have been continuously upgrading both hardware and software.

My allegiance to the profession of occupational therapy has been continuous since I became a registered occupational therapist in 1955.[5]

SHIRLEY A. WELLS, MPH, OTR

Recently Shirley A. Wells has been most readily recognized as author of an ongoing series of *OT Week* articles she wrote as part of her activities as manager of the Multicultural Affairs Program of AOTA. In that position she has developed and managed diversity and equal opportunity affairs with an emphasis on recruitment and retention of practitioners and students from diverse backgrounds, promoted cultural awareness within the association and profession, developed consumer programs and materials for ethnic populations, and facilitated leadership development among ethnic and diverse individuals. Prior to assuming the management position at AOTA in 1992, Wells was a faculty member at Texas Tech University, where she developed teaching modules, cofounded the Texas Tech University School of Allied Health Project Magic Troop, and was president of the School of Allied Health Faculty Council.

Wells began her professional career as a pediatric occupational therapist in public school positions, with the Bureau of Indian Affairs, in rehabilitation hospitals, and in MHMR state schools. Among her honors was being named as one of the Outstanding Young Women of America.

When asked how she went about making futuristic, strategic decisions, she replied, "I view each prospect in terms of the skills and knowledge I can gain from the opportunity. I look for opportunities that will force me to not only learn new skills but also use those skills I already possess. I want to be pushed to be creative, productive and test my limits. I need to feel that I have something to offer, that I can change things for the better and that I can help someone else."[6]

Summary

This chapter has emphasized that leaders are needed and that some can already be found in every occupational therapy role category: OTR and COTA practitioners, researchers, educators, supervisors, administrators, consultants, faculty members, program directors, and entrepreneurs. It was noted that each occupational therapy practitioner described as an example or referenced in this book is appreciated as a leader in the profession.

Because all leaders could not be introduced here, six contemporary leaders were selected who have consistently displayed the characteristics of effective leadership that were described in Part One and repeated in this chapter. Some of these leaders have been more visible or are better known to many of their peers, to date, than others; however, each continuously works diligently in behalf of colleagues and the profession. Together, these individuals and their counterparts, all the other leaders within the occupational therapy profession, are an awesome force for good in healthcare services delivery.

REFERENCES

1. Byers-Connon, S: Personal communication, July, 1996.
2. Hopkins, HL: Personal communication, July, 1996.
3. Rogers, JC: Personal communication, Aug, 1996.
4. Ryan, SE: Personal communication, July, 1996.
5. Sammons, F: Personal communication, June, 1996.
6. Wells, SA: Personal communication, July, 1996.

CHAPTER 22

Putting It All Together: A Synthesis

CHAPTER OBJECTIVES

- To realize that history teaches leadership, management, marketing, and adaptation to change.
- To acknowledge the infinite number of opportunities that exist within change and problems.
- To see why reading, listening, and learning must become lifelong habits.
- To realize that the sound advice of experienced occupational therapists should be valued and used.
- To recognize how the processes of occupational therapy treatment, leadership, management, and marketing can be taught in an occupational therapy curriculum in an integrated fashion.
- To remember specific steps and approaches that can be taken by students as they begin practice.
- To value and use a marketing approach in daily occupational therapy practice.

There is a logical progression of thought that can be followed and parallels that can be detected in the processes of occupational therapy, marketing, management, and leadership. By visualizing and building on the already understood process of occupational therapy treatment, the therapist can find all four processes converging. As occupational therapy is deliberately and artfully practiced, so are the other three. Achievement of ultimate goals, whether in occupational therapy, marketing, management, or leadership, is based not on chance or hunches but on a succession of deliberately planned steps.

What does the future hold for occupational therapists? It will be new, better, exciting, and gratifying if occupational therapists are able to understand and adapt to change—global, technological, cultural, organizational—as opportunity. The potential is there, but an open mind and innovation are the keys needed to unlock it.

History Teaches Leadership, Management, Marketing, and Adaptation to Change

History has proved that there is after all nothing new about leadership or management skills or the marketing process or adapting to change. During biblical times, Moses questioned his leadership potential. Socrates, in his discourse with Nicomachides, also had firm opinions related to management and leadership characteristics as he answered a question about whether an individual could manage an army just as easily as a small chorus. His opinion was that "over whatever a man may preside, he will, if he knows what he needs and is able to provide it, be a good president, whether he have the direction of a chorus, a family, a city or an army." He further opined that "the conduct of private affairs differes [sic] from that of public concerns only in magnitude" and that those who don't know how to manage will err whether they are conducting private *or* public affairs.[1] Concern about leadership and management matters have been of great interest and concern to thoughtful people for a long time. It is logical for occupational therapists, as thinking and resourceful professionals, not only to be interested but also to do something about it. Why not adopt the Socratic attitude and improve leadership skills, whether leading 3 or 30,000?

Moving on to the 19th century, an observation about the notion of change and opportunity was made by Charles Dickens in *A Tale of Two Cities:*

It was the best of times,
    it was the worst of times.
    It was the age of wisdom,
    it was the age of foolishness.
    It was the season of light,
    it was the season of darkness.
    It was the spring of hope,
    it was the winter of despair.

We had everything before us,
we had nothing before us. . . .

The association between change and opportunity, as well as the hope and the anticipation that are implied, has engaged minds for centuries. Both adaptation and resistance to change have been equally perplexing for just as long.

As for the topic of marketing, in 1850 a factory owner in the United States made an early observation about the effectiveness of marketing when he commented that he had no problem in directing his organization. His reason was that the products manufactured were so well suited to the needs of the customers that a boy employed in the office who was adept at bookkeeping could do whatever was necessary to keep things moving in the business. Even though it was not given a name, the marketing process was obviously in place and had been effective.

Throughout this book have been suggestions about the value of paying attention to the past while also looking to the future. We remember Kierkegaard's admonition that "life must be lived forward, but can only be understood backwards."[2]

What This Book Has Proposed

This book has sought to present a unifying and universal thread—the marketing process—around which to strengthen the teaching and learning of curricular requirements. The focus for decision making in healthcare delivery is shifting universally to the client and the healthcare payer. The role of the occupational therapist must shift as well if it is to continue to be an essential resource for consumers and healthcare payers. What more logical way to do this than to use a marketing approach?

Here, at the conclusion of this book, the difference between selling and marketing, so commonly misunderstood by occupational therapists, is again clarified. Although marketing is appearing more prominently in the healthcare system, many still confuse it with selling. As a result, they dismiss the marketing concept as unethical and inappropriate. Therefore, to be certain that marketing has been fully explained, here is a brief recapitulation of marketing as a social process.

SELLING VS. MARKETING

The selling concept assumes that prospective users will not purchase products or services unless they are approached with sizable selling and promotional efforts. Underlying this assumption is that health services are sold, not bought, and that there is no particular concern about repeat business.

Compared to selling, conscious use of the marketing concept originated only about 40 years ago in the commercial business sector. Marketing, in contrast to selling, is a management concept that deals with exchange relationships. It presumes that the central task of an organization or system is to determine the wants, needs, and values of target markets and to pattern the organization and its products to provide satisfaction to those target markets. The first requirement is that the organization develop an active marketing research plan to identify those wants, needs, or values.

Market research focuses on development of information to improve decision making. The objective is to better understand the consumer's behavior, attitudes, usage criteria, and other factors so as to meet the perceived needs of consumers more efficiently. Thus limited resources are not wasted by a hit-or-miss approach.

THE MARKETING PLAN

All activities that are related to one's consumers are guided by the marketing plan. In marketing consumer goods, the four elements of a marketing plan are called the four Ps: product, promotion, place, and price. Healthcare marketing, in contrast, might use an acronym CAPS: Considerations or costs exchanged for health care, Access and availability, Promotion, and Service development.[3] Considerations or costs include things of value in addition to money, such as time waiting, opportunity costs, handing control of one's body over to another, discomfort, or perceived lowering of social status or self-esteem. Access or availability is similar to "place" in goods marketing. Promotion in goods marketing is primarily personal selling and advertising, but in healthcare marketing the focus is on public relations and atmospherics, with some increase in use of advertising. Service development is similar to product development in goods marketing.[3]

A marketing plan describes selected markets, the timing and amount of financial and human resources assigned to each market segment, and a forecast of the expected results. All effective organizations use marketing to plan, transact, and facilitate voluntary exchanges with their previously targeted constituencies or publics. The action taken, in most cases, is to focus efforts on specific market segments with the goal of becoming the provider of choice for those whose needs, attitudes, and preferences most closely approximate the capabilities and resources of their own organizations.

Finally, marketers ask themselves the all-important question, "What is my business [or product or service]?" Defining what you have to offer is often the least-understood part of marketing. What are you offering that is unique or that distinguishes your service from all others? Who will buy your product or service? Why would they buy it? What is it that they are buying? How will you provide it? Occupational therapists must first believe in, understand, and be able to clearly describe their product—occupational therapy—before they can make judgments about new and advantageous applications. So, exactly what are you offering?

In summary, the marketing concept begins with ascertaining the existing or potential consumer needs, planning a coordinated set of programs and services to fulfill them, and as a result creating satisfaction of your organization's own goals by providing consumer satisfaction, support for the organization (e.g., referrals, volunteers), consumer loyalty, and repeat usage. For a detailed review of the marketing concept, its tools, and its techniques, reread Part Two.

What Must Be Taught in Occupational Therapy Programs

Caregiving in the managed care environment demands more than personal rapport and love of working with patients. Increasingly more complex reimbursement guidelines have to be learned, data collected, numbers crunched, and cost reductions made without sacrificing high-quality care. The occupational therapy student today needs knowledge about critical thinking, divergent and innovative problem solving, systems management processes, budgeting, reimbursement, third-party payers, managed care, Medicare, contracts, outcomes documentation, personnel management, management of productivity, marketing, networking, and ethical decision making.

In an effort to corroborate these assertions, I conducted an informal survey in several states among occupational therapists newly graduated and in their first positions. I asked them what they considered the most essential information that must be added or emphasized in today's occupational therapy curricula. Of the variety of opinions expressed, five occurred universally: Change is inevitable, active participation in professional organizations is everyone's responsibility, appreciating the marketing process is essential, understanding cultural differences is critical, and comprehending and negotiating politics are necessary.

As healthcare team members, in institutional or community practice, with excellent generalist backgrounds and flexible approaches, occupational therapists are eminently well qualified to serve as leaders of interdisciplinary teams. Being able to globally assess the total person and use interpersonal skills to advantage gives occupational therapists a head start as team members and leaders. What is needed is the self-confidence, empowerment, and motivation to take hold of this advantage. Students can and should be supported and strengthened in these areas.

Integrated Teaching of Occupational Therapy, Leadership, Management, and Marketing

A primary assertion of this book was that occupational therapy practitioners can be taught leadership, marketing, and management by first demonstrating how to visualize those basic processes as similar in many ways to the occupational therapy treatment process itself. In this way the perception that the intricacies of management, leadership, and marketing have to be learned as additional subjects, as add-ons to occupational therapy education coursework, can be altered. A summary of the similarities and parallels among the processes of occupational therapy treatment, marketing, management, and leadership can be seen in Table 22–1. Each process uses a systems approach, for all begin with active listening, conclude with the measurement of outcomes, acknowledge feedback, are followed by revisions and adjustments in goals and methods, and then cyclically and systematically begin again.

An Educator's View

In addition to the assertions in this book, there is an additional perspective I wish to include here. What should be taught to today's occupational therapy students was said best by Gail Fidler[4] in 1977:

> Educating for a profession requires that both content and the process of learning have as their primary focus the development of:
>
> A concept of self as responsible, accountable to self and others.
> An attitude of inquiry.
> The ability to use logic, to value and apply objective scholarly analysis, disciplined thinking and reasoning.
> The ability to make evaluative judgments, to view "the whole" . . . to see parts as they relate to the whole, and to assess, evaluate and judge.
> A commitment to the continuing development, sophistication and accountability of the profession.
> A mastery of the body of knowledge and professional skills essential for entry level competency.

Final Tips for Students

DO YOU HAVE VISION?

Kanter considered those who bring about change or innovation as entrepreneurs: "Entrepreneurs are above all visionaries. They are willing to continue single-minded pursuit of a clearly articulated vision, even when the line of least effort or resistance would make it easy to give up."[5] Begin with a vision, that natural outgrowth of a creative mind, followed by systematically planned clear objectives based on "what I do best" (my product), building on previous success but unencumbered by those parts of the past that are no longer relevant or useful, aware of all environmental trends, and prepared to make future-oriented decisions. I hope the content of this book has shown that opportunities and horizons are unlimited for those who are open, alert, and aware.

SUCCESS IS POSSIBLE REGARDLESS
OF AN ORGANIZATION'S SIZE

Corroboration of the major premises discussed throughout this book was once more affirmed in the March 6, 1996, issue of *Fortune*, which listed the most admired corporations of America.[6] There was virtually no relationship between the size of a company or its assets and the sheen of its reputation, although financial performance did correlate strongly with reputation. To reach this conclusion, a research firm studied the assets, profits, and 10-year annual return of the Fortune 1000, including the service industries. Their results showed that at least half of a company's reputation comes from intangibles, such as how their employees are treated and the strength of its management team. The increasing effect of globalization was also evident, with 15 of the biggest U.S. subsidiaries of overseas companies joining the list.

The eight key attributes of a company's image and reputation were identified as the quality of the management; the quality of the services provided; the ability to attract, develop, and keep talented people; financial soundness; innovativeness; value as a long-term investment; how company assets were used; and community and environmental responsibility. Successful companies invested much thought, effort, and money in seeing that consumers as well as employees were satisfied. For example, in one service company cited, although employee turnover in that particular region was usually 43 percent a year, its rate was only 12 percent as a result of its commitment to satisfying the needs and wants of its employees. Too many employers just continue saying the "right words" and giving plaques to people while stifling the greatest gift their employees have, their creativity. That is not what is meant by giving people opportunity and job satisfaction.[6]

In occupational therapy, as well, the strength of small business is evident, with Susan M. Stockdell, OTR, CHT, as one example. This Arizonan was one of 36 Arizona business executives selected as regional finalists for the 1993 Entrepreneur of the Year Award sponsored by Ernst & Young, Inc. Magazine, and Merrill Lynch. Acknowledging that her business is relatively small, Stockdell credited cost-effectiveness and quality care for making it the regional center of excellence in functional outcomes.[7]

When asked her opinion about why her private practice of 14 years in Denver continues successfully, Mary K. Hubbell, OTR, confided that from the start she has always realized the value of marketing. Since the initial establishment of her business, she has incorporated ethical procedures, strong values, sound business techniques, and a marketing approach into her occupational therapy practice.[8]

LOOK FOR THE OPPORTUNITIES HIDING
BEHIND THE PROBLEMS

By now you are fully aware that there is a revolution in the American work scene. What strikes one immediately is that it is a whole new world of work out

TABLE 22–1

Occupational Therapy, Leadership, Management, and Marketing: Parallel Processes

The process of > ↓	Occupational Therapy Treatment	Marketing as a Social Process
Employs > ↓	Art & science	Art & science
& Has an eclectic basis of >	Psychology Sociology Biologic sciences Modalities	Psychology Sociology Marketing Management tools
↓		
& Is sensitive to needs of > ↓	Clients	Publics/constituencies
Practitioner uses > ↓	Treatment goals	Marketing objectives
& First > ↓	Actively listens	Actively listens
For > ↓	Needs, wants & preferences	Needs, wants & preferences
Then analyzes>	Clients' status re strengths & weaknesses	Constituencies' status re levels of exchanges
↓		
& Performs >	An environmental survey	An environmental survey/marketing audit
↓		
& Sets > ↓	Goals & objectives	Goals & objectives
Using > ↓	Creativity	Creativity
&> ↓	Adaptation	Adaptation
To form a > ↓	Treatment plan	Marketing plan
Which is implemented by using > ↓	Purposeful activity/modalities	A marketing mix of tools & techniques
Monitored by >	Assessment of client progress toward goals	Evaluation of changes in status of exchanges
↓		
Which provides > ↓	Outcome information	Outcome information
& Is followed by >	Treatment plan revisions	Adjusting of marketing mix

TABLE 22–1

Occupational Therapy, Leadership, Management, and Marketing: Parallel Processes *(Continued)*

Management	Leadership
Art & science	Art & science
Psychology Sociology Management Functions Business tools	Psychology Sociology Power bases Group process
Organizational members	Followers
Organizational goals	Vision/goals
Actively listens	Actively listens
Needs, wants & preferences	Needs, wants & preferences
Organizational strengths & weaknesses	Followers' strengths & weaknesses
An environmental survey	An environmental survey
Goals & objectives	Goals & objectives
Creativity	Creativity
Adaptation	Adaptation
Strategic plan	Strategic plan
Management functions & techniques	Power & motivation as tools
Management control measures	Evaluation of success level achieved toward goal/vision
Outcome information	Outcome information
Revision in methods used	Adjustment of methods & approaches

there: Flexibility and creativity are more important for success than endurance and loyalty. Leadership and acceptance within one's peer group is more important than building relationships with higher-level managers. Holding a high priority among the attitudes and proficiencies expected of occupational therapy practitioners is customer service.

Managed care is here to stay, and occupational therapists will do well to diligently study its ramifications, challenges, and opportunities. The two goals of managed care are to contain costs and improve the quality of care. A synonym for *managed care* has been suggested: *managed cost.* As a result, occupational therapists now need to expand their vision and enthusiastically move ahead. Occupational therapists should work proactively with staff in insurance companies and managed care companies by building relationships and using their marketing skills to develop these connections.

Outcomes data, the ubiquitous term with which everyone should by now be familiar, obviously play a steadily growing role in verification for reimbursement of occupational therapy services. Occupational therapists can help themselves gain proficiency in gathering such data through the many sources and prototypes being developed to address this need. One example is an outcomes research project inaugurated by the Home Health and Community Special Interest Section of AOTA.

Look for those opening doors instead watching the closing ones, and make your own opportunities. Why not create and develop niches in the airline industry, the architecture and building fields, or manufacturing industries?

MAKE LIFELONG HABITS OF READING, LISTENING, AND LEARNING

An occupational therapy practitioner should make a lifelong habit of reading a wide range of literature, adding knowledge and skills by learning and listening whenever possible. Attend as many state, regional, and national occupational therapy conferences as you can to hear about the newest trends and happenings in the profession. For example, had you been a participant at the 1995 Great Southern Occupational Therapy conference, you would have learned that occupational therapy practitioners, who know what people need and where they can receive care, can become medical case managers paid by insurance companies.[9] Legal consultation is another available avenue; occupational therapists can serve as expert witnesses in Americans with Disabilities Act (ADA) complaints, Social Security disability, personal injury, or medical record review cases. Attendees were also advised to explore self-employment options such as conducting home assessments or providing services for stress management, relaxation, time management, and smoking cessation. Operating children's activity centers or forming partnerships with the workplace as "productivity enhancers" (those who facilitate an employee's return to work or help corporations reconceptualize ways to make job restructurings and reassignments work) were among the innovative, yet realistic, suggestions made.

Throughout the conference, comments supported the relevance of this book to today's practice. Statements such as "the days of traditional rehab therapy are rapidly fading" were heard many times, but at the same time occupational therapists were observed to already have problem-solving knowledge and skills to apply to new situations. Another speaker declared that occupational therapy practitioners need to determine and prioritize what clients need from them. Predictions were made that direct treatment by occupational therapists will decrease because some of the less skilled tasks customarily performed by occupational therapists will be transferred to other staff members. Employers will more often be found restricting payment for some services to those staff members having qualifications at that lower skill level. The need to give priority to client-centered care was often reiterated.[9] There is no limit to what an occupational therapy practitioner can learn through attending even a single conference.

As a team leader or a manager, learn and practice how to develop a proactive attitude in anticipation of strategic planning. Identify what information is needed, which issues merit attention, and where to find the information needed. Assign topics to focus groups and interested persons so that all relevant information can be investigated and findings shared. Then decisions will be made based on as thorough a foundation as possible. It is your personal responsibility to initiate such action where you live and work, in your local professional groups, and in your state organization. It is your own pulse to which you should pay attention, your own problems for which to seek solutions, because the trends begin with you in your own environment, and you have the power to address them there. Then share your conclusions with colleagues. Through this sharing, you will help and be helped.

According to your preference, use hard copy publications or electronic resources to develop awareness and to communicate. Communication is the key component, for occupational therapists will be doing more cognitive work: the assessment and planning of client care. Assistants and aides will handle much of the routine work. Therapists will be required to do more supervision and management and less direct client care. Effective intraprofessional teamwork is not only smart but also critical to future success, and it, too, can be learned.

Look for continuing education offerings in the areas in which you are deficient. Courses, workshops, and weekend seminars are offered by a variety of organizations. Clinicians tend to limit their choices to seminars that deal with treatment issues while ignoring those that deal with management or marketing. Look for both.

DEVELOP A FOCUSED RESUME

Spend time developing a clear, focused resume. It is usually your first—and often only—introduction to a potential employer. Computer-friendly resumes are being used more widely. For that reason, keep in mind that they are less liable to get lost in a computer or online system if you remember a few suggestions:

■ Select key words carefully. Resumes may be scanned for key words, terms, or phrases during searches of databases to match a specific need.

For example, using a noun such as *case manager* rather than a verb such as *developed* or *initiated* may be more effective.

- Keep it simple. Avoid colored paper or unusual typefaces. Use white paper and a common font.

- Be sure to put your most relevant and best information first. Many computer screens display only a dozen or so lines of text at one time, so use a strong beginning. Give a concise and accurate summary, along with a listing of your skills.

- Mail the resume flat, as folds in the pages may cause information to get lost while the resume is scanned.[10]

Conclusions

This book has provided basic information about leadership, marketing, and management and offered suggestions on how to develop personal leadership strengths. It concludes here with a summary of qualities that students should begin to develop as they progress toward becoming effective occupational therapy practitioners, managers, and leaders:

1. Tolerant of uncertainty, welcoming changes, challenges, and problems as inevitable.

2. Accepting conflict as a fact of life that you must recognize and handle in the early stages.

3. Considerate, protecting the interests of those for whom and to whom you are responsible.

4. Autonomous, providing structure so that your employees and team members understand their responsibilities and your expectations.

5. Visionary, including awareness of what is going on inside and outside your personal world and thus being able to anticipate and predict the outcomes of your decisions.

6. Productive, with the ability to enhance and ensure high-quality production while encouraging good interpersonal relationships.

7. Self-confident, allowing employees to release their creativity while encouraging high performance.

8. Persuasive, communicating ideas with enthusiasm and conviction.

9. Courageous, remembering that "the buck stops here" with yourself.

10. Motivated, serving as a role model for your followers to simultaneously achieve organizational and personal goals.

11. A risk taker, willing to assume responsibility for new ventures after having investigated all pertinent information.

Healing is always a personal matter and understandably the ultimate concern of an occupational therapy client. Always remember that healing is the true "business" of occupational therapy. Keeping that in mind may help you focus personal and professional strategic decision making as you make progress toward professional leadership. The basic tools with which graduates emerge to practice are a well-honed mind and the ability to live with change, adapting to the needs of the times while adhering to the principles for which occupational therapy stands. Occupational therapy education is intended to provide wings, not weights.

So, what skills do *you* need to polish as you start to cultivate the qualities and strengths suggested in this book? Begin with increasing awareness of yourself as well as others; build your confidence by acting like a winner and projecting assurance; enhance your problem-solving and analytical abilities; develop your creativity by keeping a flexible, open, inquisitive mind; constantly hone your technical and psychosocial skills through the lifelong learning habit; stay alert and informed; and don't learn by surprise. Finally, a marketing perspective needs that rare commodity, common sense, much the same as does occupational therapy. Its simplicity is its uniqueness. Now, begin, and good luck!

How sweet it is to stand on the edge of tomorrow.[2]

Summary

This chapter has highlighted and synthesized the central elements of this book. A tabular representation of the manner in which occupational therapists can visualize the parallel and comparative processes inherent in occupational therapy, leadership, management, and marketing was presented. Final comments were offered to demonstrate to graduating occupational therapy students that they are entering practice with a fine potential for leadership and are expected to use their potential to enthusiastically continue the tradition of occupational therapy.

REFERENCES

1. Plato and Xenophon; Watson, JS(trans): Socratic Discourses. Dutton, New York, 1910, book III, ch. IV, pp 80–81.
2. Schuller, RH: Prayer: My Soul's Adventure with God. Thomas Nelson, Nashville, 1993.
3. Cooper, PD, and Robinson, LM: Health Care Marketing Management. Aspen, Rockville, Md, 1982.
4. Fidler, G: From plea to mandate. Am J Occup Ther 31(10), Nov/Dec, 1977.
5. Kanter, RM: The Change Masters. Simon & Schuster, New York, 1983, p 239.
6. Fisher, AB: Corporate reputations: Comebacks and comeuppances. Fortune 133(4):90, Mar 6, 1996.
7. Newsmakers, OT Week 7:30, July 29, 1993.
8. Hubbell, MK: Personal communication, Apr, 1995.
9. Hettinger, J: Great Southern tests the cutting edge. OT Week 9(48), Nov 30, 1995.
10. Gray, BB: Computer-friendly resumes. Nursing and Allied Healthweek—Dallas/Fort Worth, May 6, 1996.

Index

Page numbers followed by "f" indicate figures; page numbers followed by "t" indicate tables.